2016

The Year Book of NEONATAL AND PERINATAL MEDICINE®

ELSEVIER
MOSBY

ELSEVIER
MOSBY

Editor: Kerry Holland
Developmental Editor: Susan Showalter

2016 EDITION

Composition by TNQ Books and Journals Pvt Ltd, India

Editorial Office:
Elsevier
Suite 1800
1600 John F. Kennedy Blvd.
Philadelphia, PA 19106-3399

International Standard Serial Number: 8756-5005
International Standard Book Number: 978-0-323-44688-4

Editorial Board

Contributing Editors

Janelle Aby, MD
Clinical Professor, Pediatrics, Stanford University; Medical Director, Well Newborn Nursery, Lucile Packard Children's Hospital, Stanford, California

David H. Adamkin, MD
Professor of Pediatrics; Director of Division of Neonatology; Director of Nutritional Research; Rounsavall Chair of Neonatal Medicine; Co-Director of Neonatal Fellowship, University of Louisville, Louisville, Kentucky

William Benitz, MD
Philip Sunshine Professor of Neonatology, Division of Neonatal and Developmental Medicine, Stanford University School of Medicine, Lucile Packard Children's Hospital, Stanford, California

Varsha Bhatt-Mehta, PharmD, MS, FCCP
Clinical Professor, College of Pharmacy, Department of Pediatrics and Communicable Diseases, Medical School, University of Michigan, Ann Arbor, Michigan

Vinod K. Bhutani, MD, FAAP
Division of Neonatal and Developmental Medicine, Department of Pediatrics, Stanford University School of Medicine, Stanford, California

Patrick D. Brophy, MD, MHCDS
The Jean E. Robillard MD Chair in Pediatric Nephrology, Professor and Director Pediatric Nephrology, Dialysis & Transplantation, University of Iowa Children's Hospital, Iowa City, Iowa

Heather H. Burris, MD, MPH
Assistant Professor of Pediatrics, Division of Newborn Medicine, Boston Children's Hospital; Attending Neonatologist, Department of Neonatology, Beth Israel Deaconess Medical Center, Boston, Massachusetts

Steven M. Donn, MD
Professor of Pediatrics, Division of Neonatal-Perinatal Medicine, C.S. Mott Children's Hospital, University of Michigan Health System, Ann Arbor, Michigan

Avroy Fanaroff, MD, FRCPE, FRCP&CH
Emeritus Eliza Henry Barnes Chair of Neonatology, Rainbow Babies & Children's Hospital; Emeritus Professor, Department of Pediatrics, Case Western Reserve University School of Medicine, Cleveland, Ohio

Jonathan M. Fanaroff, MD, JD
Associate Professor of Pediatrics, Case Western Reserve University School of Medicine; Director, Rainbow Center for Pediatric Ethics; Co-Director, Neonatal Intensive Care Unit, Rainbow Babies & Children's Hospital, Cleveland, Ohio

Adam Frymoyer, MD
Clinical Assistant Professor, Division of Neonatal and Developmental Medicine, Department of Pediatrics, Stanford University School of Medicine, Stanford, California

Terrie E. Inder, MD, MBCHB
Chair, Department of Pediatric Newborn Medicine, Brigham and Women's Hospital; Mary Ellen Avery Professor of Pediatrics in the Field of Newborn Medicine, Harvard Medical School, Boston, Massachusetts

Alan H. Jobe, MD, PhD
Professor of Pediatrics, Cincinnati Children's Hospital, University of Cincinnati, Cincinnati, Ohio

Stephanie Kukora, MD
Clinical Lecturer in Pediatrics, Division of Neonatal-Perinatal Medicine, C.S. Mott Children's Hospital, University of Michigan Health System, Ann Arbor, Michigan

Naomi Tricot Laventhal, MD
Assistant Professor, University of Michigan Health System, Department of Pediatrics and Communicable Diseases, Division of Neonatal-Perinatal Medicine, C&W Mott Hospital, Ann Arbor, Michigan

M. Jeffrey Maisels, MD, DSc
Chair Emeritus and Professor; Director, Academic Affairs, Department of Pediatrics, Oakland University William Beaumont School of Medicine, Royal Oak, Michigan

Camilia R. Martin, MD, MS
Assistant Professor of Pediatrics, Harvard Medical School; Associate Director, NICU, Department of Neonatology; Director of Cross-Disciplinary Research Partnerships, Division of Translational Research, Beth Israel Deaconess Medical Center, Boston, Massachusetts

Gilbert I. Martin, MD
Director Emeritus NICU, Citrus Valley Medical Center, West Covina, California; Clinical Professor of Pediatrics, Loma Linda University Medical Center, Loma Linda, California

Richard J. Martin, MD
Drusinsky–Fanaroff Chair in Neonatology; Professor of Pediatrics, Reproductive Biology, and Physiology, Case Western Reserve University; Director, Neonatal Research Programs, Rainbow Babies & Children's Hospital, Cleveland, Ohio

Christopher C. McPherson, PharmD
Departments of Pharmacy and Pediatric Newborn Medicine, Brigham and Women's Hospital, Boston, Massachusetts

Thomas F. McElrath, MD, PhD
Division of Maternal Fetal Medicine, Brigham & Women's Hospital, Harvard Medical School, Boston, Massachusetts

Josef Neu, MD
Professor of Pediatrics, University of Florida College of Medicine, Gainesville, Florida

Mary L. Nock, MD
Associate Professor of Pediatrics, Case Western Reserve University School of Medicine; Director, Neonatal-Perinatal Medicine Fellowship Program; Co-Director, NICU, Rainbow Babies and Children's Hospital, Cleveland, Ohio

Robin K. Ohls, MD
Professor of Pediatrics; Director, Neonatal Research, University of New Mexico, Albuquerque, New Mexico

Lu-Ann Papile, MD
Professor Emerita, Division of Neonatology, University of New Mexico, Albuquerque, New Mexico

Richard B. Parad, MD, MPH
Associate Professor of Pediatrics, Harvard Medical School, Brigham and Women's Hospital; Department of Pediatric Newborn Medicine, Connors Center for Women, Boston, Massachusetts

Kenneth Pituch, MD
David G. Dickinson Professor of Pediatrics and Communicable Diseases; Medical Director, Pediatric Palliative Care Programs, C.S. Mott Children's Hospital, Dexter, Michigan

Richard A. Polin, MD
William T. Speck Professor of Neonatology; Director, Division of Neonatology, Children's Hospital of New York; Professor of Pediatrics, Columbia University College of Physicians and Surgeons, New York, New York

Patricia L. Robertson, MD
Professor of Pediatrics and Neurology, University of Michigan School of Medicine, C.S. Mott Children's Hospital, Ann Arbor, Michigan

Kate P. Stanley, MD
Clinical Assistant Professor of Pediatrics, Division of Neonatal-Perinatal Medicine, C.S. Mott Children's Hospital, University of Michigan Health System, Ann Arbor, Michigan

Eileen Stork, MD
Professor of Pediatrics, Case Western Reserve University; Director, Neonatal ECMO Program, Rainbow Babies & Children's Hospital, Cleveland, Ohio

Win Tin, FRCPCH
Professor of Paediatrics and Neonatal Medicine, The James Cook University Hospital, Middlesbrough, United Kingdom; Professor of Paediatrics and Neonatal Medicine, University of Durham, Durham, United Kingdom

Linda J. Van Marter, MD, MPH
Associate Professor of Pediatrics, Harvard Medical School; Vice-Chair, Department of Pediatric Newborn Medicine, Brigham and Women's Hospital, Boston, Massachusetts

Betty R. Vohr, MD
Professor of Pediatrics, Warren Alpert Medical School of Brown University; Medical Director, Follow-Up Clinic, Women & Infants Hospital of Rhode Island, Providence, Rhode Island

Kristi Watterberg, MD
Professor of Pediatrics/Neonatology, University of New Mexico School of Medicine, Albuquerque, New Mexico

Thomas E. Wiswell, MD
Professor of Pediatrics, University of Central Florida School of Medicine, Orlando, Florida

Table of Content

Journals Represented

Journals represented in this YEAR BOOK are listed below.

Acta Paediatrica
AJNR American Journal of Neuroradiology
American Journal of Human Genetics
American Journal of Obstetrics and Gynecology
American Journal of Perinatology
Annals of Surgery
Annals of the American Thoracic Society
Archives of Disease in Childhood
Archives of Disease in Childhood Fetal and Neonatal Edition
British Journal of Obstetrics and Gynaecology
British Medical Journal
Child's Nervous System
Childs Nervous System
Clinical Pediatrics
Developmental Medicine and Child Neurology
Epilepsia
European Journal of Obstetrics, Gynecology and Reproductive Biology
European Respiratory Journal
Journal of Clinical Microbiology
Journal of Molecular Diagnostics
Journal of Pediatric Gastroenterology and Nutrition
Journal of Pediatric Orthopaedics
Journal of Pediatric Surgery
Journal of Pediatrics
Journal of Perinatology
Journal of the American Medical Association
Journal of the American Medical Association Pediatrics
Journal of Thoracic and Cardiovascular Surgery
JPEN Journal of Parenteral and Enteral Nutrition
Lancet
Lancet Neurology
Liver Transplantation
Medicine
Nature Medicine
New England Journal of Medicine
Nutrient
Obesity
Obstetrics & Gynecology
Ophthalmology
Pediatric Infectious Disease Journal
Pediatric Radiology
Pediatric Research
Pediatrics
Proceedings of the National Academy of Sciences of the United States of America
Prostaglandins Leukotrienes and Essential Fatty Acids
Science
Ultrasound in Obstetrics & Gynecology

Standard Abbreviations

The following terms are abbreviated in this edition: acquired immunodeficiency syndrome (AIDS), cardiopulmonary resuscitation (CPR), central nervous system (CNS), cerebrospinal fluid (CSF), computed tomography (CT), deoxyribonucleic acid (DNA), electrocardiography (ECG), health maintenance organization (HMO), human immunodeficiency virus (HIV), intensive care unit (ICU), intramuscular (IM), intravenous (IV), magnetic resonance (MR) imaging (MRI), ribonucleic acid (RNA), and ultrasound (US).

Note

To facilitate the use of the Year Book of Neonatal and Perinatal Medicine® as a reference tool, all illustrations and tables included in this publication are now identified as they appear in the original article. This change is meant to help the reader recognize that any illustration or table appearing in the Year Book of Neonatal and Perinatal Medicine® may be only one of many in the original article. For this reason, figure and table numbers will often appear to be out of sequence within the Year Book of Neonatal and Perinatal Medicine®.

Introduction

The 2016 Year Book of Neonatal and Perinatal Medicine includes over 200 commentaries, almost 10% greater than 2015. The articles for comment have been selected, the comments written, and we have just finally organized the sections. The editors have completed their tasks and it remains for you the readers to enjoy the fruits of our labor. A few key articles have commentaries from multiple editors and it is always interesting to see the different perspectives and interpretation of the same publication. Our challenge remains to include all the landmark publications, and a high percentage of the randomized trials and Cochrane reviews. We continue to be frustrated by the publication of randomized trials with insufficient power to answer the question that has been posed. The 2016 Year Book includes an article on "Choosing wisely," an effort to reduce or eliminate tests and treatments that could not be justified on the basis of efficacy, safety, or cost. This volume also contains much information on the use of antenatal corticosteroids, periviability, the neonatal biome, the impact and diagnosis of neonatal hypoglycemia, many aspects of human milk, as well as the emerging advances in genetics. The adjuvant therapies for hypoxic ischemic encephalopathy are discussed extensively as are the importance of G6PD as a cause of jaundice and the mechanism of action of phototherapy. Advances in genetics and the application of the human genome will highlight the transition from evidence-based medicine to precision or personalized medicine. Mitochondrial replacement therapy is near at hand and remains the focus of safety, ethical, and legal concerns, as do all gene therapies.

We remain indebted to our many colleagues who assist us with their comments. Their wisdom and insight not only educate us but also make the volume that much more interesting and entertaining.

Elsevier continues to provide us with the technical and moral support as well as the editorial assistance. We thank their staff and Susan Showalter in particular for so ably helping us with the project.

Avroy A. Fanaroff, MD

William E. Benitz, MD

Steven M. Donn, MD

Josef Neu, MD

Lu-Ann Papile, MD

Linda J. Van Marter, MD, MPH

The editors are sad to inform you that this will be the final rendition of the Year Book of Neonatal and Perinatal Medicine, as the Year Book series has been discontinued by the publisher. It has been our pleasure working on this publication, and we hope that you the readers have enjoyed the product as much as we have enjoyed producing it. Sayonara.

1 The Fetus

The maternal microbiota drives early postnatal innate immune development

Gomez de Agüero M, Ganal-Vonarburg SC, Fuhrer T, et al (Univ of Bern, Switzerland; Swiss Federal Inst of Technology (ETH) Zürich, Switzerland; et al)

Science 351:1296-1302, 2016

Postnatal colonization of the body with microbes is assumed to be the main stimulus to postnatal immune development. By transiently colonizing pregnant female mice, we show that the maternal microbiota shapes the immune system of the offspring. Gestational colonization increases intestinal group 3 innate lymphoid cells and $F4/80^+CD11c^+$ mononuclear cells in the pups. Maternal colonization reprograms intestinal transcriptional profiles of the offspring, including increased expression of genes encoding epithelial antibacterial peptides and metabolism of microbial molecules. Some of these effects are dependent on maternal antibodies that potentially retain microbial molecules and transmit them to the offspring during pregnancy and in milk. Pups born to mothers transiently colonized in pregnancy are better able to avoid inflammatory responses to microbial molecules and penetration of intestinal microbes.

▶ Classical dogma is that postnatal colonization of the newborn with microbes is the main stimulus to immune development in the newborn. This study used pregnant germ free mice to determine whether maternal microbiota affect the immune system of the offspring. Pregnant mice were colonized with a genetically engineered *Escherichia coli* HA 107, which does not persist in the intestine and allows the pregnant dams to become germ free again before term and naturally deliver germ free pups. The offspring of these animals were compared to noncolonized control offspring. Maternal colonization increased innate lymphoid immune cells and mononuclear cells in the pups. Maternal colonization also reprogrammed intestinal expression of genes encoding epithelial antibacterial peptides as well as metabolism of microbial molecules. The pups born to mothers transiently colonized in pregnancy had a greater capability to avoid inflammatory responses to microbial molecules and penetration of intestinal microbes.

Several postnatal immune cell types are found to differ in offspring of pregnant dams exposed to the *E coli* HA 107. The authors concluded from their studies that the maternal microbiota plays an important role in preparing the newborn for host-microbial mutualism. In their system, they do not find live microbes in the fetal maternal unit, and the effects they see are thought to be due to ligands for the Ahr signaling pathway, that are derived from the maternal microbiota.

This study is of major interest, but is highly reductionist from the real life situation where the pregnant mother is exposed to a large variety of microbes. Several studies suggest that the maternal fetal unit is not sterile and there is exposure of both the fetus and the placenta to a variety of live and dead microbes that may be derived from the vagina, the maternal intestine or oral cavity.[1] The fetal intestine is colonized with microbes prenatally. The viability of these microbes and their effect in the fetal intestine still remains to be evaluated. Nevertheless, the current study demonstrates a relationship between the prenatal maternal microbial environment that has major effects on postnatal innate immunity and tolerance. So the question of whether the maternal fetal unit actually consists of a third component (the maternal fetal microbiome) that forms a triad "holobiont"[2] (mother, fetus and microbes), whose well-being is highly responsive to its environment and can have long-lasting consequences in development of the immune system or even the overall health of the individual throughout the life of the individual via epigenetics.

J. Neu, MD

References

1. Neu J. Developmental aspects of maternal-fetal, and infant gut microbiota and implications for long-term health. *Matern Health Neonatol Perinatol.* 2015;1:6.
2. Rosenberg E, Zilber-Rosenberg I. Microbes drive evolution of animals and plants: the hologenome concept. *MBio.* 2016;7:e01395.

Effects of prenatal antiepileptic drug exposure on newborn brain activity

Videman M, Tokariev A, Stjerna S, et al (Univ of Helsinki, Finland)

Epilepsia 57:252-262, 2016

Objective.—Prenatal exposure to antiepileptic drugs (AEDs) is associated with an increased risk of cognitive dysfunction at early school age. Our aim was to investigate whether signs of adverse drug effects on brain function could be detected already during the first 2 weeks of life.

Methods.—We studied prospectively 56 full-term newborns with prenatal exposure to AEDs and 67 unexposed newborns for the following characteristics: Background information, AED exposure data, pregnancy outcome, neuropsychological evaluation of the mothers, clinical neurologic status with Hammersmith Neonatal Neurological Examination and early cortical activity using electroencephalography (EEG). For EEG assessment, we developed and provide automated quantitation algorithms of several earlier described features: oscillatory bouts at theta and alpha frequencies, frequency spectra, interhemispheric synchrony, and interburst intervals (IBIs).

Results.—The AED-exposed newborns had lower limb and axial tone and were less irritable than the unexposed newborns. EEG assessment disclosed significant differences in alpha bouts, in the frequency spectra, as well as in the spatial distributions of interhemispheric synchrony and IBIs.

Significance.—The results indicate that fetal AED exposure may affect early neonatal neurologic status and several features of early cortical activity. The findings suggest that interference of activity-dependent network development may be a possible mechanism to explain the link from fetal AED exposure to later neurocognitive sequelae.

▶ Accumulating data from animal and human studies indicate that the prenatal environment plays a significant role in shaping children's neurocognitive development. There is, however, a paucity of data linking fetal exposure to pharmaceutical agents and longer term neurodevelopmental outcomes such as presented by Videman who showed that fetal antiepileptic drug exposure is associated with several neurologic and neurophysiologic changes that can be observed during the early neonatal period. These agents may interfere with both development and function.

Clinically the most impairing and devastating effects on the brain are produced by alcohol during fetal development. Gerace reported that prolonged incubation with ethyl alcohol and its subsequent withdrawal from the medium induce an impairment of excitatory synaptic transmission and possibly an incorrect formation of neuronal circuits in developing hippocampus in vitro, which is suggestive of mechanisms that may lead to mental retardation in fetal alcohol spectrum disorders.

Prenatal marijuana exposure (PME) is linked to neurobehavioral and cognitive impairments. Grewen[1] studying unsedated sleep found significant changes in the brain structure of marijuana exposed infants who may also have been exposed to cocaine, nicotine, and alcohol. They reported altered striatal connectivity to areas involved in visual spatial and motor learning, attention, and fine-tuning of motor outputs involved in movement and language production. These structural changes may contribute to neurobehavioral deficits reported in this at-risk group. Other areas involved rendered these infants more vulnerable to drug use and dependency.

Another means of monitoring fetal brain development is the 4-dimensional (4D) ultrasound. Transforming a 3-dimensional image into real-time heralded the era of the 4D ultrasonography. This provides continuous monitoring of fetal face and other surface areas, such as the extremities. Prospectively monitoring facial expressions has provided evidence of maturational changes, permits study of fetal behavior, and is a tool to examine the impact of noxious agents on the developing brain. Kurjak has been the pioneer and the tests are referred to as the Kurjak Antenatal Neurodevelopmental Test (KANET).[2]

To monitor fetal behavior and brain maturation, Sato et al[3] examined the facial expressions of 23 healthy fetuses using 4D ultrasound at 20 to 24 weeks. Each fetus was recorded continuously for 15 minutes. The frequencies of mouthing, yawning, smiling, tongue expulsion, scowling, sucking, and blinking were assessed and the data combined with those expressions observed at 25 to 34 weeks of gestation in 2 previous studies (n = 34) to determine the correlation between gestational age and each of the facial expressions.

Mouthing was significantly more frequent than the other 6 facial expressions at 20 to 24 weeks. Yawning was significantly more frequent than smiling, scowling, and blinking, and sucking was significantly more frequent than smiling, scowling, and blinking. The frequency of yawning, smiling, tongue expulsion, scowling, and blinking increased with gestational age, but mouthing movement and sucking frequencies remained constant between 20 and 34 weeks. With advancing gestational age, development and maturation of the brain is manifest by an increase in the frequency of complicated facial expressions such as smiling and scowling.

Reissland[4] using the same technology and compared the facial expressions in fetuses of smokers and nonsmokers. They noted that the rates of fetal mouth movement and facial self-touch differ significantly between smokers and nonsmokers. There are now the means to study behavioral as well as anatomic features of the developing brain and central nervous system.

It would be interesting to apply this technique accompanied by in utero imaging of the brain to epileptic mothers and note if there are detectable structural and behavioral differences, which correlate with the longer term outcome differences.

A. A. Fanaroff, MD

References

1. Gerace E, Landucci E, Totti A, et al. Alterations of excitatory synaptic transmission in immature organotypic hippocampal slice cultures. *Alcohol Clin Exp Res.* 2016;40:706-716.
2. Kurjak A, Stanojević M, Predojević M, Laušin I, Salihagić-Kadić A. Neurobehavior in fetal life. *Semin Fetal Neonatal Med.* 2012;17:319-323.
3. Sato M, Kanenishi K, Hanaoka U, Noguchi J, Marumo G, Hata T. 4D ultrasound study of fetal facial expressions at 20–24 weeks of gestation. *Int J Gynaecol Obstet.* 2014;126:275-279.
4. Reissland N, Francis B, Kumarendran K, Mason J. Ultrasound observations of subtle movements: a pilot study comparing foetuses of smoking and nonsmoking mothers. *Acta Paediatr.* 2015;104:596-603.

Neurodevelopmental outcome at 2 years in twin-twin transfusion syndrome survivors randomized for the Solomon trial

van Klink JMM, Slaghekke F, Balestriero MA, et al (Leiden Univ Med Ctr, the Netherlands; V Buzzi Children's Hosp, Milan, Italy; et al)
Am J Obstet Gynecol 214:113.e1-7, 2016

Background.—The preferred treatment for twin-twin transfusion syndrome is fetoscopic laser coagulation of inter-twin vascular anastomoses on the monochorionic placenta. Severe postoperative complications can occur when inter-twin vascular anastomoses remain patent including twin-anemia polycythemia sequence or recurrent twin-twin transfusion syndrome. To minimize the occurrence of residual anastomoses, a modified laser surgery technique, the Solomon technique, was developed in which the entire vascular equator is coagulated. In the Solomon randomized controlled trial (NTR1245), the Solomon technique was associated with a significant reduction in twin-anemia polycythemia sequence and recurrence of twin-twin transfusion syndrome when compared with the standard laser surgery technique. Although a significant improvement in perinatal outcome was shown after the Solomon technique, the clinical importance should also be ascertained with long-term follow-up evaluation of the surviving children.

Objective.—The purpose of this study was to compare the long-term neurodevelopmental outcome in surviving children with twin-twin transfusion syndrome who were included in the Solomon randomized trial and treated with either the Solomon technique or standard laser surgery technique.

Study Design.—Routine standardized follow-up evaluation in survivors, at least 2 years after the estimated date of delivery, was performed at 2 of the 5 centers that participated in the Solomon trial: Buzzi Hospital Milan (Italy) and Leiden University Medical Center (The Netherlands). The primary outcome of this follow-up study was survival without long-term neurodevelopmental impairment at age 2 years. *Neurodevelopmental impairment* was defined as cerebral palsy, cognitive and/or motor development score of <85, bilateral blindness, or deafness. Cognitive and motor development was evaluated with the use of Bayley-III. All analyses per fetus, neonate, or child were conducted with the generalized estimated equation module to account for the effect that observations between cotwins are not independent.

Results.—The primary outcome (survival without neurodevelopmental impairment) was detected in 95 of 141 cases (67%) in the Solomon group and in 99 of 146 cases (68%) in the standard group (P =.92). Neurodevelopmental impairment in long-term survivors who were included for follow-up evaluation was detected in 12 of 107 cases (11%) in the Solomon and in 10 of 109 cases (9%) in the standard group (P = .61). Neurodevelopmental impairment was due to cerebral palsy in 1 case (1%; spastic unilateral) in the Solomon group and in 2 cases (2%; spastic unilateral and spastic bilateral) in the standard group (P = .58). Cognitive development <85 cases was detected in 2 of 105 children (2%) in the Solomon group and in 6 of 106 children (6%) in the standard group (P =.23). Motor development <85 occurred in 8 of 103 children (8%) in the Solomon group and 3 of 104 children (3%) in the standard group (P =.23).

Conclusion.—We found no difference in survival without neurodevelopmental impairment between the Solomon and standard laser techniques. In view of the reduction of short-term complications and the absence of increased adverse long-term effects, these data support the use of the Solomon technique in the treatment of twin-twin transfusion syndrome.

▶ Monochorionic twin pregnancies can be complicated by twin-to-twin transfusion syndrome (TTTS). Currently the most popular form of fetal surgery and the best treatment option for TTTS is fetoscopic laser coagulation of the vascular anastomoses between donor and recipient. After standard laser therapy, up to 33% residual anastomoses may still be present and be responsible for recurrent TTTS and twin anemia polycythemia sequence (TAPS). To reduce the number of residual anastomoses and their complications, the Solomon technique, where the whole vascular equator is coagulated, was introduced. In the initial trial, the Solomon technique was associated with a reduction in TAPS (3% vs 16%) for the standard treatment and recurrence of TTTS (1% vs 7%).[1] Further experience has been positive. The incidence of recurrent TTTS after the Solomon technique ranges from 0% to 3.9% compared with 5.3% to 8.5% after the selective technique. The incidence of TAPS after the Solomon technique ranged from 0% to 2.9% compared with 4.2% to 15.6% after the selective technique. The Solomon technique may improve dual survival rates ranging from 64% to 85% compared with 46% to 76% for the selective technique. There was no difference reported in procedure-related complications such as intrauterine infection and preterm premature rupture of membranes. The Solomon technique has thus become the treatment of choice for TTTS.[2,3]

It remained to look at the longer outcome of these pregnancies. This initial follow-up study of subjects from 2 of the original Solomon centers by van Klink shows equivalent neurodevelopmental outcomes in the Solomon group when compared with the standard laser therapy group. It would have been nice to have a twin control group that had not had laser surgery too. However, these results overall are encouraging and the 94% retention rate for follow-up is spectacular.

Akkerman[4] provides perspective on the advances in the treatment of TTTS over the past 25 years. From 34 studies including 3868 monochorionic twin pregnancies, the mean survival of both twins increased significantly from 35% to 65% and for at least 1 twin from 70% to 88% over the past 25 years. Mean gestational age at birth remained stable over the years at 32 weeks' gestation. They also showed a significantly improved perinatal survival with the evolution of the laser technique from nonselective to selective, selective sequential and the Solomon technique. They attribute the improved outcome to several factors including " evolution of the laser technique, learning curve effect, better referral and improved early neonatal care."

A. A. Fanaroff, MD

References

1. Slaghekke F, Lopriore E, Lewi L, et al. Fetoscopic laser coagulation of the vascular equator versus selective coagulation for twin-to-twin transfusion syndrome: an open-label randomized controlled trial. *Lancet.* 2014;21:2144-2151.
2. Slaghekke F, Oepkes D. Solomon technique versus selective coagulation for twin-twin transfusion syndrome. *Twin Res Hum Genet.* 2016;19:217-221.
3. Dhillon RK, Hillman SC, Pounds R, Morris RK, Kilby MD. Comparison of Solomon technique with selective laser ablation for twin-twin transfusion syndrome: a systematic review. *Ultrasound Obstet Gynecol.* 2015;46:526-533.
4. Akkermans J, Peeters SH, Klumper FJ, Lopriore E, Middeldorp JM, Oepkes D. Twenty-five years of fetoscopic laser coagulation in twin-twin transfusion syndrome: a systematic review. *Fetal Diagn Ther.* 2015;38:241-253.

Trends in Care Practices, Morbidity, and Mortality of Extremely Preterm Neonates, 1993-2012

Stoll BJ, for the Eunice Kennedy Shriver National Institute of Child Health and Human Development Neonatal Research Network (Emory Univ School of Medicine, Atlanta, GA; et al)
JAMA 314:1039-1051, 2015

Importance.—Extremely preterm infants contribute disproportionately to neonatal morbidity and mortality.

Objective.—To review 20-year trends in maternal/neonatal care, complications, and mortality among extremely preterm infants born at Neonatal Research Network centers.

Design, Setting, Participants.—Prospective registry of 34 636 infants, 22 to 28 weeks' gestation, birth weight of 401 to 1500 g, and born at 26 network centers between 1993 and 2012.

Exposures.—Extremely preterm birth.

Main Outcomes and Measures.—Maternal/neonatal care, morbidities, and survival. Major morbidities, reported for infants who survived more than 12 hours, were severe necrotizing enterocolitis, infection, bronchopulmonary dysplasia, severe intracranial hemorrhage, cystic periventricular leukomalacia, and/or severe retinopathy of prematurity. Regression models assessed yearly changes and were adjusted for study center, race/ethnicity, gestational age, birth weight for gestational age, and sex.

Results.—Use of antenatal corticosteroids increased from 1993 to 2012 (24% [348 of 1431 infants]) to 87% (1674 of 1919 infants]; $P < .001$), as did cesarean delivery (44% [625 of 1431 births] to 64% [1227 of 1921]; $P < .001$). Delivery room intubation decreased from 80% (1144 of 1433 infants) in 1993 to 65% (1253 of 1922) in 2012 ($P < .001$). After increasing in the 1990s, postnatal steroid use declined to 8% (141 of 1757 infants) in 2004 ($P < .001$), with no significant change thereafter. Although most infants were ventilated, continuous positive airway pressure without ventilation increased from 7% (120 of 1666 infants) in 2002 to 11% (190 of 1756 infants) in 2012 ($P < .001$). Despite no improvement from 1993 to 2004, rates of late-onset sepsis declined between 2005 and 2012 for infants of each gestational age (median, 26 weeks [37% {109 of 296} to 27% {85 of 320}]; adjusted relative risk [RR], 0.93 [95% CI, 0.92-0.94]). Rates of other morbidities declined, but bronchopulmonary dysplasia increased between 2009 and 2012 for infants at 26 to 27 weeks' gestation (26 weeks, 50% [130 of 258] to 55% [164 of 297]; $P < .001$). Survival increased between 2009 and 2012 for infants at 23 weeks' gestation (27% [41 of 152] to 33% [50 of 150]; adjusted RR, 1.09 [95% CI, 1.05-1.14]) and 24 weeks (63% [156 of 248] to 65% [174 of 269]; adjusted RR, 1.05 [95% CI, 1.03-1.07]), with smaller relative increases for infants at 25 and 27 weeks' gestation, and no change for infants at 22, 26, and 28 weeks' gestation. Survival without major morbidity increased approximately 2% per year for infants at 25 to 28 weeks' gestation, with no change for infants at 22 to 24 weeks' gestation.

Conclusions and Relevance.—Among extremely preterm infants born at US academic centers over the last 20 years, changes in maternal and infant care practices and modest reductions in several morbidities were observed, although bronchopulmonary dysplasia increased. Survival increased most markedly for infants born at 23 and 24 weeks' gestation and survival without major morbidity increased for infants aged 25 to 28 weeks. These findings may be valuable in counseling families and developing novel interventions.

Trial Registration.—clinicaltrials.gov Identifier: NCT00063063.

▶ Globally, 2.9 million infants die in the first month of life, and an additional 2.6 million are stillborn. Four of 5 newborn deaths result from 3 preventable or treatable conditions: (1) complications from prematurity and low birth weight, (2) complications during childbirth (including birth asphyxia), and (3) infection. Proven low-cost interventions, health commodities, and medicines can prevent more than two-thirds of newborn deaths. Proficiency in the care of the preterm neonate is paramount to ensuring safe and quality outcomes. Gaps in coverage, equity, and quality of care around birth and postnatal care for small and ill newborn infants exist in health facilities in many low- and middle-income countries. These gaps include insufficient numbers of trained caregivers, poor birth attendant skills, poor quality of services, and lack of access to even basic technology and medications. Practical, competency-based training for providers, and implementation of quality improvement mechanisms for clinical services can help address these barriers to optimal care and thus to child survival.[1-3]

In addition to the article from Stoll abstracted here, there have been 3 articles concerning the outcome of low birth weight, low gestational age infants from the *Eunice Kennedy Shriver* National Institute of Child Health and Human Development Neonatal Research Network (NICHD) generic database.[4-6] These manuscripts address important issues such as center variability,[4] the impact of proactive care at the borders of viability,[5] and the causes and timing of death.[6]

Stoll et al, in what should be considered a classic publication reviewed 20-year trends in maternal/neonatal care, complications, and mortality among 34 636 infants 22 to 28 weeks' gestation, birth weight of 401 to 1500 g, and born between 1993 and 2012 at Neonatal Research Network centers. Survival increased between 2009 and 2012 for infants at 23 weeks' gestation (27%–33%) and 24 weeks (63%–65%); with smaller relative increases for infants at 25 and 27 weeks' gestation, and no change for infants at 22, 26, and 28 weeks' gestation. Survival without major morbidity increased approximately 2% per year for infants at 25 to 28 weeks' gestation, with no change for infants at 22 to 24 weeks' gestation.

They noted that the use of antenatal corticosteroids increased from 24% in 1993 to 87% in 2012, as did cesarean delivery, from 44% to 64%. In other words, there was more active care. Importantly, delivery room intubation decreased from 80% in 1993 to 65% in 2012. After increasing in the 1990s, postnatal steroid use, after proven to be harmful, declined to 8% in 2004, with no significant change thereafter. Although most infants were ventilated, continuous positive airway pressure without ventilation increased from 7% in 2002 to 11% in 2012. Despite no improvement from 1993 to 2004, rates of late-onset sepsis declined between 2005 and 2012 for infants of each gestational age. This reflects increased attention to quality improvement, surgical placement, and management of central lines. After accepting high rates of infection in immature babies as inevitable, we have come to recognize that better management of central lines, together with more aggressive enteral feeding so that lines can be removed sooner, can substantially reduce hospital acquired infections. Rates of other morbidities declined, but bronchopulmonary dysplasia increased between 2009 and 2012 for infants at 26 to 27 weeks' gestation.

In summary, the improvements in outcomes over the past decade have been incremental rather than dramatic. There are still many problems to solve and no magic bullets on the horizon. To obtain the best results, units need to practice evidence-based medicine with a culture dedicated to exceptional care of these fragile infants.

Rysavy[4] reported that overall rates of survival and survival without severe impairment ranged from 5.1% and 3.4%, respectively, among children born at 22 weeks' gestation to 81.4% and 75.6%, respectively, among those born at 26 weeks' gestation. Hospital rates of active treatment accounted for 78% and 75% of the between-hospital variation in survival and survival without severe impairment, respectively, among children born at 22 or 23 weeks' gestation, and accounted for 22% and 16%, respectively, among those born at 24 weeks' gestation, but the rates did not account for any of the variation in outcomes among those born at 25 or 26 weeks' gestation. Markers of a proactive approach to perinatal and neonatal management include interventions by obstetricians (antenatal corticosteroids and cesarean deliveries for fetal distress) and neonatologists (delivery room resuscitation, optimal cord management, and intensive care).

Smith[5] reported on the NICHD Neonatal Network centers experience and approach to infants born at 22 to 24 weeks' gestation. This included a cohort of 3631 infants 22 to 24 weeks' gestation and 5227 infants 25 to 27 weeks' gestation. Among the 22- to 24-week infants, use of antenatal corticosteroids ranged from 28% to 100%, cesarean delivery from 13% to 65%, and resuscitation from 30% to 100% by center. Centers with higher rates of antenatal corticosteroid use in 22- to 24-week infants had reduced rates of death, death or retinopathy of prematurity, death or late-onset sepsis, death or necrotizing enterocolitis, and death or neurodevelopmental impairment in 25- to 27-week infants.

They concluded that physicians' willingness to provide care to extremely low gestation infants as measured by frequency of use of antenatal corticosteroids, willingness to perform a cesarean delivery, and willingness to actively resuscitate is associated with improved survival.

Backes[7] on the basis of a single-center experience, confirmed the above findings, noting that at 23 weeks' gestation, proactive, interdisciplinary care enabled more than half of the neonates to survive, and approximately half of children evaluated at 18 months exhibited no or mild impairment. Patel[6] noted that the number of deaths per 1000 live births was 275 (95% confidence interval [CI]: 264–285) from 2000 through 2003 and 285 (95% CI: 275–295) from 2004 through 2007; the number decreased to 258 (95% CI: 248–268) in the 2008–2011 period ($P = .003$ for the comparison across 3 periods). There were significantly fewer pulmonary-related deaths attributed to the respiratory distress syndrome and bronchopulmonary dysplasia in 2008–2011 than in 2000–2003 or 2004–2007. Compared with 2000–2003, in 2008–2011, there were decreases in deaths attributed to immaturity, infection, and central nervous system injury, but there were increases in deaths attributed to necrotizing enterocolitis. Overall, 40.4% of deaths occurred within 12 hours after birth, and 17.3% occurred after 28 days.

Taking the view from above, we can be encouraged by the declining rates of mortality and morbidity. Nonetheless, there is no room for complacency. The increase in the number of infants surviving with bronchopulmonary dysplasia and dying from necrotizing enterocolitis needs urgent attention. Attention to the resuscitation and management on the first day of life is vital to further improve outcomes.

A. A. Fanaroff, MD

References

1. UNICEF. WHO. Every newborn: an action plan to end preventable newborn deaths. 2013. www.everynewborn.org.
2. Dickson KE, Simen-Kapeu A, Kinney MV, et al. for the Lancet Every Newborn Study Group. Health-systems bottlenecks and strategies to accelerate scale-up in countries. *Lancet.* 2014;384:438-454.
3. Bhutta ZA, Das JK, Bahl R, et al. for the Lancet Newborn Interventions Review Group and The Lancet Every Newborn StudyGroup. Can available interventions end preventable deaths in mothers, newborn babies, and stillbirths, and at what cost? *Lancet.* 2014;384:347-370.
4. Rysavy MA, Li L, Bell EF, et al. Eunice Kennedy Shriver National Institute of Child Health and Human Development Neonatal Research Network. Between-hospital variation in treatment and outcomes in extremely preterm infants. *N Engl J Med.* 2015;372:1801-1811.
5. Patel RM, Kandefer S, Walsh MC, et al. Eunice Kennedy Shriver National Institute of Child Health and Human Development Neonatal Research Network. Causes and timing of death in extremely premature infants from 2000 through 2011. *N Engl J Med.* 2015;372:331-340.
6. Smith PB, Ambalavanan N, Li L, et al. Generic Database Subcommittee; Eunice Kennedy Shriver National Institute of Child Health Human Development Neonatal Research Network. Approach to infants born at 22 to 24weeks' gestation: relationship to outcomes of more-mature infants. *Pediatrics.* 2012;129:e1508-e1516.
7. Backes CH, Rivera BK, Haque U, et al. A Proactive approach to infants born at 23 weeks gestation. *Obstet Gynecol.* 2015;126:939-946.

Trends in Care Practices, Morbidity, and Mortality of Extremely Preterm Neonates, 1993-2012

Stoll BJ, for the Eunice Kennedy Shriver National Institute of Child Health and Human Development Neonatal Research Network (Emory Univ School of Medicine, Atlanta, GA; et al)

JAMA 314:1039-1051, 2015

Importance.—Extremely preterm infants contribute disproportionately to neonatal morbidity and mortality.

Objective.—To review 20-year trends in maternal/neonatal care, complications, and mortality among extremely preterm infants born at Neonatal Research Network centers.

Design, Setting, Participants.—Prospective registry of 34,636 infants, 22 to 28 weeks' gestation, birth weight of 401 to 1500 g, and born at 26 network centers between 1993 and 2012.

Exposures.—Extremely preterm birth.

Main Outcomes and Measures.—Maternal/neonatal care, morbidities, and survival. Major morbidities, reported for infants who survived more than 12 hours, were severe necrotizing enterocolitis, infection, bronchopulmonary dysplasia, severe intracranial hemorrhage, cystic periventricular leukomalacia, and/or severe retinopathy of prematurity. Regression models assessed yearly changes and were adjusted for study center, race/ethnicity, gestational age, birth weight for gestational age, and sex.

Results.—Use of antenatal corticosteroids increased from 1993 to 2012 (24% [348 of 1431 infants]) to 87% (1674 of 1919 infants]; $P < .001$), as did cesarean delivery (44% [625 of 1431 births] to 64% [1227 of 1921]; $P < .001$). Delivery room intubation decreased from 80% (1144 of 1433 infants) in 1993 to 65% (1253 of 1922) in 2012 ($P < .001$). After increasing in the 1990s, postnatal steroid use declined to 8% (141 of 1757 infants) in 2004 ($P < .001$), with no significant change thereafter. Although most infants were ventilated, continuous positive airway pressure without ventilation increased from 7% (120 of 1666 infants) in 2002 to 11% (190 of 1756 infants) in 2012 ($P < .001$). Despite no improvement from 1993 to 2004, rates of late-onset sepsis declined between 2005 and 2012 for infants of each gestational age (median, 26 weeks [37% {109 of 296} to 27% {85 of 320}]; adjusted relative risk [RR], 0.93 [95% CI, 0.92-0.94]). Rates of other morbidities declined, but bronchopulmonary dysplasia increased between 2009 and 2012 for infants at 26 to 27 weeks' gestation (26 weeks, 50% [130 of 258] to 55% [164 of 297]; $P < .001$). Survival increased between 2009 and 2012 for infants at 23 weeks' gestation (27% [41 of 152] to 33% [50 of 150]; adjusted RR, 1.09 [95% CI, 1.05-1.14]) and 24 weeks (63% [156 of 248] to 65% [174 of 269]; adjusted RR, 1.05 [95% CI, 1.03-1.07]), with smaller relative increases for infants at 25 and 27 weeks' gestation, and no change for infants at 22, 26, and 28 weeks' gestation. Survival without major morbidity increased approximately 2% per year for infants at 25 to 28 weeks' gestation, with no change for infants at 22 to 24 weeks' gestation.

Conclusions and Relevance.—Among extremely preterm infants born at US academic centers over the last 20 years, changes in maternal and infant care practices and modest reductions in several morbidities were observed, although bronchopulmonary dysplasia increased. Survival increased most markedly for infants born at 23 and 24 weeks' gestation and survival without major morbidity increased for infants aged 25 to 28 weeks. These findings may be valuable in counseling families and developing novel interventions.

Trial Registration.—clinicaltrials.gov Identifier: NCT00063063.

▶ In this report from the *Eunice Kennedy Shriver* National Institute of Child Health and Human Development Neonatal Research Network, Stoll et al provide an important historical overview of outcomes for infants born before 29 weeks gestation over the past 2 decades. Although much of the recent controversy about management of infants at the margin of viability has focused on those born before 24 weeks' gestation, the remarkable trends described here took place in more mature infants. The prevalent belief that survival rates have increased notwithstanding, changes in survival have been few and small. Survival rates at 22 weeks are unchanged at a dismal 7%. The modest increases in survival at 23 and 24 weeks between 2003–2007 and 2008–2012, from 26% to 32% and 55% to 62%, respectively, were statistically significant ($P = .064$, chi-squared for trend across the 4 five-year epochs and 0.004 for change between most recent 2 epochs at 23 weeks, and $P < .001$ for both comparisons at 24 weeks) but too small in magnitude to influence a substantial change in practice. No changes in mortality across the 4 epochs were apparent at 25 through 27 weeks ($P > .05$ by chi-squared for trend), and only a small increase from 92 to 94% at 28 weeks. Regression analysis focused on the interval from 2009 to 2012, adjusting for study center, maternal race/ethnicity, infant gestational age, small size for gestational age, and sex, demonstrated significant increases in survival among infants born at 23, 24, 25, and 27 weeks gestation within that era (adjusted relative risks of survival 1.09, 1.05, 1.01, and 1.01 per year, respectively), suggesting that we may be in the midst of a transitional period to improved survival rates, particularly at 23 and 24 weeks gestation. Sadly, those trends are not matched by major improvements in rates of survival without major morbidity, which have not changed over the past 20 years for infants born at 23 or 24 weeks' gestation. Rates of survival without major morbidity increased by an average of 2% per year (relative to prior year) in infants born at 25 through 28 weeks gestation, increasing from 13% to 17% at 25 weeks, 19% to 27% at 26 weeks, 28% to 43% at 27 weeks, and 35% to 56% at 28 weeks. Those improvements occurred between the past 2 half-decades for infants born at 25 weeks, in the first 3 for those born at 26 weeks, and between the first 2 and last 2 epochs for the 27- and 28-week cohorts, suggesting that the reasons for improved outcomes may vary between the least mature and more mature preterm infants. Although we can take considerable satisfaction about these improved outcomes, particularly for infants born at 27 or 28 weeks' gestation, it should be evident that there is still a large opportunity for continued improvement.

These data provide little support for the concept that improving rates and quality of survival among the most immature infants (<26 or 27 weeks) demand a reevaluation of attitudes and practices related to decision making about their care. The regression models suggest a very recent trend toward improved survival rates, but survival without major morbidity has not followed suit so far. The case for stronger advocacy for more active intervention for these infants rests on the expectation that outcomes can be improved by more proactive management, as suggested by experience accruing from single institutions or overseas. Parent counseling, both before and after birth of an extremely premature infant, should account for that possibility and should not overlook either the real potential for healthy survival at 23 to 24 weeks nor the persistent nontrivial risks of death or disability at 25 or 26 weeks' gestation.

W. E. Benitz, MD

2 Epidemiology and Pregnancy Complications

Antenatal Betamethasone for Women at Risk for Late Preterm Delivery

Gyamfi-Bannerman C, for the NICHD Maternal–Fetal Medicine Units Network
(Columbia Univ, NY; et al)

N Engl J Med 374:1311-1320, 2016

Background.—Infants who are born at 34 to 36 weeks of gestation (late preterm) are at greater risk for adverse respiratory and other outcomes than those born at 37 weeks of gestation or later. It is not known whether betamethasone administered to women at risk for late preterm delivery decreases the risks of neonatal morbidities.

Methods.—We conducted a multicenter, randomized trial involving women with a singleton pregnancy at 34 weeks 0 days to 36 weeks 5 days of gestation who were at high risk for delivery during the late preterm period (up to 36 weeks 6 days). The participants were assigned to receive two injections of betamethasone or matching placebo 24 hours apart. The primary outcome was a neonatal composite of treatment in the first 72 hours (the use of continuous positive airway pressure or high-flow nasal cannula for at least 2 hours, supplemental oxygen with a fraction of inspired oxygen of at least 0.30 for at least 4 hours, extracorporeal membrane oxygenation, or mechanical ventilation) or stillbirth or neonatal death within 72 hours after delivery.

Results.—The primary outcome occurred in 165 of 1427 infants (11.6%) in the betamethasone group and 202 of 1400 (14.4%) in the placebo group (relative risk in the betamethasone group, 0.80; 95% confidence interval [CI], 0.66 to 0.97; $P = 0.02$). Severe respiratory complications, transient tachypnea of the newborn, surfactant use, and bronchopulmonary dysplasia also occurred significantly less frequently in the betamethasone group. There were no significant between-group differences in the incidence of chorioamnionitis or neonatal sepsis. Neonatal hypoglycemia was more common in the betamethasone group than in the placebo group (24.0% vs. 15.0%; relative risk, 1.60; 95% CI, 1.37 to 1.87; $P < 0.001$).

Conclusions.—Administration of betamethasone to women at risk for late preterm delivery significantly reduced the rate of neonatal respiratory complications. (Funded by the National Heart, Lung, and Blood Institute and the Eunice Kennedy Shriver National Institute of Child Health and Human Development; ClinicalTrials.gov number, NCT01222247.)

▶ This well-designed and executed *Eunice Kennedy Shriver* National Institute of Child Health and Human Development study reports modest, but significant, improvement in the incidence of respiratory morbidity among late preterm infants born to mothers who received antenatal betamethasone. This was a large multicenter prospective placebo (saline) controlled trial involving more than 2800 subjects who received betamethasone or saline injections before anticipated late preterm delivery with a primary outcome of respiratory morbidity in the newborn within the first 72 hours of life. The majority of infants delivered between 350/7 to 366/7 weeks' gestation.

Five hundred and ninety-six (42%) infants whose mothers received betamethasone, and 629 (45%) control infants, required admission to an intermediate care unit or neonatal intensive care unit (NICU; $P = .009$). However, the control infants spent significantly more time (≥3 days) in the intermediate care nursery or NICU (37%) compared with treated newborns (32.9%), $P = .03$, relative risk [RR] 0.89 (95% confidence interval [CI] 0.80–0.98).

The composite of respiratory distress syndrome (RDS), transient tachypnea of the newborn (TTN), or apnea favored the treatment group ($P = .004$) and was largely due to a lower rate of TTN in betamethasone-treated infants. The incidence of RDS, oddly enough, was not reduced by antenatal steroid treatment, but bronchopulmonary dysplasia (BPD), defined as oxygen requirement at 28 days, was lower in the treatment group: 2 versus 9 infants, $P = .04$. The authors note that similar findings were reported in the ASTECS Trial, a British multicenter study in which women were prospectively randomized to receive antenatal betamethasone or no glucocorticoids 48 hours before elective cesarean delivery at term.[1] In this more mature cohort of infants, there was a significant reduction in the rate of admission to NICUs for respiratory complications in the betamethasone group (RR: 0.46: 95% CI: 0.23–0.93.), owing primarily to fewer cases of TTN.

Nearly a quarter of the treated infants developed hypoglycemia (defined as a blood glucose <40 mg/dL), compared with 15% incidence in the controls, $P < .001$. The authors claim this was a transient issue that did not prolong hospitalization. I do not think this has been reported in previous trials because it was not looked for. Clearly, glucose monitoring will be required for infants exposed to antenatal steroids in the future.

Surprising to me is the fact that the median length of hospital stay (LOS; 7–8 days) was not different between the betamethasone-treated late preterms and their placebo comrades. The higher rate of BPD in control infants (n = 9) compared with treated infants (n = 2) may have skewed the mean LOS but, given how few infants carry the diagnosis of BPD in this large cohort, the median LOS was clearly more appropriate.

There were no extracorporeal membrane oxygenation (ECMO) patients in either arm of this study, which, I think, reflects the many improvements in respiratory care of the term and late preterm newborn over the past 20 years.[2-4] Among these are surfactant, inhaled nitric oxide, and permissive hyperapnea/gentle ventilation in the sicker infants with hypoxic respiratory failure. Increased use of noninvasive ventilation, that is, continuous positive airway pressure, nasal intermittent mandatory ventilation, and high flow nasal cannulae may also be of added benefit. In the 1990s, term and late preterm infants with respiratory failure figured prominently in the Extracorporeal Life Support Organization Registry of neonatal ECMO patients, but far less so today.[5]

Lastly, a financial analysis of dollars saved through the use of antenatal betamethasone and its resultant decrease in neonatal respiratory morbidity would be most welcome.

E. K. Stork, MD

References

1. Stutchfield P, Whitaker R, Russell I, on behalf of the Antenatal Steroids for Term Elective Caesarean Section [ASTECS] Research Team. Antenatal betamethasone and incidence of neonatal respiratory distress after elective caesarean section: pragmatic randomised trial. *BMJ*. 2005;331:662-666.
2. Ramachandrappa A, Rosenberg ES, Wagoner S, Jain L. Morbidity and mortality in late preterm infants with severe hypoxic respiratory failure on extra-corporeal membrane oxygenation. *J Pediatr.* 2011;159:192-198.
3. Keszler M, Carbone MT, Cox C, Schumacher RE. Severe respiratory failure after elective repeat cesarean delivery: a potentially preventable condition leading to extracorporeal membrane oxygenation. *Pediatrics*. 1992;89:670-672.
4. Gouyon J-B, Iacobelli S, Ferdynus C, Bonsante F. Neonatal problems of late and moderate preterm infants. *Semin Fetal Neonatal Med.* 2012;17:146-152.
5. Extracorporeal Life Support Organization [ELSO] Registry, January 2016. Registry of neonatal ECMO cases.

Antenatal Betamethasone for Women at Risk for Late Preterm Delivery

Gyamfi-Bannerman C, for the NICHD Maternal—Fetal Medicine Units Network (Columbia Univ, NY)
N Engl J Med 374:1311-1320, 2016

Background.—Infants who are born at 34 to 36 weeks of gestation (late preterm) are at greater risk for adverse respiratory and other outcomes than those born at 37 weeks of gestation or later. It is not known whether betamethasone administered to women at risk for late preterm delivery decreases the risks of neonatal morbidities.

Methods.—We conducted a multicenter, randomized trial involving women with a singleton pregnancy at 34 weeks 0 days to 36 weeks 5 days of gestation who were at high risk for delivery during the late preterm period (up to 36 weeks 6 days). The participants were assigned to receive two injections of betamethasone or matching placebo 24 hours apart. The primary outcome was a neonatal composite of treatment in the first 72 hours (the use of continuous positive airway pressure or high-flow nasal cannula for at least 2 hours, supplemental oxygen with a fraction of inspired oxygen of at least 0.30 for at least 4 hours, extracorporeal membrane oxygenation, or mechanical ventilation) or stillbirth or neonatal death within 72 hours after delivery.

Results.—The primary outcome occurred in 165 of 1427 infants (11.6%) in the betamethasone group and 202 of 1400 (14.4%) in the placebo group (relative risk in the betamethasone group, 0.80; 95% confidence interval [CI], 0.66 to 0.97; $P = 0.02$). Severe respiratory complications, transient tachypnea of the newborn, surfactant use, and bronchopulmonary dysplasia also occurred significantly less frequently in the betamethasone group. There were no significant between-group differences in the incidence of chorioamnionitis or neonatal sepsis. Neonatal hypoglycemia was more common in the betamethasone group than in the placebo group (24.0% vs. 15.0%; relative risk, 1.60; 95% CI, 1.37 to 1.87; $P < 0.001$).

Conclusions.—Administration of betamethasone to women at risk for late preterm delivery significantly reduced the rate of neonatal respiratory complications. (Funded by the National Heart, Lung, and Blood Institute and the Eunice Kennedy Shriver National Institute of Child Health and Human Development; ClinicalTrials.gov number, NCT01222247.)

▶ I recall that as a resident in the late 1990s, the question of elective delivery between 34 and 36 weeks was usually preceded by a question regarding whether an amniocentesis for fetal lung maturity (FLM) had been performed. Although the use of the FLM now seems quaint in its obsolescence, the intention at the time was to gain some insight into the potential well-being of the electively delivered near-term neonate. Care in this interval is not typically marked by the morbidity of the earlier gestational weeks but, by dint of sheer numbers, represents a significant drain on perinatal resources. The problem is as vexing in contemporary practice as it was in the day of the FLM. Gyamfi-Bannerman et al. represent the most recent attempt to improve outcomes for infants delivered 34 to 36 + 6 weeks. Their large multicenter study administered a standard course of betamethasone or placebo to women at high risk of delivering in this interval. They found the administration of the betamethasone was associated with a significant reduction in the incidence of their primary respiratory outcome composite. Within that composite, the need for mechanical ventilation, stillbirth or neonatal death, or the fraction of inspired oxygen ≥0.30 for ≥4 hours was not different between the groups. The difference seems to have been mostly driven by a reduced need for continuous positive airway pressure (CPAP) or high-flow nasal cannula for ≥2 continuous hours. There was also a higher incidence of neonatal hypoglycemia in infants of mothers who received betamethasone. Are the advantages of reduced CPAP sufficient to warrant adoption of this treatment into standard obstetrical practice? Absent improvement in the need for mechanical ventilation or any of the more severe morbidities within the composite and given the possibility of glycemic instability, the utility of the treatment is less clear. Add to this the ongoing concerns for potential adverse long-term developmental outcomes after betamethasone exposure, and the utility is even less evident. For these reasons, at my home institution, we have not yet adopted the use of betamethasone after 34 weeks. Until additional follow-up information is available, the problem of care in this interval will remain vexing.

T. F. McElrath, MD, PhD

Antenatal Betamethasone for Women at Risk for Late Preterm Delivery

Gyamfi-Bannerman C, for the NICHD Maternal–Fetal Medicine Units Network (Columbia Univ, NY; et al)

N Engl J Med 374:1311-1320, 2016

Background.—Infants who are born at 34 to 36 weeks of gestation (late preterm) are at greater risk for adverse respiratory and other outcomes than those born at 37 weeks of gestation or later. It is not known whether betamethasone administered to women at risk for late preterm delivery decreases the risks of neonatal morbidities.

Methods.—We conducted a multicenter, randomized trial involving women with a singleton pregnancy at 34 weeks 0 days to 36 weeks 5 days of gestation who were at high risk for delivery during the late preterm period (up to 36 weeks 6 days). The participants were assigned to receive two injections of betamethasone or matching placebo 24 hours apart. The primary outcome was a neonatal composite of treatment in the first 72 hours (the use of continuous positive airway pressure or high-flow nasal cannula for at least 2 hours, supplemental oxygen with a fraction of inspired oxygen of at least 0.30 for at least 4 hours, extracorporeal membrane oxygenation, or mechanical ventilation) or stillbirth or neonatal death within 72 hours after delivery.

Results.—The primary outcome occurred in 165 of 1427 infants (11.6%) in the betamethasone group and 202 of 1400 (14.4%) in the placebo group (relative risk in the betamethasone group, 0.80; 95% confidence interval [CI], 0.66 to 0.97; $P = 0.02$). Severe respiratory complications, transient tachypnea of the newborn, surfactant use, and bronchopulmonary dysplasia also occurred significantly less frequently in the betamethasone group. There were no significant between-group differences in the incidence of chorioamnionitis or neonatal sepsis. Neonatal hypoglycemia was more common in the betamethasone group than in the placebo group (24.0% vs. 15.0%; relative risk, 1.60; 95% CI, 1.37 to 1.87; $P<0.001$).

Conclusions.—Administration of betamethasone to women at risk for late preterm delivery significantly reduced the rate of neonatal respiratory complications. (Funded by the National Heart, Lung, and Blood Institute and the Eunice Kennedy Shriver National Institute of Child Health and Human Development; ClinicalTrials.gov number, NCT01222247.)

▶ The benefits of antenatal steroid therapy for threatened preterm delivery have been well documented for infants born at less than 34 weeks of gestation.

Additionally, a large randomized, controlled trial (RCT) found that antenatal steroid therapy provided benefit for infants born by cesarean section without labor at early-term gestation (37-38 weeks).[1] Now, Gyamfi-Bannerman and colleagues of the National Institute of Child Health and Human Development Maternal—Fetal Medicine Units Network have bridged the gestational age gap by reporting benefits for late preterm infants. In this multicenter, randomized, clinical trial, the investigators evaluated the effects of 1 course (2 doses) of antenatal betamethasone in 2827 women with singleton pregnancies between 34 and 36 weeks of gestation at high risk of preterm delivery. Women with gestational diabetes were excluded.

The primary outcome for the study was a composite respiratory neonatal outcome, described in the abstract, which occurred significantly less often in the treated group than in the placebo group (14.4% vs 11.6%). The benefit was particularly apparent for infants with planned cesarean section (Appendix online: 16.2% vs 26.2%, relative risk, 0.62; [95% confidence interval, 0.43-0.90]). The authors also found other benefits, including significant decreases in resuscitation at birth (18.7% vs 14.5%), median time to first feeding (5.5 vs 9.9 hours), and neonatal intensive care unit admission ≥3 days (32.9% vs 37%). The only apparent short-term adverse effect was an increase in hypoglycemia (24% vs 15%) not associated with longer hospital stay. The authors conclude that administration of betamethasone to women at risk for late preterm delivery significantly reduced the rate of neonatal respiratory complications.

These results have important implications not only for potentially decreasing costs and improving outcomes for late-preterm infants but also for substantially increasing the number of fetuses exposed to glucocorticoids. Importantly, the study inclusion criteria (preterm labor with ≥3-cm dilation or 75% cervical effacement or rupture of membranes; or any other indication either through induction or cesarean section between 24 hours and 7 days as determined by the obstetrical provider) defined a patient population at very high risk for preterm delivery: only 16% of these women delivered at term, and only 3% delivered at ≥ 39 weeks of gestation. With the significant benefits demonstrated in this RCT, therapeutic creep may result in treatment of increasing numbers of pregnancies that are at lower risk of preterm delivery. Although 1 long-term study of adult outcomes of patients enrolled in an RCT of antenatal corticosteroid exposure was generally reassuring,[2,3] this RCT provides a unique and important opportunity to further evaluate long-term effects of antenatal steroid exposure in a large population; funding agencies should be urged to do so.

L. A. Papile, MD

References

1. Stutchfield P, Whitaker R, Russell I. Antenatal betamethasone and incidence of neonatal respiratory distress after elective caesarean section: pragmatic randomised trial. *BMJ*. 2005;331:662.
2. Dalziel SR, Lim VK, Lambert A, et al. Antenatal exposure to betamethasone: psychological functioning and health related quality of life 31 years after inclusion in randomised controlled trial. *BMJ*. 2005;331:665.

3. Dalziel SR, Walker NK, Parag V, et al. Cardiovascular risk factors after antenatal exposure to betamethasone: 30 year follow-up of a randomised controlled trial. *Lancet*. 2005;365:1856-1862.

Antenatal Betamethasone for Women at Risk for Late Preterm Delivery

Gyamfi-Bannerman C, for the NICHD Maternal—Fetal Medicine Units Network (Columbia Univ, NY; et al)

N Engl J Med 374:1311-1320, 2016

Background.—Infants who are born at 34 to 36 weeks of gestation (late preterm) are at greater risk for adverse respiratory and other outcomes than those born at 37 weeks of gestation or later. It is not known whether betamethasone administered to women at risk for late preterm delivery decreases the risks of neonatal morbidities.

Methods.—We conducted a multicenter, randomized trial involving women with a singleton pregnancy at 34 weeks 0 days to 36 weeks 5 days of gestation who were at high risk for delivery during the late preterm period (up to 36 weeks 6 days). The participants were assigned to receive two injections of betamethasone or matching placebo 24 hours apart. The primary outcome was a neonatal composite of treatment in the first 72 hours (the use of continuous positive airway pressure or high-flow nasal cannula for at least 2 hours, supplemental oxygen with a fraction of inspired oxygen of at least 0.30 for at least 4 hours, extracorporeal membrane oxygenation, or mechanical ventilation) or stillbirth or neonatal death within 72 hours after delivery.

Results.—The primary outcome occurred in 165 of 1427 infants (11.6%) in the betamethasone group and 202 of 1400 (14.4%) in the placebo group (relative risk in the betamethasone group, 0.80; 95% confidence interval [CI], 0.66 to 0.97; $P = 0.02$). Severe respiratory complications, transient tachypnea of the newborn, surfactant use, and bronchopulmonary dysplasia also occurred significantly less frequently in the betamethasone group. There were no significant between-group differences in the incidence of chorioamnionitis or neonatal sepsis. Neonatal hypoglycemia was more common in the betamethasone group than in the placebo group (24.0% vs. 15.0%; relative risk, 1.60; 95% CI, 1.37 to 1.87; $P < 0.001$).

Conclusions.—Administration of betamethasone to women at risk for late preterm delivery significantly reduced the rate of neonatal respiratory complications. (Funded by the National Heart, Lung, and Blood Institute and the Eunice Kennedy Shriver National Institute of Child Health and Human Development; ClinicalTrials.gov number, NCT01222247.)

▶ Publication of this randomized, controlled trial of antenatal glucocorticoids in mothers expected to deliver a late-preterm infant was followed almost immediately by a recommendation from the Society for Maternal-Fetal Medicine for adoption of this practice into routine care. That recommendation was based on confirmation of previously suspected, but not well-documented, beneficial effects on pulmonary function in late-preterm babies. In addition to a lower rate of the rather complicated composite primary outcome, for which the number needed to treat (NNT) to avoid one such event was 35, betamethasone treatment was associated with significant reductions in severe respiratory complications ($P < .001$, NNT = 25); transient tachypnea ($P = .002$, NNT = 31); respiratory distress syndrome, transient tachypnea, or apnea as a composite ($P = .004$, NNT = 26); resuscitation at birth ($P = .003$, NNT = 24); surfactant use ($P = .03$, NNT = 80); care in a neonatal intensive care unit for 3 or more days ($P = .03$, NNT = 25); and bronchopulmonary dysplasia ($P = .04$, NNT = 200). Similar benefits were recently described in infants born by elective cesarean section at term,[1] strengthening these conclusions. Those benefits must be balanced against an increased rate of hypoglycemia, defined as a serum glucose measurement of < 40 mg/dL at any time, from 15% in controls to 24% in betamethasone-exposed neonates ($P < .0001$, number needed to harm = 11). Hypoglycemia was not associated with any reported adverse events or with prolongation of hospitalization, but betamethasone treatment exposed 18 babies to hypoglycemia for each averted case of bronchopulmonary dysplasia. Other effects were limited to short-term perturbations during the transitional period. Both hypoglycemia and bronchopulmonary dysplasia are associated with long-term neurodevelopmental impairments, so net long-term impacts are unknown. Long-term respiratory or neurodevelopmental outcomes are not reported, so the ultimate benefit of antenatal betamethasone treatment in these late preterm infants remains uncertain. Although this treatment may be a useful addition to our armamentarium, adoption as a mandated standard of care may be premature. As it becomes common practice, monitoring of betamethasone-exposed babies for hypoglycemia in the immediate postpartum period and for late neurodevelopmental effects as they reach school age will be essential.

W. E. Benitz, MD

Reference

1. Nada AM, Shafeek MM, El Maraghy MA, et al. Antenatal corticosteroid administration before elective caesarean section at term to prevent neonatal respiratory morbidity: a randomized controlled trial. *Eur J Obstet Gynecol Reprod Biol.* 2016;199:88-91.

Antenatal corticosteroid administration before elective caesarean section at term to prevent neonatal respiratory morbidity: a randomized controlled trial

Nada AM, Shafeek MM, El Maraghy MA, et al (Cairo Univ, Egypt; Natl Res Centre, Cairo, Egypt; Ain Shams Univ, Cairo, Egypt)

Eur J Obstet Gynecol Reprod Biol 199:88-91, 2016

Objective.—To assess the effect of prophylactic corticosteroid administration before elective caesarean section at term (between 38 and

38^{+6} weeks) in reducing neonatal respiratory morbidity and admission to a neonatal intensive care unit (NICU) with respiratory complications.

Methods.—Women in this study ($n = 1290$) were randomized into two groups: the dexamethasone group ($n = 645$) and the control group ($n = 645$). Women in the dexamethasone group received three doses of intramuscular dexamethasone 8 mg, 12 h apart, 48 h before caesarean section. Women in the control group received intramuscular saline as a placebo in the same dosage as the dexamethasone group. Primary outcome: Comparison of NICU admission rates and the occurrence of neonatal respiratory morbidity between the two groups.

Results.—The NICU admission rate for respiratory morbidity was significantly lower in the dexamethasone group compared with the control group [10/616 (1.6%) vs 24 (3.9%), respectively; $p = 0.014$]. Antenatal administration of dexamethasone was significantly associated with almost 2.5-fold reduction in the risk of NICU admission for respiratory morbidity (relative risk 0.41, 95% confidence interval 0.2–0.86; number needed to treat ≅43).

Conclusion.—Antenatal corticosteroids reduce the incidence of NICU admission with respiratory morbidity after elective caesarean section at term.

▶ This is the latest and the largest prospective randomized single-center trial of antenatal steroid (dexamethasone) treatment for the prevention of neonatal respiratory distress in singleton term infants undergoing elective caesarean delivery. Twelve hundred patients were enrolled over 3 years ending in December 2014 and were evenly divided between the dexamethasone treatment group and the saline control group. After randomization, 3 doses of intramuscular dexamethasone or saline were administered 48 hours before delivery. The entire cohort was delivered between 380/7 and 386/7 weeks' gestation, mean 384/7 weeks. The majority (91%) of women enrolled were repeat caesarean deliveries, with 70% delivered under general anesthesia. Compared with the saline control group in which 24 of 611 (3.9%) were admitted to neonatal intensive care unit (NICU) for respiratory morbidity, treated infants had a 2-fold reduction in NICU admission—10 of 616 (1.6%)—for respiratory distress, $P = .014$. The majority of those admitted for respiratory symptoms carried a diagnosis of transient tachypnea of the newborn (TTN), which was decreased by half in the treatment arm: 41 controls (6.7%) versus 19 treated (3.1%) patients, $P = .003$. RDS was diagnosed in only 14 patients, 10 controls, and 4 treated infants, which proved to be nonsignificant, $P = .10$.

This study confirms the findings of the British ASTECS multicenter randomized study published 11 years ago in the BMJ, where 998 women were enrolled more than 7 years to receive 2 doses of betamethasone or usual care (ie, no placebo injection) within 48 hours before cesarean delivery with a primary outcome of special care/NICU admission for respiratory distress (1). Thirty-five infants required special care nursery admission, 24 (5.1%) in the control group, and 11 (2.4%) in the treatment arm, $P = .021$, relative risk 0.46 in favor of treatment. This study enrolled all term infants from 37 through

42 weeks' gestation at delivery, which allowed calculation of a logistic regression model predicting the probability of admission to a special care baby unit with respiratory distress from the gestational age of the infant. At 37 weeks' gestation, the predicted probability of admission to a special care unit was 11.4% in the control group and 5.2% in the treatment arm; at 38 weeks was 6.2% and 2.8%, whereas at 39 weeks, it was 1.5% and 0.6%. The ASTECS Research team also claimed to be the first to report that antenatal steroids prevent TTN, with a nearly 50% reduction in TTN cases in the betamethasone arm of the study (19 controls, 10 treated infants).

TTN, which was responsible for the majority of cases admitted to special care nurseries in both studies, has been attributed to a variety of causes. The ASTECS group believes that delay in transition of the secretory fetal lung to one of sodium and fluid absorption is responsible for the "wet lung" of TTN. Upregulation of endogenous steroids in mother and fetus during the stress of labor are thought to enhance the expression of epithelial channel genes, which code for active fluid absorption. Without this natural stress response, some infants delivered by cesarean delivery may have inadequate steroid levels to orchestrate the "flip of the switch" in a timely manner. In the article by Nada et al, surfactant deficiency and/or dysfunction are proposed as major determinants of respiratory distress in term infants diagnosed with TTN. Antenatal steroids, as we all know, accelerate the production of pulmonary surfactant.

To date, antenatal steroid use before term elective cesarean delivery has not been embraced in the United States, although I understand it is used routinely in Great Britain, largely because of the ASTECS Study.[1,2] I doubt that the newest paper by Nada et al will change practice this side of the pond unless a financial analysis of savings incurred by avoiding TTN proves worthwhile.

E. K. Stork, MD

References

1. Stutchfield P, Whitaker R, Russell Ion behalf of the Antenatal Steroids for Term Elective Caesarean Section [ASTECS] Research Team. Antenatal betamethasone and incidence of neonatal respiratory distress after elective caesarean section: pragmatic randomised trial. *BMJ*. 2005;331:662-666.
2. Gyamfi-Bannerman C, Thom EA, Blackwell SC, et al. NICHD Maternal-Fetal Medicine Units Network. Antenatal betamethasone for women at risk for late preterm delivery. *N Engl J Med*. 2016;374:1311-1320.

Accurate prediction of gestational age using newborn screening analyte data

Wilson K, Hawken S, Potter BK, et al (Ottawa Hosp Res Inst, Ontario, Canada; Univ of Ottawa, Ontario, Canada; et al)
Am J Obstet Gynecol 214:513.e1-9, 2016

Background.—Identification of preterm births and accurate estimates of gestational age for newborn infants is vital to guide care. Unfortunately, in developing countries, it can be challenging to obtain estimates of gestational age. Routinely collected newborn infant screening metabolic analytes vary by gestational age and may be useful to estimate gestational age.

Objective.—We sought to develop an algorithm that could estimate gestational age at birth that is based on the analytes that are obtained from newborn infant screening.

Study Design.—We conducted a population-based cross-sectional study of all live births in the province of Ontario that included 249,700 infants who were born between April 2007 and March 2009 and who underwent newborn infant screening. We used multivariable linear and logistic regression analyses to build a model to predict gestational age using newborn infant screening metabolite measurements and readily available physical characteristics data (birthweight and sex).

Results.—The final model of our metabolic gestational dating algorithm had an average deviation between observed and expected gestational age of approximately 1 week, which suggests excellent predictive ability (adjusted R-square of 0.65; root mean square error, 1.06 weeks). Two-thirds of the gestational ages that were predicted by our model were accurate within ±1 week of the actual gestational age. Our logistic regression model was able to discriminate extremely well between term and increasingly premature categories of infants (c-statistic, >0.99).

Conclusion.—Metabolic gestational dating is accurate for the prediction of gestational age and could have value in low resource settings.

▶ The evolution of assessment of gestational age (GA) has been well documented. Traditionally, clinicians resorted to the Battaglia and Lubchenco charts,[1] and then the Dubowitz examination, which incorporated a scoring system including clinical and neurologic features.[2] This was then modified by Ballard using a subset of the Dubowitz physical and neurological examination, and because it was quicker, it was used extensively. Ballard updated the scoring system in 1991 to include extremely preterm infants.[3] Donovan et al, however, evaluated the new Ballard Score (NBS).[4] They found that at each week from 22 to 28 weeks' GA by accurate menstrual history, NBS estimates exceeded GA by dates by 1.3 to 3.3 weeks, and estimates varied widely (range of widths of 95% CIs for the observations, 6.8–11.9 weeks).

They suggested that refinement of GA scoring systems is needed to optimize clinical benefit. Ultrasound soon became the gold standard to determine gestational age, but this of course has limited availability in resource-limited countries. Over the past few years, investigators have been probing analytes from blood spots to determine metabolic profiles related to gestational ages. Wilson [5] published an article titled "Metabolomics of Prematurity: Analysis of Patterns of Amino Acids, Enzymes, and Endocrine Markers by Categories of Gestational Age." The cohorts included 373 819 children born at term (> 36 weeks gestation), 26 483 near-term children (33–36 weeks' gestation), 4354 very premature children (28–32 weeks' gestation), and 1146 extremely premature children (< 28 weeks gestation). The levels of 3 amino acids (arginine, leucine, and valine) were at least 50% different between the cohorts of extremely premature and term children. The levels of 17-hydroxyprogesterone increased with greater prematurity, while thyrotropin-stimulating hormone values consistently decreased with increasing prematurity. None of the 3 enzyme markers we examined showed a trend in levels across categories of prematurity. An algorithm was developed and applied to the total Ontario, Canada, birth population. They were able to discriminate well between near term (late preterm is our preferred terminology) and term infants. Ryckman[6] in a parallel study from Iowa using screening analytes, created a newborn metabolic regression model. GA was predicted within 1 week for 78% of the individuals and within 2 weeks of gestation for 95% of the individuals. This model yielded an area under the curve of 0.899 (95% confidence interval 0.895–0.903) in differentiating those born preterm (< 37 weeks) from those born term (≥ 37 weeks). In the subset of infants born small for gestational age, the average difference between gestational ages predicted by the newborn metabolic model, and the recorded gestational age was 1.5 weeks. In contrast, the average difference between gestational ages predicted by the model including only newborn weight and the recorded gestational age was 1.9 weeks. It is thus possible to use the newborn screening blood spots to determine GA. As these models are refined, they will become even more accurate and most helpful in countries with limited resources.

A. A. Fanaroff, MD

References

1. Battaglia FC, Lubchenco LO. A practical classification of newborn infants by weight and gestational age. *J Pediatr.* 1967;71:159-163.
2. Dubowitz LM, Dubowitz V, Goldberg C. Clinical assessment of gestational age in the newborn infant. *J Pediatr.* 1970;77:1-10.
3. Ballard J, Khoury J, Wednig K, et al. New Ballard Score expanded to include extremely premature infants. *J Pediatr.* 1991;119:411.
4. Donovan EF, Tyson JE, Ehrenkranz RA, et al. Inaccuracy of Ballard scores before 28 weeks' gestation. National Institute of Child Health and Human Development Neonatal Research Network. *J Pediatr.* 1999;135:147-152.
5. Wilson K, Hawken S, Ducharme R, et al. Metabolomics of prematurity: analysis of patterns of amino acids, enzymes, and endocrine markers by categories of gestational age. *Pediatr Res.* 2014;75:367-373.
6. Ryckman KK, Berberich SL, Dagle JM. Predicting gestational age using neonatal metabolic markers. *Am J Obstet Gynecol.* 2016;214:515.e1-e13.

A Randomized Trial of a Cervical Pessary to Prevent Preterm Singleton Birth

Nicolaides KH, Syngelaki A, Poon LC, et al (King's College Hosp, UK; et al)
N Engl J Med 374:1044-1052, 2016

Background.—Preterm birth is the leading cause of neonatal and infant death and of disability among survivors. It is unclear whether a pessary inserted around the cervix reduces the risk of preterm singleton birth.

Methods.—We conducted a multicenter, randomized, controlled trial comparing pessary placement with expectant management (control) in girls and women who were pregnant with singletons (singleton pregnancies) and who had a cervical length of 25 mm or less at 20 weeks 0 days to 24 weeks 6 days of gestation. Participants in either group who had a cervical length of 15 mm or less, at randomization or at subsequent visits, received treatment with vaginal progesterone. The primary outcome was spontaneous delivery before 34 weeks of gestation.

Results.—In an intention-to-treat analysis, there was no significant difference between the pessary group (465 participants) and the control group (467 participants) in the rate of spontaneous delivery before 34 weeks (12.0% and 10.8%, respectively; odds ratio in the pessary group, 1.12; 95% confidence interval, 0.75 to 1.69; $P = 0.57$). There were no significant differences in the rates of perinatal death (3.2% in the pessary group and 2.4% in the control group, $P = 0.42$), adverse neonatal outcome (6.7% and 5.7%, respectively; $P = 0.55$), or neonatal special care (11.6% and 12.9%, respectively; $P = 0.59$). The incidence of new or increased vaginal discharge was significantly higher in the pessary group than in the control group.

Conclusions.—Among girls and women with singleton pregnancies who had a short cervix, a cervical pessary did not result in a lower rate of spontaneous early preterm delivery than the rate with expectant management. (Funded by the Fetal Medicine Foundation; Current Controlled Trials number, ISRCTN01096902.)

► The challenge of reducing the number and rate of preterm births on a worldwide basis remains significant. Although the rate in the United States has inched down and birth defects are now the leading cause of death, preterm births still contribute disproportionality to neonatal mortality. Romero,[1] a leading investigator in this field, has identified one of the problems. Preterm birth is regarded as a single condition, but he is of the opinion that it should be considered as 2 conditions at the minimum. Two thirds of preterm births occur after the spontaneous onset of labor, and the remaining one third after "indicated" preterm birth. The causes of spontaneous preterm labor and "indicated" preterm birth are different.

This leads to the consideration of the use of vaginal progesterone to reduce preterm births. A cause of spontaneous preterm birth is a decline in progesterone action, which induces cervical ripening. A sonographic short cervix, < 25 mm (identified in the midtrimester) is a powerful predictor of spontaneous preterm delivery. Indeed, short cervical length, as measured by transvaginal ultrasound in the second trimester, represents the single most predictive risk factor for spontaneous preterm birth.

Randomized clinical trials and individual patient meta-analyses have shown that vaginal progesterone reduces the rate of preterm delivery at < 33 weeks of gestation by 44%, along with the rate of admission to the neonatal intensive care unit, respiratory distress syndrome, requirement for mechanical ventilation, and composite neonatal morbidity/mortality score. Vaginal progesterone is as effective as cervical cerclage in reducing the rate of preterm delivery in women with a singleton gestation, history of preterm birth, and a short cervix (< 25 mm). To prevent 1 case of spontaneous preterm birth < 33 weeks of gestation, 11 patients with a short cervix would need to be treated (based on an individual patient meta-analysis).[2] Vaginal progesterone reduces the rate of spontaneous preterm birth in women with a short cervix, both with and without a prior history of preterm birth. In patients with a prior history of preterm birth, vaginal progesterone is as effective as cervical cerclage to prevent preterm delivery.

The study by Nikolaides et al came to a disappointing conclusion. Explanations included the failure to the originally planned 1600 and the skewed distribution of cervical lengths at enrollment. The observed distribution of cervical lengths differed from that used for the power calculations (29% and 71% for respective lengths of 1—15 mm and 16—25 mm, rather than the expected 14% and 86%); correspondingly, the observed rate of spontaneous delivery before 34 weeks was 11%, rather than the expected 6%. Many of the subjects received vaginal progesterone additionally, particularly those with very short cervices, and the open nature of the trial, so that the pessary could have been removed at different times when contractions began. Despite the failure of the cervical pessary in this trial, the evidence for the use of vaginal progesterone remains strong. It remains important to identify all women at risk hence the call by Romero for "Routine assessment of the risk of preterm birth with cervical ultrasound coupled with vaginal progesterone for women with a short cervix is cost-effective, and the implementation of such a policy is urgently needed."[3]

A. A. Fanaroff, MD

References

1. Romero R, Nicolaides K, Conde-Agudelo A, et al. Vaginal progesterone decreases preterm birth ≤34 weeks of gestation in women with a singleton gestation and a short cervix: an updated meta-analysis including data from the optimum study. *Ultrasound Obstet Gynecol.* 2016.
2. Romero R, Yeo L, Chaemsaltong P, et al. Progesterone to prevent spontaneous preterm birth. *Semin Fetal Neonatal Med.* 2014;19:15-26.
3. Romero R, Yeo L, Miranda J, Hassan SS, Conde-Agudelo A, Chaiworapongsa T. A blueprint for the prevention of preterm birth: vaginal progesterone in women with a short cervix. *J Perinat Med.* 2013;41:27-44.

A Proactive Approach to Neonates Born at 23 Weeks of Gestation

Backes CH, Rivera BK, Haque U, et al (State Univ Wexner Med Ctr, Columbus, OH; Univ of Washington School of Medicine, Seattle)
Obstet Gynecol 126:939-946, 2015

Objective.—To evaluate in-hospital survival, survival without major morbidity, and neurodevelopmental impairment for neonates born at 23 weeks of gestation provided proactive, coordinated, and comprehensive perinatal and neonatal management.

Methods.—This was a retrospective cohort study conducted at a single, tertiary care center between 2004 and 2013. Enrollment was limited to mother–neonate dyads at 23 weeks of gestation who were provided a proactive approach defined as documented evidence of antenatal corticosteroid administration, willingness to provide cesarean delivery for fetal distress, and neonatal resuscitation and intensive care. Among survivors, major morbidities (predischarge) and neurodevelopmental assessments at corrected ages of 18–22 months were examined.

Results.—Among 152 live births identified, 101 neonates received proactive care, of whom 60 (59%) survived to hospital discharge. Preterm premature rupture of membranes (adjusted odds ratio [OR] 0.29, 95% confidence interval [CI] 0.09–0.94), fetal growth restriction (OR 0.16, 95% CI 0.03–0.89), delivery room cardiopulmonary resuscitation (OR 0.07, 95% CI 0.02–0.32), and prolonged intubation sequence (OR 0.15, 95% CI 0.05–0.45) were associated with lower neonatal survival. Among neonatal intensive care unit survivors, 62% had at least one major morbidity. Among 50 survivors with assessment at 18–22 months, six (12%) were unimpaired, 20 (40%) had mild impairment, and 24 (48%) had moderate or severe neurodevelopmental impairment.

Conclusion.—Proactive, interdisciplinary care enabled more than half of the neonates born at 23 weeks of gestation to survive, and approximately half of children evaluated at 18 months exhibited no or mild impairment. This information should be considered when providing prognostic advice to families with threatened preterm birth at 23 weeks of gestation (Fig 1).

▶ This description of outcomes of preterm infants born at 23 weeks' gestation and provided proactive support throughout labor, delivery, resuscitation, and initial neonatal intensive care at a single children's hospital is 1 of several reports that suggest that better outcomes may be achievable by more consistent and aggressive interventions for babies at this extreme of prematurity. Indeed, infants managed with a proactive approach were more likely to survive (60 of 101) than those who were not (16 of 51; unadjusted odds ratio 3.2, $P = .001$). Qualitatively, that is not dissimilar to results reported from the *Eunice Kennedy Shriver* National Institute of Child Health and Human Development Neonatal Research Network,[1] in which infants who received active treatment were also more likely to survive (71 of 213) than those who were not (107 of 542; unadjusted odds ratio 2.0, $P = .0001$). Although the Network data revealed a strong relationship between rates of active treatment and survival rates at participating hospitals, survival in this single-hospital experience was greater in both groups. There should be little doubt that institutional commitment to aggressive management of these extremely preterm infants will increase survival rates. The high rate of neurodevelopmental impairment in survivors remains sobering, however, as only 12% of the survivors, or approximately 7% of the proactively managed infants, in this cohort who were evaluated at 18 to 22 months were free of impairments (40% had mild and 48% moderate or

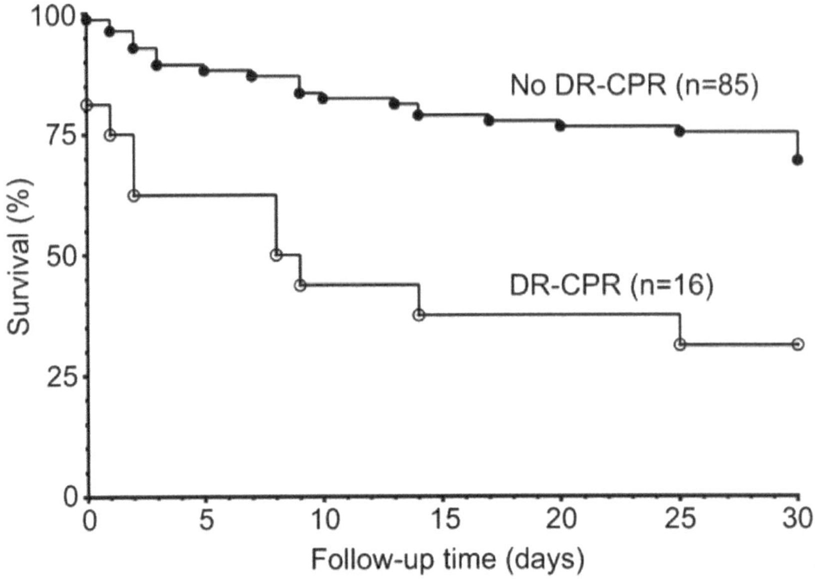

FIGURE 1.—Kaplan-Meier survival plot stratified according to receipt of delivery room cardiopulmonary resuscitation (DR-CPR, n = 16) or no delivery room cardiopulmonary resuscitation (no DR-CPR, n = 85). DR-CPR defined as chest compressions ± epinephrine. *P* < .01. (Reprinted from Backes CH, Rivera BK, Haque U, et al. A proactive approach to neonates born at 23 weeks of gestation. *Obstet Gynecol.* 2015;126:939-946, with permission from The American College of Obstetricians and Gynecologists.)

severe impairments). The relative value of potential benefits and risks at the outset of care in such infants remains a highly individualized matter.

This report affirms another important observation: the need for chest compressions or epinephrine in the delivery room (DR CPR) is a bad prognostic sign (Fig 1), with a 100% positive predictive value for death (81%) or neurodevelopmental impairment (19%). Nearly all (15 of 16) infants who received DR CPR required more than 3 intubation attempts, but such prolonged intubation sequences were not as strongly predictive of neonatal intensive care unit death (23 of 35, or 66%), suggesting that repeated intubation attempts may have reflected failure to detect exhaled carbon dioxide in infants who had no effective cardiac output or pulmonary perfusion. In any case, this serves as a reminder that these very immature babies are not appropriate learning opportunities for inexperienced intubators.

W. E. Benitz, MD

Reference

1. Rysavy MA, Li L, Bell EF, et al. Between-hospital variation in treatment and outcomes in extremely preterm infants. *N Engl J Med.* 2015;372:1801-1811.

#3: Periviable birth

American College of Obstetricians and Gynecologists and the Society for Maternal—Fetal Medicine ()

Am J Obstet Gynecol 213:604-614, 2015

Approximately 0.5% of all births occur before the third trimester of pregnancy, and these very early deliveries result in the majority of neonatal deaths and more than 40% of infant deaths. A recent executive summary of proceedings from a joint workshop defined periviable birth as delivery occurring from 20 0/7 weeks to 25 6/7 weeks of gestation. When delivery is anticipated near the limit of viability, families and health care teams are faced with complex and ethically challenging decisions. Multiple factors have been found to be associated with short-term and long-term outcomes of periviable births in addition to gestational age at birth. These include, but are not limited to, nonmodifiable factors (eg, fetal sex, weight, plurality), potentially modifiable antepartum and intrapartum factors (eg, location of delivery, intent to intervene by cesarean delivery or induction for delivery, administration of antenatal corticosteroids and magnesium sulfate), and postnatal management (eg, starting or withholding and continuing or withdrawing intensive care after birth). Antepartum and intrapartum management options vary depending upon the specific circumstances but may include short-term tocolytic therapy for preterm labor to allow time for administration of antenatal steroids, antibiotics to prolong latency after preterm premature rupture of membranes or for intrapartum group B streptococci prophylaxis, and delivery, including cesarean delivery, for concern regarding fetal well-being or fetal malpresentation. Whenever possible, periviable births for which maternal or neonatal intervention is planned should occur in centers that offer expertise in maternal and neonatal care and the needed infrastructure, including intensive care units, to support such services. This document describes newborn outcomes after periviable birth, provides current evidence and recommendations regarding interventions in this setting, and provides an outline for family counseling with the goal of incorporating informed patient preferences. Its intent is to provide support and guidance regarding decisions, including declining and accepting interventions and therapies, based on individual circumstances and patient values.

▶ Periodic flurries of consensus reports and practice guidelines typically reflect 2 realities: the standard of practice is changing, and it is not yet clear where it will settle. This consensus statement from the American College of Obstetricians and Gynecologists and the Society for Maternal-Fetal Medicine, coupled with recent similar commentaries from a *Eunice Kennedy Shriver* National Institute of Child Health and Human Development (NICHD) Workshop[1] and the American Academy of Pediatrics (AAP)[2] are part of such a cluster. Appropriately, this statement focuses primarily on decisions about antepartum obstetrical interventions (steroids, magnesium, antibiotics, fetal monitoring, and cesarean delivery), while that from the AAP is weighted toward decisions about management of the baby (aggressiveness of resuscitation and initiation of intensive care). All 3 advocate presentation of current, accurate prognostic data—often a difficult task—to support joint decision making with parents to the extent that is possible. Remarkably, the least controversial part of these statements seems to be the most substantial change: there is now a consensus that aggressive prenatal measures (excepting cesarean delivery at <25 weeks), immediate resuscitation, and initiation and provision of ongoing intensive care are recommended for all infants born at 24 weeks or more. Fewer than 15 years ago, all infants born before 26 weeks' gestation were included in the zone of uncertainty.[3] These guidelines reflect solidification of attitudinal changes that were already becoming established about a decade ago.[4]

Uncertainty about the future state centers on recommendations for management of infants born before 24 weeks' gestation. Many practitioners felt that the matrix of recommendations proposed by the NICHD Workshop was too prescriptive, primarily with respect to "Recommended" use of steroids, magnesium, antibiotics, monitoring, and cesarean delivery, and (with qualification) aggressive newborn resuscitation beginning at a threshold of 23 weeks. This statement from the obstetrical community backs away from that a bit, reserving "Recommended" for those measures only at 24 weeks or more, and substituting "Consider" for the same measures at 23 weeks. The statements differ slightly in recommendations for anticipated births at 22 weeks' gestation, with this ACOG/SFM statement advising against all interventions (with the exception of "Consider" for use of antibiotics to prolong latency and for neonatal resuscitation), and the Workshop Summary adding recommendations to "Consider" antenatal steroids "if delivery after 23 weeks is anticipated" and aggressive resuscitation "based on individual circumstances." Both statements agree that before 22 weeks, the only intervention to consider is antibiotic treatment for premature rupture of membranes, with all others not recommended. The AAP statement avoids prescriptive guidance altogether. These inconsistencies reflect the tension between recognition of increased rates of survival and persistence of alarming rates of neurosensory impairments for 22 and 23 weeks' gestation babies. The most recent US data suggest rates of moderate to severe morbidity in 90% to 100% of survivors born at 22 or 23 weeks' gestation. Whatever framework is adopted at any facility, and no matter what value a family may attach to such outcomes, it must be remembered that their pursuit always comes at a cost, including substantial risks to the mother (succinctly outlined in this report) and suffering sustained by the baby during and after the stay in the neonatal intensive care unit. Our high level of discomfort with these difficult choices is very appropriate.

W. E. Benitz, MD

References

1. Raju TN, Mercer BM, Burchfield DJ, et al. Periviable birth: executive summary of a joint workshop by the Eunice Kennedy Shriver National Institute of Child Health and Human Development, Society for Maternal-Fetal Medicine, American Academy of Pediatrics, and American College of Obstetricians and Gynecologists. *Am J Obstet Gynecol.* 2014;210:406-417.

2. Cummings J, Committee on Fetus and Newborn. Antenatal counseling regarding resuscitation and intensive care before 25 weeks of gestation. *Pediatrics*. 2015; 103:588-595.
3. MacDonald H. Perinatal care at the threshold of viability. *Pediatrics*. 2002;110: 1024-1027.
4. Peerzada JM, Richardson DK, Burns JP. Delivery room decision-making at the threshold of viability. *J Pediatr*. 2004;145:492-498.

#3: Periviable birth

American College of Obstetricians and Gynecologists and the Society for Maternal—Fetal Medicine ()
Am J Obstet Gynecol 213:604-614, 2015

Approximately 0.5% of all births occur before the third trimester of pregnancy, and these very early deliveries result in the majority of neonatal deaths and more than 40% of infant deaths. A recent executive summary of proceedings from a joint workshop defined periviable birth as delivery occurring from 20 0/7 weeks to 25 6/7 weeks of gestation. When delivery is anticipated near the limit of viability, families and health care teams are faced with complex and ethically challenging decisions. Multiple factors have been found to be associated with short-term and long-term outcomes of periviable births in addition to gestational age at birth. These include, but are not limited to, nonmodifiable factors (eg, fetal sex, weight, plurality), potentially modifiable antepartum and intrapartum factors (eg, location of delivery, intent to intervene by cesarean delivery or induction for delivery, administration of antenatal corticosteroids and magnesium sulfate), and postnatal management (eg, starting or withholding and continuing or withdrawing intensive care after birth). Antepartum and intrapartum management options vary depending upon the specific circumstances but may include short-term tocolytic therapy for preterm labor to allow time for administration of antenatal steroids, antibiotics to prolong latency after preterm premature rupture of membranes or for intrapartum group B streptococci prophylaxis, and delivery, including cesarean delivery, for concern regarding fetal well-being or fetal malpresentation. Whenever possible, periviable births for which maternal or neonatal intervention is planned should occur in centers that offer expertise in maternal and neonatal care and the needed infrastructure, including intensive care units, to support such services. This document describes newborn outcomes after periviable birth, provides current evidence and recommendations regarding interventions in this setting, and provides an outline for family counseling with the goal of incorporating informed patient preferences. Its intent is to provide support and guidance regarding decisions, including declining and accepting interventions and therapies, based on individual circumstances and patient values (Fig 1, Tables 1 and 2).

▶ Preterm birth remains an important cause of neonatal morbidity and mortality globally. As noted in the consensus statement, approximately 0.5% of all births

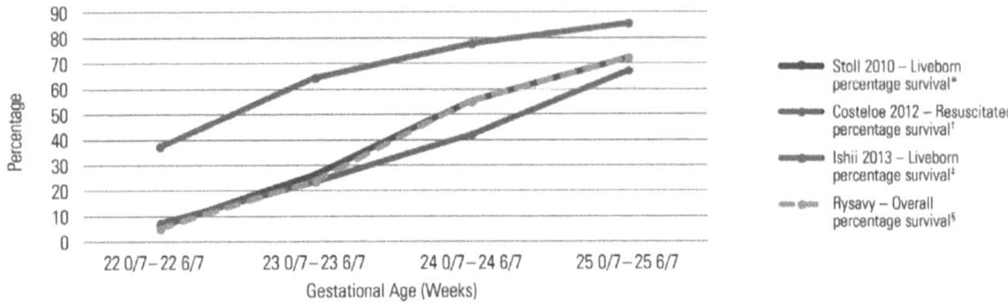

*Stoll BJ, Hansen NI, Bell EF, Shankaran S, Laptook AR, Walsh MC, et al. Neonatal outcomes of extremely preterm infants from the NICHD Neonatal Research Network. Eunice Kennedy Shriver National Institute of Child Health and Human Development Neonatal Research Network. Pediatrics 2010;126:443–56.

†Costeloe KL, Hennessy EM, Haider S, Stacey F, Marlow N, Draper ES. Short term outcomes after extreme preterm birth in England: comparison of two birth cohorts in 1995 and 2006 (the EPICure studies). BMJ 2012;345:e7976.

‡Ishii N, Kono Y, Yonemoto N, Kusuda S, Fujimura M. Outcomes of infants born at 22 and 23 weeks' gestation. Neonatal Research Network, Japan. Pediatrics 2013;132:62–71.

§Rysavy MA, Li L, Bell EF, Das A, Hintz SR, Stoll BJ, et al. Between-hospital variation in treatment and outcomes in extremely preterm infants. Eunice Kennedy Shriver National Institute of Child Health and Human Development Neonatal Research Network. N Engl J Med 2015;372:1801–11.

FIGURE 1.—Percentage of survival by gestational age. (Reprinted from American College of Obstetricians and Gynecologists and the Society for Maternal–Fetal Medicine. #3: Periviable birth. *Am J Obstet Gynecol.* 2015;213:604-614.)

occur before the third trimester of pregnancy, and these very early deliveries result in the majority of neonatal deaths and more than 40% of infant deaths. An increasing number of extremely low birth weight infants (ELBW) neonates now survive with proactive care. Their survival depends on fetal and neonatal adaptations of multiple organ systems. "Miracle" ELBW infants who survive without disability are examples of developmental plasticity. Miracle baby stories in the popular press and other media are a regular occurrence and often the first source from which the general public learn about extremely premature babies. Often overly optimistic and dramatic, they may lead to unrealistic expectations on the part of the families and provide hope where continuing care is considered futile by the treating team.

Better survival can be anticipated with advancing gestational age, higher birth weights, female sex, and birth by cesarean delivery. Kangaroo care and strategies to enhance neurodevelopment improve the chances of survival without morbidity. The data continue to demonstrate that intensive care units with larger volumes of low birth weight babies have better outcomes, and a multidisciplinary approach with continued training of the personnel is important for the best outcomes. There are no magic bullets but application of best care practices and evidence gives the best results. These include but are not limited to antenatal corticosteroids, avoidance of hypothermia in the delivery room, optimal cord clamping, postnatal surfactant treatment for infants with respiratory distress syndrome, gentle ventilation, early nutritional support including colostrum, prevention of major morbidities including severe intraventricular hemorrhage and bronchopulmonary dysplasia together with avoidance of infection.

Tables 1 and 2 from units in Japan, the United Kingdom, and the United States demonstrate the wide variety in outcomes.[1-7,8] Survival rates from Japan as reported by Ishii,[1] are superior to the United States and United Kingdom for these periviable infants. Fig 1 powerfully demonstrates the difference in outcomes if only the live births are counted (Stoll) or all births (Rysavy). The morbidity data shows similar trends. We should be encouraged by the finding

TABLE 1.—Factors that Affect the Reliability of Estimates of Survival or the Actual Outcomes Among Periviable Births

Variable	Effect
Factors affecting reliability of estimates of probability of clinical outcomes	
Data source	International, national, regional, and single-institution data reflect variations in regional and local practices.
Cohort selection	Exclusion of newborns not surviving to NICU admission results in inclusion of those with higher potential for survival and higher reported rates of survival. Inclusion of nonresuscitated infants or stillbirths reduces overall reported rates of survival. Inclusion of anomalous infants may decrease reported survival estimates.
Gestational age assignment	In vitro fertilization and ovulation induction provide accurate gestational age assignment. Dating by last menstrual period assumes accurate recollection of this date as well as conception on day 14. Ultrasonography initially performed at less than 24 weeks of gestation estimates gestational age within 5 to 14 days.[a]
Factors potentially affecting clinical outcomes	
Nonmodifiable risk factors	Race and ethnicity, plurality (singleton versus multiple gestation), infant sex, birthweight, gestational age
Modifiable obstetric practices	Antenatal interventions (eg, corticosteroids, tocolysis, antibiotics for preterm PROM, or magnesium for neuroprotection), site and mode of delivery
Modifiable neonatal practices	Initial resuscitation and subsequent care (eg, approaches to ventilation and oxygenation, nutritional support, and treatment of newborn infections)
Approaches to comfort care	Influenced by institutional and physician philosophies, parental wishes, and religious convictions
Regional/hospital legal and practice guidelines	Policies concerning neonatal resuscitation

NICU, neonatal intensive care unit; *PROM*, premature rupture of membranes.
Modified from Raju et al.[2]
Editor's Note: Please refer to original journal article for full references.
[a]Method for estimating due date. Committee Opinion No. 611. American College of Obstetricians and Gynecologists. ObstetGynecol 2014;124:863–6.[23]
Reprinted from American College of Obstetricians and Gynecologists and the Society for Maternal–Fetal Medicine. #3: Periviable birth. *Am J Obstet Gynecol.* 2015;213:604-614.

TABLE 2.—Recommendations for Periviable Birth

Recommendations	Grade of Recommendations
Based on anticipated neonatal or maternal complications, antepartum transport to a center with advanced levels of neonatal or maternal care is recommended when feasible and appropriate.	Best practice
Prenatal and postnatal counseling regarding anticipated short-term and long-term neonatal outcome should take into consideration anticipated gestational age at delivery, as well as other variables that may alter the likelihood of survival and adverse newborn outcomes (eg, fetal sex, multiple gestation, the presence of suspected major fetal malformations, antenatal corticosteroid administration, birth weight, and response to initial newborn resuscitation).	Best practice
Family counseling should be provided by a multidisciplinary team that includes obstetrician-gynecologists and other obstetric providers, maternal-fetal medicine specialists, if available, and neonatologists who can address their individual and shared considerations and perspectives. Maternal and neonatal outcomes should be considered. Follow-up counseling should be provided when there is relevant new information about the maternal and fetal status or the newborn's evolving condition.	Best practice
A predelivery plan, made with the parents, family, or both, should be recognized as a general plan of approach, which may be modified as the neonate's condition and response is evaluated by the neonatal providers. A recommendation regarding assessment for resuscitation is not meant to indicate that resuscitation should always either be undertaken or deferred, or that every possible intervention need be offered. A stepwise approach concordant with neonatal circumstances and condition and with parental wishes is appropriate. Care should be reevaluated regularly and potentially redirected based on the evolution of the clinical situation.	Best practice

Recommendations regarding specific interventions, tailored to gestational age and other clinical data, and taking into account individual family preferences and values, are summarized in Table 3.
Editor's Note: Please refer to original journal article for full references.
Reprinted from American College of Obstetricians and Gynecologists and the Society for Maternal–Fetal Medicine. #3: Periviable birth. *Am J Obstet Gynecol*. 2015;213:604-614.

that in addition to having a high survival rate, Ishi's cohort has lower morbidity than the USA multicenter Neonatal Research Network data. Overall the consensus report provides a lot of useful information and ideas for the management of these periviable infants. The approach to these infants will of necessity be different in developed nations as opposed to developing nations.

A. A. Fanaroff, MD

References

1. Ishii N, Kono Y, Yonemoto N, Kusuda S, Fujimura MNeonatal Research Network, Japan. Outcomes of infants born at 22 and 23 weeks' gestation. *Pediatrics*. 2013;132:62-71.
2. Stoll BJ, Hansen NI, Bell EF, et al. Eunice Kennedy Shriver National Institute of Child Health and Human Development Neonatal Research Network. Neonatal outcomes of extremely preterm infants from the NICHD Neonatal Research Network. *Pediatrics*. 2010;126:443-456.
3. Rysavy MA, Li L, Bell EF, et al. Eunice Kennedy Shriver National Institute of Child Health and Human Development Neonatal Research Network. Between-hospital variation in treatment and outcomes in extremely preterm infants. *N Engl J Med*. 2015;372:1801-1811.
4. Costeloe KL, Hennessy EM, Haider S, Stacey F, Marlow N, Draper ES. Short term outcomes after extreme preterm birth in En- gland: comparison of two birth cohorts in 1995 and 2006 (the EPICure studies). *BMJ*. 2012;345:e7976.
5. Wood NS, Marlow N, Costeloe K, Gibson AT, Wilkinson AREPICure Study Group. Neurologic and developmental disability after extremely preterm birth. *N Engl J Med*. 2000;343:378-384.
6. Moore GP, Lemyre B, Barrowman N, Daboval T. Neurodevelopmental outcomes at 4 to 8 years of children born at 22 to 25 weeks' gestational age: a meta-analysis. *JAMA Pediatr*. 2013;167:967-974.
7. Marlow N, Wolke D, Bracewell MA, Samara MEPICure Study Group. Neurologic and developmental disability at six years of age after extremely pre-term birth. *N Engl J Med*. 2005;352:9-19.

Trends in Stillbirth by Gestational Age in the United States, 2006–2012

MacDorman MF, Reddy UM, Silver RM (Univ of Maryland, College Park; Univ of Utah Health Sciences Ctr, Salt Lake City)
Obstet Gynecol 126:1146-1150, 2015

Objective.—To evaluate stillbirth trends by gestational age.

Methods.—National Center for Health Statistics' fetal death and live birth data files were used to analyze the 2006 and 2012 cohorts of deliveries and compute gestational age-specific stillbirth rates at 20 weeks of gestation or greater using two methods: traditional (eg, stillbirths at 38 weeks of gestation/live births and stillbirths at 38 weeks of gestation) and prospective (stillbirths at 38 weeks of gestation/number of women still pregnant at 38 weeks of gestation). Changes in rates and in the percent distribution of stillbirths and live births were assessed.

Results.—In 2006 and 2012, the stillbirth rate was 6.05 stillbirths per 1,000 deliveries. There was little change in the percent distribution of stillbirths by gestational age from 2006 to 2012. However, the percent distribution of live births by gestational age changed considerably: births at 34–38 weeks of gestation decreased by 10–16%, and births at 39 weeks of gestation increased by 17%. Traditionally computed stillbirth rates were unchanged at most gestational ages, but rose at 24–27, 34–36, 37, and 38 weeks of gestation. However, rates were influenced by decreases in births at those gestational ages; the pattern of stillbirths by gestational age was unchanged. In contrast, there were no differences in prospective stillbirth rates at 21–42 weeks of gestation.

Conclusion.—The lack of change in prospective stillbirth rates from 2006 to 2012 suggests that preventing nonmedically indicated deliveries before 39 weeks of gestation did not increase the U.S. stillbirth rate.

▶ Soon after a national campaign was mounted in the middle of the last decade to reduce iatrogenic neonatal morbidities through avoidance of elective cesarean sections and induced labor before 39 weeks of gestation, concerns were raised that reduced morbidities might be offset by higher stillbirth rates. One report suggested that 1 additional infant might be stillborn for every 11 infants who avoided neonatal intensive care unit admission.[1] Although other analyses yielded conflicting results, the necessity for population-based surveillance for unintended consequences of the new practice guidelines was apparent. This report and another published in the same issue of Obstetrics & Gynecology[2] provide such ongoing surveillance from national vital statistics databases. Happily, both reports fail to identify the feared increase in the stillbirth rate as elective deliveries prior to 39 weeks of gestation decreased. These observations are succinctly represented in the Figure, which reflects a shift in births from 34 to 38 weeks of gestation to 39 weeks of gestation without a corresponding increase in stillbirths during those intervals. These reassuring reports support continuation of efforts to avoid non–medically indicated delivery before 39 weeks of gestation. However, the low power of even such large studies to detect changes in very low frequency events like stillbirth at term should not be overlooked; this population-based analysis was sufficiently powered to detect a difference in prospective stillbirth rates of 6% or more, yet smaller increments might still be of concern. While we can breathe more easily with these data in hand, ongoing surveillance is required to determine whether further reductions in elective births before 39 weeks, as recent national guidelines from the American College of Obstetricians and Gynecologists and the Joint Commission are fully implemented, will produce an identifiable increment in late stillbirths.

W. E. Benitz, MD

References

1. Ehrenthal DB, Hoffman MK, Jiang X, et al. Neonatal outcomes after implementation of guidelines limiting elective delivery before 39 weeks of gestation. *Obstet Gynecol.* 2011;118:1047-1055.
2. Little SE, Zera CA, Clapp MA, et al. A multi-state analysis of early-term delivery trends and the association with term stillbirth. *Obstet Gynecol.* 2015;126:1138-1145.

Cause of Preterm Birth as a Prognostic Factor for Mortality

Delorme P, Goffinet F, Ancel P-Y, et al (Paris Descartes Univ, France; St. Joseph Hosp, Paris, France; Hôtel Dieu Hosp, Paris, France; et al)

Obstet Gynecol 127:40-48, 2016

Objective.—To investigate the association of the cause of preterm birth on in-hospital mortality of preterm neonates born from 24 to 34 weeks of gestation.

Methods.—L'Etude épidémiologique sur les petits ages gestationnels (EPIPAGE)-2 is a prospective, nationwide, population-based cohort of very preterm births. After dividing causes of preterm birth into six mutually exclusive groups, we analyzed the association of each cause with in-hospital deaths of preterm neonates born alive with adjustment for organizational, maternal, and obstetric factors.

Results.—The analysis included 3,138 singleton live births from 24 to 34 weeks of gestation with a newborn in-hospital mortality rate of 5.0% (95% confidence interval 4.5-5.7). Preterm labor was the most frequent cause of preterm birth (n = 1,293 [43.5%]) followed by preterm premature rupture of membranes (n = 765 [23.9%]), hypertensive disorders without suspected fetal growth restriction (n = 397 [12.7%]), hypertensive disorders with suspected fetal growth restriction (n = 408 [10.9%]), placental abruption after an uncomplicated pregnancy (n = 92 [3.0%]), and suspected fetal growth restriction without hypertensive disorders (n = 183 [5.9%]). Neonates born because of suspected fetal growth restriction with or without hypertensive disorders (adjusted odds ratio [OR] 3.0 [1.9–4.7] and adjusted OR 2.3 [1.1–4.6], respectively) had higher adjusted risks of in-hospital death than those born after preterm labor. Risks of in-hospital mortality for preterm births caused by preterm premature rupture of membranes (adjusted OR 1.3 [0.9–1.9]), hypertensive disorders without fetal growth restriction (adjusted OR 0.7 [0.4–1.4]), or placental abruption (adjusted OR 1.6 [0.7–3.7]) were similar to those born after preterm labor.

Conclusion.—Among neonates born alive before 34 weeks of gestation, only those born because of suspected fetal growth restriction have a higher mortality risk than those born after preterm labor.

▶ Prediction of mortality in preterm infants to aid in counseling of parents or incipient parents has moved from use of mortality tables based solely on birth weight or estimated gestational age to use of prediction formulas derived from multivariate regression models,[1,2] but concerns about uncertainty and inaccuracies in predictions persist. One reason for those problems may be that traditional models treat all preterm babies the same, without regard to the reasons for their premature birth. This analysis of a national data set from France is the second to draw attention to importance of etiology in stratification of mortality risk in preterm infants. Identification of significantly greater mortality risks in infants with fetal growth restriction, whether associated with maternal hypertension or not, recapitulates earlier observations associating higher mortality with low birth weight for gestational age (SGA).[2] This is not entirely new, and SGA is a component of the predictive score developed by the Canadian Neonatal Network, but low birth weight for gestation is at most an implicit variable in the *Eunice Kennedy Shriver* National Institute of Child Health and Human Development Neonatal Network Calculator.[1] The context of these observations—consideration of the impact of etiology of prematurity—may still be important, however. A similar analysis of data from the Italian Neonatal Network revealed an interaction between gestational age and cause of preterm birth, with infants born to women with hypertensive disorders at greater risk for death (compared with those whose mothers had chorioamnionitis) before 27 weeks, but at lower risk at 30 weeks.[3] Data from the present study do not include information about chorioamnionitis exposure, so its role in the French sample is unknown. Together, these studies suggest that the etiology of prematurity and its interactions with gestational age may be useful variables for inclusion in regression models and formulas for prediction of mortality in preterm infants. The reason why a preterm baby is with us in the nursery rather than still in utero seems to matter.

W. E. Benitz, MD

References

1. Tyson JE, Parikh NA, Langer J, et al. Intensive care for extreme prematurity—moving beyond gestational age. *N Engl J Med.* 2008;358:1672-1681.
2. Ge WJ, Mirea L, Yang J, et al. Prediction of neonatal outcomes in extremely preterm neonates. *Pediatrics.* 2013;132:e876-e885.
3. Gagliardi L, Rusconi F, Bellu R, et al. Association of maternal hypertension and chorioamnionitis with preterm outcomes. *Pediatrics.* 2014;134:e154-e161.

Trends in Morbidity and Mortality of Extremely Preterm Multiple Gestation Newborns

Yeo KT, for the Australian and New Zealand Neonatal Network (Royal Hosp for Women, Randwick, Australia; et al)
Pediatrics 136:263-271, 2015

Objectives.—To examine the risk of mortality and major morbidities in extremely preterm multiple gestation infants compared with singletons over time.

Methods.—This is a retrospective study of 15 402 infants born ≤27 weeks' gestation, admitted to NICUs in the Australian and New Zealand Neonatal Network from 1995 to 2009. Mortality and major morbidities were compared between singletons and multiples across three 5-year epochs.

Results.—Extreme preterm multiples were more likely to have lower birth weight; higher maternal age; and higher rates of assisted conception, antenatal steroid use, and cesarean delivery compared with singletons. The mortality rate was significantly higher in multiples compared with singletons even as there was a trend of decreasing gestational-age stratified mortality in multiples over the time period investigated. The rates of major morbidities or composite adverse outcomes were not different between multiples and singletons across all epochs. The adjusted odds ratio (AOR) for mortality in multiples was significantly higher in multiples compared with singletons (AOR 1.20, 95% confidence interval [CI] 1.08–1.34). There were no differences in the adjusted odds for poor outcomes in multiples compared with singletons in the most recent epoch: mortality (AOR 1.00, 95% CI 0.84–1.19), major morbidity (0.95, 95% CI 0.81–1.10), and composite adverse outcome (0.96, 95% CI 0.83–1.11).

Conclusions.—Over the 15-year period, the odds for mortality in extremely preterm NICU infants of multiple gestation was significantly higher compared with singletons. The adjusted odds of poor outcomes in multiples were not significantly different from that of singletons in the most recent epoch.

▶ The differential perinatal risks associated with multiple gestations have been familiar for decades. Although much of that difference is attributable to the increased likelihood of premature delivery, preterm multiples historically have higher mortality rates than singletons at equivalent gestational ages. At one time, a reasonable rule was that the mortality risk in multiple gestations approximated that for singletons at a gestational age 1 week less mature for each additional fetus present. That difference has been eroding and increasingly limited to the lowest gestational ages. This report suggests that even that residual differential risk has now disappeared. These data show downward trends in mortality rates in all 4 study groups ($P < .001$ by χ^2 for trend for each group). For singletons, mortality rate decreased only between epochs 1 and 2 among those born at 26 to 27 weeks (χ^2, $P = .037$) and only between epochs 2 and 3 ($P = .003$) for those born at 23 to 25 weeks of gestation. Among multiples, mortality rates declined only between epochs 2 and 3 ($P < .001$ at 23 to 25 weeks and $P = .002$ at 26 to 27 weeks). Increasing survival seems to have propagated to earlier gestational ages, with effects in multiples trailing those in singletons by about 5 years. It is, therefore, likely that the widely used National Institute of Child Health and Human Development Preterm Outcomes Calculator, based on data accrued from 1998 to 2003, now overestimates both the risk of death and the disadvantage conferred by multiple gestations.

Unfortunately, the regression model developed by these authors does not offer a more current alternative. Their model describes a significantly higher mortality risk in multiples across all eras (adjusted odds ratio, 1.20; 95% confidence interval, 1.08-1.34) but did not include either the epoch of care or any terms for interactions between epoch, gestational age, or plurality. Such an analysis or a regression model specific to the most recent epoch would be more valuable. The utility of these data would also have been enhanced by more complete reporting of outcomes for each week of gestation rather than pooling infants with gestational ages spanning a 3-week interval (23-25 weeks) during which outcomes are rapidly evolving. Because of that data pooling, these outcome statistics (for mortality or major morbidity) should not be used to inform counseling of parents confronting anticipated birth of a preterm infant at this early stage of gestation.

W. E. Benitz, MD

Zika Virus and Pregnancy: What Obstetric Health Care Providers Need to Know

Meaney-Delman D, Rasmussen SA, Staples JE, et al (Centers for Disease Control and Prevention, Atlanta, GA)
Obstet Gynecol 127:642-648, 2016

Zika virus is a flavivirus transmitted by *Aedes (Stegomyia)* species of mosquitoes. In May 2015, the World Health Organization confirmed the first local transmission of Zika virus in the Americas in Brazil. The virus has spread rapidly to other countries in the Americas; as of January 29, 2016, local transmission has been detected in at least 22 countries or territories, including the Commonwealth of Puerto Rico and the U.S. Virgin Islands. Zika virus can infect pregnant women in all three trimesters. Although pregnant women do not appear to be more susceptible to or more severely affected by Zika virus infection, maternal–fetal transmission has been documented. Several pieces of evidence suggest that maternal Zika virus infection is associated with adverse neonatal outcomes, most notably microcephaly. Because of the number of countries and territories with local Zika virus transmission, it is likely that obstetric health care providers will care for pregnant women who live in or have traveled to an area of local Zika virus transmission. We review information on Zika virus, its clinical presentation, modes of transmission, laboratory testing, effects during pregnancy, and methods of prevention to assist obstetric health care providers in caring for pregnant women considering travel or with a history of travel to areas with ongoing Zika virus transmission and pregnant women residing in areas with ongoing Zika virus transmission.

▶ Zika virus is the new HIV and is in the news on a daily basis. Although most reports on microcephaly and other fetal disorders have come from Brazil, this problem is rapidly becoming global. Since first appearing in the Americas in May 2015, Zika virus has spread rapidly throughout the region and is likely to continue to spread. Data on pregnant women infected with Zika virus are limited. The Zika virus may be transmitted to the fetus throughout pregnancy. The full spectrum of outcomes that might be associated with congenital Zika virus infection is unknown; however, microcephaly, brain atrophy, cerebellar hypoplasia, ventricular enlargement, and intracranial calcifications have been reported in neonates who have tested positive for Zika virus infection. Freitas[1] reported on the ocular findings in infants with suspected Zika virus infections. Thirty-four percent of patients with microcephaly had severe ocular findings. Bilateral findings were found in 7 of 10 patients presenting with ocular lesions, most common of which were focal pigment mottling of the retina and chorioretinal atrophy, followed by optic nerve abnormalities, bilateral iris coloboma, and lens subluxation. Congenital infection due to presumed Zika virus exposure is associated with vision-threatening findings, which include bilateral macular and perimacular lesions, as well as optic nerve abnormalities in most cases.

Many of the findings are similar to congenital cytomegalovirus infection, and it appears as if the microcephaly is associated with first trimester transmission. Although Zika virus has been identified in tissues from stillborn infants, it is unclear whether it was responsible for the pregnancy loss.

The Centers for Disease Control and Prevention (CDC) has published helpful interim guidelines for health care providers and all women concerning Zika virus.[2,3] Because there is neither a vaccine nor are there medications available to prevent Zika virus transmission, the CDC recommends that all pregnant women consider postponing travel to areas of ongoing Zika virus transmission if possible (updated information on travel advisories is available here: http://wwwnc.cdc.gov/travel/notices).

It is the responsibility of perinatal health care providers to familiarize themselves with the signs and symptoms of Zika virus, the laboratory testing available, and the guidelines outlined here to appropriately counsel their patients. The CDC will issue updates as more information becomes available.[4]

A. A. Fanaroff, MD

References

1. De Paula Freitas B, Oliveira Dias J, Prazeres J, et al. Ocular findings in infants with microcephaly associated with presumed zika virus congenital infection in salvador, Brazil. *JAMA Ophthalmol.* 2016;134:529-535.
2. Oduyebo T, Petersen E, Rasmussen SA, et al. Update: interim guidelines for health care providers caring for pregnant women and women of reproductive age with possible Zika virus exposure United States, 2016. *MMWR Morb Mortal Wkly Rep.* 2016;65:122-127.
3. Petersen EE, Staples JE, Meaney-Delman D, Fischer M, Ellington SR, Callaghan WM, et al. Interim guidelines for pregnant women during a Zika virus outbreak United States, 2016. *MMWR Morb Mortal Wkly Rep.* 2016;65:30-33.
4. http://www.cdc.gov/zika/hc-providers/index.html.

Clinical features and neuroimaging (CT and MRI) findings in presumed Zika virus related congenital infection and microcephaly: retrospective case series study

de Fatima Vasco Aragao M, van der Linden V, Brainer-Lima AM, et al (Mauricio de Nassau Univ, Recife, Pernambuco, Brazil; Barão de Lucena Hosp, Recife, Brazil; Univ of Pernambuco, Recife, Brazil; et al)

BMJ 353:i1901, 2016

Objective.—To report radiological findings observed in computed tomography (CT) and magnetic resonance imaging (MRI) scans of the first cases of congenital infection and microcephaly presumably associated with the Zika virus in the current Brazilian epidemic.

Design.—Retrospective study with a case series.

Setting.—Association for Assistance of Disabled Children (AACD), Pernambuco state, Brazil.

Participants.—23 children with a diagnosis of congenital infection presumably associated with the Zika virus during the Brazilian microcephaly epidemic.

Main Outcome Measures.—Types of abnormalities and the radiological pattern of lesions identified on CT and MRI brain scans.

Results.—Six of the 23 children tested positive for IgM antibodies to Zika virus in cerebrospinal fluid. The other 17 children met the protocol criteria for congenital infection presumably associated with the Zika virus, even without being tested for IgM antibodies to the virus—the test was not yet available on a routine basis. Of the 23 children, 15 underwent CT, seven underwent both CT and MRI, and one underwent MRI. Of the 22 children who underwent CT, all had calcifications in the junction between cortical and subcortical white matter, 21 (95%) had malformations of cortical development, 20 (91%) had a decreased brain volume, 19 (86%) had ventriculomegaly, and 11 (50%) had hypoplasia of the cerebellum or brainstem. Of the eight children who underwent MRI, all had calcifications in the junction between cortical and subcortical white matter, malformations of cortical development occurring predominantly in the frontal lobes, and ventriculomegaly. Seven of the eight (88%) children had enlarged cisterna magna, seven (88%) delayed myelination, and six each (75%) a moderate to severe decrease in brain volume, simplified gyral pattern, and abnormalities of the corpus callosum (38% hypogenesis and 38% hypoplasia). Malformations were symmetrical in 75% of the cases.

Conclusion.—Severe cerebral damage was found on imaging in most of the children in this case series with congenital infection presumably associated with the Zika virus. The features most commonly found were brain calcifications in the junction between cortical and subcortical white matter associated with malformations of cortical development, often with a simplified gyral pattern and predominance of pachygyria or polymicrogyria in the frontal lobes. Additional findings were enlarged cisterna magna, abnormalities of corpus callosum (hypoplasia or hypogenesis), ventriculomegaly, delayed myelination, and hypoplasia of the cerebellum and the brainstem.

▶ At the time of this writing, we are still in the early months of experience with the newly recognized association between congenital microcephaly and intrauterine Zika virus infection. Although initial reports in late 2015 were greeted with appropriate skepticism, based on the scantiness of confirmatory clinical and epidemiologic data, reports such as this have largely supplanted that skepticism with deepening concern about this growing epidemic. This report provides the first detailed description of neuroimaging findings in congenital Zika virus infection, highlighting the characteristic and unusual location of cerebral calcifications at the junction between cortical and subcortical white matter.

Clinical and neuroimaging reports are now supported by neuropathologic and immunologic data from affected infants and epidemiologic investigations, including a recent report showing a striking temporal correlation between the Zika outbreak in Salvador, Brazil in late 2014 and birth of infants with microcephaly 30 to 33 weeks later.[1] There is now consensus that this association is causal, and that the risk of adverse fetal outcomes is greatest when Zika virus infections occur during the first trimester.

Much of the public health response to date has focused on advice to women who are or might become pregnant and their obstetric care providers.[2] Some advice to those who care for affected infants has also been provided,[3] but many questions about treatment of these infants remain unanswered. We do not yet know, for example, what the best confirmatory diagnostic testing strategy is, which neuroimaging studies are indicated and what diagnostic or prognostic information they provide, what evaluation for other etiologies of microcephaly are appropriate, or whether there may be long-term risks for babies with evidence of congenital or perinatal infection in the absence of microcephaly. Answers to these and myriad other questions will only become available with addition of data and experience. We need to pay close attention to ongoing updates provided by the Centers for Disease Control and Prevention (http://www.cdc.gov/zika/hc-providers/qa-pediatrician.html), American Medical Association (http://www.ama-assn.org/ama/pub/physician-resources/public-health/zika-resource-center.page), and American Academy of Pediatrics (https://www.aap.org/en-us/advocacy-and-policy/aap-health-initiatives/Children-and-Disasters/Pages/ZikaVirus.aspx). In our mobile world, there will be few perinatal centers that will not be touched by these concerns.

W. E. Benitz, MD

References

1. Paploski IA, Prates AP, Cardoso CW, et al. Time lags between exanthematous illness attributed to Zika Virus, Guillain-Barre Syndrome, and microcephaly, Salvador, Brazil. *Emerg Infect Dis.* 2016;22.
2. Meaney-Delman D, Rasmussen SA, Staples JE, et al. Zika virus and pregnancy: what obstetric health care providers need to know. *Obstet Gynecol.* 2016;127: 642-648.
3. Centers for Disease Control and Prevention. *Questions and Answers for Healthcare Providers Caring for Infants and Children with Possible Zika Virus Infection.* Atlanta, GA: National Center for Emerging and Zoonotic Infectious Diseases (NCEZID); Division of Vector-Borne Diseases (DVBD); 2016, http://www.cdc.gov/zika/hc-providers/qa-pediatrician.html.

Zika Virus and Birth Defects — Reviewing the Evidence for Causality

Rasmussen SA, Jamieson DJ, Honein MA, et al (Ctrs for Disease Control and Prevention, Atlanta, GA; et al)

N Engl J Med 374:1981-1987, 2016

The Zika virus has spread rapidly in the Americas since its first identification in Brazil in early 2015. Prenatal Zika virus infection has been linked to adverse pregnancy and birth outcomes, most notably microcephaly and other serious brain anomalies. To determine whether Zika virus infection during pregnancy causes these adverse outcomes, we evaluated available data using criteria that have been proposed for the assessment of potential teratogens. On the basis of this review, we conclude that a causal relationship exists between prenatal Zika virus infection and microcephaly and other serious brain anomalies. Evidence that was used to support this causal relationship included Zika virus infection at times during prenatal development that were consistent with the defects observed; a specific, rare phenotype involving microcephaly and associated brain anomalies in fetuses or infants with presumed or confirmed congenital Zika virus infection; and data that strongly support biologic plausibility, including the identification of Zika virus in the brain tissue of affected fetuses and infants. Given the recognition of this causal relationship, we need to intensify our efforts toward the prevention of adverse outcomes caused by congenital Zika virus infection. However, many questions that are critical to our prevention efforts remain, including the spectrum of defects caused by prenatal Zika virus infection, the degree of relative and absolute risks of adverse outcomes among fetuses whose mothers were infected at different times during pregnancy, and factors that might affect a woman's risk of adverse pregnancy or birth outcomes. Addressing these questions will improve our ability to reduce the burden of the effects of Zika virus infection during pregnancy.

▶ The devastating effects of Zika virus infection during pregnancy have been widely communicated in both medical publications and conventional public media. This scholarly review explores the scientific evidence for the association between Zika virus of a pregnant woman and the evolution of microcephaly and brain malformation in her fetus. Using several models of causal analysis, the authors conclude that sufficient evidence exists linking Zika virus infection during pregnancy and fetal microcephaly. They also discuss next steps in this investigation, including understanding the full spectrum of effects (suspecting the phenotype will expand), qualifying the relative and absolute risks to infants born to women infected at different times during pregnancy, and identifying factors that modify the risk. Two additional publications of relevance and interest include the first case report of a Zika virus in the United States: a Finnish woman living in Washington, DC, who traveled to Mexico, Guatemala, and Belize in November 2015 and presented to a hospital 1 day after returning home with ocular pain, myalgia, rash, and low-grade fever.[1] The second publication[2] is a brief summary of a World Health Organization meeting focused on Zika and its challenges, including the obstacles to producing a vaccine to prevent Zika infection. Finally, the Centers for Disease Control and Prevention offers a wealth of information and frequent updates regarding the epidemiology and guidelines for Zika virus infection prevention and management on its website.[3] Although alarmism is not useful, the threat of Zika to pregnant women is real and on our doorstep; it almost certainly will affect women admitted to US hospitals in greater numbers, and these resources provide a starting point in our preparations.

L. J. Van Marter, MD, MPH

References

1. Driggers RW, Ho CY, Korhonen EM, et al. Zika virus infection with prolonged maternal viremia and fetal brain abnormalities. *N Engl J Med.* 2016;374: 2142-2151.
2. Huang CJ, Kieny MP, Murgue B. The Zika challenge. *N Engl J Med.* 2016;374: 1801-1803.
3. Centers for Disease Control and Prevention. Zika virus information. www.cdc.gov/zika.

3 Genetics and Teratology

Screening for trisomies 21, 18 and 13 by cell-free DNA analysis of maternal blood at 10–11 weeks' gestation and the combined test at 11–13 weeks

Quezada MS, Gil MM, Francisco C, et al (King's College Hosp, London, UK)

Ultrasound Obstet Gynecol 45:36-41, 2015

Objective.—To examine in a general population the performance of cell-free DNA (cfDNA) testing for trisomies 21, 18 and 13 at 10–11 weeks' gestation and compare it to that of the combined test at 11–13 weeks.

Methods.—In 2905 singleton pregnancies, prospective screening for trisomies was performed by chromosome-selective sequencing of cfDNA in maternal blood at 10–11 weeks' gestation and by the combined test at 11–13 weeks' gestation.

Results.—Median maternal age of the study population was 36.9 (range, 20.4–51.9) years. Results from cfDNA analysis were provided for 2851 (98.1%) cases and these were available within 14 days from sampling in 2848 (98.0%) cases. The trisomic status of the pregnancies was determined by prenatal or postnatal karyotyping or clinical examination of the neonates. Of the 2785 pregnancies with a cfDNA result and known trisomic status, cfDNA testing correctly identified all 32 cases with trisomy 21, nine of 10 with trisomy 18 and two of five with trisomy 13, with false-positive rates of 0.04%, 0.19% and 0.07%, respectively. In cases with discordant results between cfDNA testing and fetal karyotype, the median fetal fraction was lower than in those with concordant results (6% vs 11%). Using the combined test, the estimated risk for trisomy 21 was ≥1/100 in all trisomic cases and in 4.4% of the non-trisomic pregnancies.

Conclusion.—The performance of first-trimester cfDNA testing for trisomies 21 and 18 in the general population is similar to that in high-risk pregnancies. Most false-positive and false-negative results from cfDNA testing could be avoided if the a priori risk from the combined test is taken into account in the interpretation of individual risk.

▶ Screening for many conditions has become an integral component of neonatal-perinatal care. Newborn screening has been expanded so that with the use of tandem mass spectrometry, most states can detect in excess of 40 disorders from a drop of blood. Central to the success of screening, especially for a disease with a low incidence, is the premise that there must be a high detection rate and low false-positive rate. Detection of an abnormal fetal karyotype lends itself well to the screening process and the old order changes, yielding to the newer less invasive, more precise technology. First-trimester screening for trisomies 21, 18, and 13 by a combination of maternal age, fetal nuchal translucency thickness, fetal heart rate, and serum-free β-human chorionic gonadotropin (β-hCG) and pregnancy-associated plasma protein A (PAPP-A) can detect about 90% of cases of trisomy 21 and 95% of those with trisomies 18 and 13, with a false-positive rate of approximately 5%. The addition of sonographic detection of the nasal bone as well as flow studies improves the detection rate for trisomies >95% with a false-positive rate decreased to <3%. The literature now abounds with studies on the use of maternal plasma (cell free DNA-cfDNA) to detect an abnormal karyotype during the first trimester.[1-3] Evidence suggests that analysis of cfDNA in maternal blood can detect about 99% of cases of trisomy 21, 97% of trisomy 18, and 92% of trisomy 13, with respective false-positive rates of 0.08%, 0.15%, and 0.2%.[1-3]

The study from Quezeda et al confirms the value of cfDNA for screening a general population. Per chance, the average age of their subjects was 5 years older than the usual London population, but they had not had any other prior screening. Of note, the median fetal fraction in the 12 cases with discordant results (6.0%; range, 4.2–8.7%) was significantly lower than in the 2730 cases with concordant normal results (11.1%; range, 4.1–40.2%) and the 43 cases with concordant abnormal results (9.6%; range, 4.7–20.4%) (Mann–Whitney U test, $P < .0001$). In the 32 cases of trisomy 21 with concordant results, the median fetal fraction was 10.1% (range, 5.4%–20.4%), and the median estimated risk from the combined test was 1/2 (range, 1/2 to 1/81). In the case with discordant results, the fetal fraction was 4.7%, and the risk from the combined test was 1 in 6966. Thus the authors recommended that in the interpretation of cfDNA results, particularly in cases with a low fetal fraction, the a priori risk should be taken into consideration.

A. A. Fanaroff, MD

References

1. Nicolaides KH, Syngelaki A, Ashoor G, Birdir C, Touzet G. Noninvasive prenatal testing for fetal trisomies in a routinely screened first-trimester population. *Am J Obstet Gynecol.* 2012;207:374.e1-6.
2. Song Y, Liu C, Qi H, et al. Noninvasive prenatal testing of fetal aneuploidies by massively parallel sequencing in a prospective Chinese population. *Prenat Diagn.* 2013;33:700-706.
3. Bianchi DW, Parker RL, Wentworth J, et al. CARE Study Group. DNA sequencing versus standard prenatal aneuploidy screening. *N Engl J Med.* 2014;370:799-808.

Newborn Screening for Cystic Fibrosis in California

Kharrazi M, Yang J, Bishop T, et al (California Dept of Public Health, Richmond; et al)

Pediatrics 136:1062-1072, 2015

Objectives.—This article describes the methods used and the program performance results for the first 5 years of newborn screening for cystic fibrosis (CF) in California.

Methods.—From July 16, 2007, to June 30, 2012, a total of 2 573 293 newborns were screened for CF by using a 3-step model: (1) measuring immunoreactive trypsinogen in all dried blood spot specimens; (2) testing 28 to 40 selected cystic fibrosis transmembrane conductance regulator (CFTR) mutations in specimens with immunoreactive trypsinogen values ≥62 ng/mL (top 1.6%); and (3) performing DNA sequencing on specimens found to have only 1 mutation in step 2. Infants with ≥2 mutations/variants were referred to CF care centers for diagnostic evaluation and follow-up. Infants with 1 mutation were considered carriers and their parents offered telephone genetic counseling.

Results.—Overall, 345 CF cases, 533 CFTR-related metabolic syndrome cases, and 1617 carriers were detected; 28 cases of CF were missed. Of the 345 CF cases, 20 (5.8%) infants were initially assessed as having CFTR-related metabolic syndrome, and their CF diagnosis occurred after age 6 months (median follow-up: 4.5 years). Program sensitivity was 92%, and the positive predictive value was 34%. CF prevalence was 1 in 6899 births. A total of 303 *CFTR* mutations were identified, including 78 novel variants. The median age at referral to a CF care center was 34 days (18 and 37 days for step 2 and 3 screening test–positive infants, respectively).

Conclusions.—The 3-step model had high detection and low false-positive levels in this diverse population.

▶ Newborn screening for cystic fibrosis (CF) has been universal for all births in all 50 US states since 2009 and has changed the face of disease presentation, natural history, and outcome. Screening algorithms vary significantly by state, but most include an initial measurement of the serum analyte immunoreactive trypsinogen (IRT), a pancreatic enzyme, from the newborn dried blood spot (DBS). For those babies with the highest IRT levels, the most common algorithm performs a second-tier DBS DNA test to screen for a panel of common CFTR mutations. Detection of 2 CF-causing mutations is diagnostic for CF, but the identification only a single mutation in hypertrypsinogenemic samples has required bringing the screen positive newborn in for sweat chloride concentration measurement for distinction between carrier versus affected status. In 2007, California initiated an innovative and controversial algorithm of IRT/DNA testing followed by a third tier of gene sequencing as part of the newborn screening (NBS) lab testing. If sequencing of the *CFTR* gene did not reveal a second mutation, the infant could be deemed a carrier and this would preclude the need for sweat testing. Carriers identified by the screen were contacted by mail and offered genetic counseling, although the uptake was low. DNA sequencing as a tertiary tier of testing to lower reported false-positive rates is a remarkable component of this new algorithm. Currently, with the IRT/DNA algorithm, *CFTR* sequencing is only performed after the sweat chloride level is confirmed to be outside the normal range. The study demonstrated a dramatic decrease in the number of sweat tests required for CF NBS, but in addition, the spectrum of genotypes identified by this algorithm was shifted toward atypical CF cases (*CFTR*-related metabolic syndrome; CRMS), detecting 2:1 CRMS to classic CF cases. These milder genotypes had not previously been identified prospectively. In the past, such children either presented later with mild CF symptoms (including infertility in males or chronic respiratory symptoms). Because it appears that only about 10% of these CRMS cases go in to develop classic CF, many of these screen-positive cases would never develop symptoms. There is poor understanding of the extreme variability in penetrance of these genotypes. With the screening of 2.5 million births over a 5-year period, this population-based experience is rich in data on the characterization of CF newborns in the California population. Ethnicity was a challenging consideration in the planning of this screening program because California (more than 50% Hispanic) requires that implemented screening tests be optimized equally for all groups. CF-causing mutations tend to vary significantly by racial and ethnic groups, and thus the initial mutation panel selected needed to be tailored for the California population rather than the general US Caucasian majority population. This California 3-step screening algorithm has introduced the concept of DNA sequencing as part of NBS, and this has opened the door for use of this technology to improve the screening of other NBS disorders, even lending support to the feasibility of primary DNA sequencing for disorders that do not reveal measurable analytes on the newborn DBS.

R. B. Parad, MD, MPH

Next-Generation Molecular Testing of Newborn Dried Blood Spots for Cystic Fibrosis

Lefterova MI, Shen P, Odegaard JI, et al (Stanford Univ Med Ctr, CA; Stanford Univ, Palo Alto, CA; et al)

J Mol Diagn 18:267-282, 2016

Newborn screening for cystic fibrosis enables early detection and management of this debilitating genetic disease. Implementing comprehensive *CFTR* analysis using Sanger sequencing as a component of confirmatory testing of all screen-positive newborns has remained impractical due to relatively lengthy turnaround times and high cost. Here, we describe CFseq, a highly sensitive, specific, rapid (<3 days), and cost-effective assay for comprehensive *CFTR* gene analysis from dried blood spots, the common newborn screening specimen. The unique design of CFseq integrates optimized dried blood spot sample processing, a novel multiplex amplification method from as little as 1 ng of genomic DNA, and multiplex next-generation sequencing of 96 samples in a single run to detect all relevant *CFTR* mutation types. Sequence data analysis utilizes publicly available software supplemented by an expert-curated compendium of >2000 *CFTR* variants. Validation studies across 190 dried blood spots demonstrated 100% sensitivity and a positive predictive value of 100% for single-nucleotide variants and insertions and deletions and complete concordance across the polymorphic poly-TG and consecutive poly-T tracts. Additionally, we accurately detected both a known exon 2,3 deletion and a previously undetected exon 22,23 deletion. CFseq is thus able to replace all existing *CFTR* molecular assays with a single robust, definitive assay at significant cost and time savings and could be adapted to high-throughput screening of other inherited conditions.

▶ Cystic fibrosis (CF) is among the most common genetic disorders and identified in approximately 1 in 4000 live births. Great progress has been made in both the treatment and recognition, with many patients living productive lives well into adulthood.

CF is an autosomal recessive disorder caused by mutations in the CF transmembrane conductance regulator gene (*CFTR*). Although a single genetic variant accounts for 70% of the cases, many single nucleotide variants have been identified.

Because CF is a common disorder with significant clinical sequelae and progressive responses to therapeutic interventionsm it meets the criteria for universal screening that was introduced in the United States 2010. Mak[1] reporting on the Canadian experience noted that Newborn Screening NBS patients were diagnosed earlier and had their first at a younger age. Pancreatic insufficiency was less common in NBS patients. The incidence of *Pseudomonas aeruginosa* and *Staphylococcus aureus* were lower in NBS patients. The NBS patients also grew better, so they concluded that "NBS programs for CF lead to improved long-term health outcomes for the CF population."[1]

Screening methodology has come a long way from the early days when CF was recognized because the babies tasted salty and had foul-smelling stools. Measuring the sweat chloride after iontophoresis would then be the confirmatory test.

Most screening programs now begin with immunoreactive trypsinogen testing of dried blood spots (DBSs) taken from newborn heel sticks. This assay is sensitive but not specific with a high rate of false-positives, necessitating follow-up testing. Sontag et al[2] reported an effort to Improve the Sensitivity and Positive Predictive Value in a Cystic Fibrosis Newborn Screening Program Using a Repeat Immunoreactive Trypsinogen and Genetic Analysis.

This methodology showed some improvement but will be replaced by next generation sequencing (NGS) as described in the article discussed here. The spectacular report from Lefterova and colleagues is written in a foreign language if you are not a geneticist. However, they explain everything beautifully and the new technology is both specific and sensitive.

I have included a key paragraph to the commentary.

"Here we describe the design, development, and validation of CFseq, a highly sensitive, specific, cost effective,and rapid clinical NGS assay that reliably sequences all exons, flanking intronic regions, and key noncoding regions of the CFTR gene from a single 3.2-mm newborn DBS punch. This performance is achieved through optimized DBS sample processing and DNA extraction, a novel multiplex PCR (mPCR)-based target amplification strategy, and standard NGS using the MiSeq platform (Illumina, San Diego, CA) coupled with a customizable automated bioinformatics pipeline for data analysis and interpretation. Importantly, the CFseq design allows for 96 samples to be pooled and run simultaneously, reducing the per-sample reagent cost to as little as one-fifth that of traditional tiered NBS testing and the turnaroundtime to as little as 3 days. With these performance parameters, this single workflow may be able to completely replace existing algorithms for CF NBS and provide comprehensive analysis for all hypertrypsinogenemic infants, while reducing cost and turnaround time and providing superior molecular diagnosis." The abstract and the results therein speak for themselves. With NGS, we are witnessing a transformation in screening methodology with major clinical benefits. Microsamples from the filter paper blood screening can be used to rapidly identify important clinical disorders.

A. A. Fanaroff, MD

References

1. Mak DY, Sykes J, Stephenson AL, Lands LC. The benefits of newborn screening for cystic fibrosis: the Canadian experience. *J Cyst Fibros.* 2016;15:302-308.
2. Sontag MK, Lee R, Wright D, Freedenberg D, Sagel SD. Improving the sensitivity and positive predictive value in a cystic fibrosis newborn screening program using a repeat immunoreactive trypsinogen and genetic analysis. *J Pediatr.* 2016 [Epub ahead of print].

Noninvasive prenatal testing: more caution in counseling is needed in high risk pregnancies with ultrasound abnormalities

Oneda B, Steindl K, Masood R, et al (Univ of Zurich Switzerland; et al)
Eur J Obstet Gynecol Reprod Biol 200:72-75, 2016

Objective.—Non-invasive prenatal testing (NIPT) is increasingly being used in prenatal aneuploidy screening. The objective of this study was to assess the positive predictive value in our cohort of 68 cases with positive NIPT result. In addition, we wondered if the use of NIPT in cases with ultrasound abnormalities is appropriate, given the limited number of chromosomes investigated.

Design.—We performed confirmative invasive testing using karyotyping, fluorescence *in situ* hybridization (FISH) and/or high-resolution chromosomal microarray analysis.

Results.—In line with the published data, the positive NIPT result was confirmed in 64.7% of cases. Inconclusive and negative NIPT results followed by cytogenetically pathologic findings were encountered in three and in five cases, respectively. Four of the five fetuses with negative

NIPT but pathologic cytogenetic findings were born with several malformations and diagnosed right after birth with severe genetic conditions. Of note, in all of those four cases, NIPT was offered despite the finding of major fetal ultrasound abnormalities and despite the fact that the family would not have opposed invasive testing or pregnancy termination.

Conclusion.—More education of health care providers and caution in counseling and interpretation of test results are needed in order to meet the challenges that this new test, which enriches our diagnostic options in prenatal testing, poses.

▶ Interrogation of the fetal genome in increasingly high resolution and the development of noninvasive methods of fetal testing using cell-free DNA in maternal plasma are the 2 themes that have dominated recent technological advances in prenatal diagnosis.

"However, technological progress is outpacing the ability of the health care providers and patients to incorporate these new tests into existing clinical care, and further complicates many of the economic and ethical dilemmas in prenatal diagnosis."[1] Noninvasive prenatal testing (NIPT), which uses massively parallel sequencing to align and count DNA fragments floating in the plasma of pregnant women, has become integrated into prenatal care. The main impact on clinical care has been a reduction in invasive procedures. The study by Oneda et al adds to the growing body of literature and addresses some key points necessary to advance the field.

Studies comparing NIPT to serum or combined screening for autosomal aneuploidy all show that NIPT has significantly lower false-positive rates (approximately 0.1%–0.2%), even in all-risk populations. Confirmatory testing for aneuploidies requires an invasive procedure such as chorionic villus sampling or amniocentesis; therefore, the low false-positive screening rate has a significant clinical impact. Bear in mind, though, that the positive predictive value (PPV) for NIPT is only in the range of 92.2% to 93% for trisomy 21, 58% to 76.6% for trisomy 18, 32.8% to 45% for trisomy 13, 23% to 38% for monosomy X and 67% for other sex chromosome aneuploidies. Microdeletions are still best diagnosed with invasive testing.

Bianchi highlights advancements in the utility of NIPT as well as unexpected challenges.[1] There have been multiple reports of NIPT cases in which initial testing suggested an abnormality that was not substantiated by diagnostic fetal testing. A significant number of the discordant positive cases have underlying biological reasons, including confined placental mosaicism, maternal mosaicism, cotwin demise, or maternal malignancy.[2-4] Nonetheless these false positives, however low the rate, result in much anxiety.

Professional societies currently recommend offering NIPT to women at increased risk of fetal chromosome aneuploidies. High risk includes cases with abnormal ultrasound findings indicating an increased risk for aneuploidy including an abnormal neck translucency. Studies are ongoing to evaluate the clinical utility of these tests in average-risk pregnancies. It is necessary to emphasize that NIPT is a screening test that focuses on a limited number of chromosomal aneuploidies. Continuing education of parents and providers is mandatory.

A. A. Fanaroff, MD

References

1. Hui L, Bianchi DW. Recent advances in the prenatal interrogation of the human fetal genome. *Trends Genet.* 2013;29:84-91.
2. Bianchi DW, Wilkins-Haug L. Integration of noninvasive DNA testing for aneuploidy into prenatal care: what has happened since the rubber met the road? *Clin Chem.* 2014;60:78-87.
3. Bianchi DW. Prepare for unexpected prenatal test results. *Nature.* 2015;522: 29-30.
4. Dar P, Curnow KJ, Gross SJ, et al. Clinical experience and follow-up with large scale single-nucleotide polymorphism-based noninvasive prenatal aneuploidy testing. *Am J Obstet Gynecol.* 2014;211:527.e1-17.

DNA Methylation in Newborns and Maternal Smoking in Pregnancy: Genome-wide Consortium Meta-analysis

Joubert BR, Felix JF, Yousefi P, et al (Natl Inst of Environmental Health Sciences, Research Triangle Park, NC; Univ Med Ctr Rotterdam, the Netherlands; Univ of California Berkeley; et al)

Am J Hum Genet 98:680-696, 2016

Epigenetic modifications, including DNA methylation, represent a potential mechanism for environmental impacts on human disease. Maternal smoking in pregnancy remains an important public health problem that impacts child health in a myriad of ways and has potential lifelong consequences. The mechanisms are largely unknown, but epigenetics most likely plays a role. We formed the Pregnancy And Childhood Epigenetics (PACE) consortium and meta-analyzed, across 13 cohorts ($n = 6,685$), the association between maternal smoking in pregnancy and newborn blood DNA methylation at over 450,000 CpG sites (CpGs) by using the Illumina 450K BeadChip. Over 6,000 CpGs were differentially methylated in relation to maternal smoking at genome-wide statistical significance (false discovery rate, 5%), including 2,965 CpGs corresponding to 2,017 genes not previously related to smoking and methylation in either newborns or adults. Several genes are relevant to diseases that can be caused by maternal smoking (e.g., orofacial clefts and asthma) or adult smoking (e.g., certain cancers). A number of differentially methylated CpGs were associated with gene expression. We observed enrichment in pathways and processes critical to development. In older children (5 cohorts, $n = 3,187$), 100% of CpGs gave at least nominal levels of significance, far more than expected by chance (p value $< 2.2 \times 10^{-16}$). Results were robust to different normalization methods used across studies and cell type adjustment. In this large scale meta-analysis of methylation data, we identified numerous loci involved in response to maternal smoking in pregnancy with persistence into later childhood and provide insights into mechanisms underlying effects of this important exposure.

▶ Previous cohort studies have repeatedly shown that maternal smoking during pregnancy is associated with cord blood DNA methylation in the aryl-hydrocarbon receptor repressor (AHRR). Joubert et al performed an extensive meta-analysis pooling data and examined associations between maternal smoking and epigenome-wide DNA methylation in umbilical cord blood. The Pregnancy and Childhood Epigenetics (PACE) consortium included 13 cohorts (n = 6685 mother-infant pairs). They found 2965 CpG sites that were differentially methylated in offspring of smokers versus nonsmokers, 2017 of which are from genes not previously related to smoking. Many of the genes have been described in diseases that can be caused by maternal smoking including asthma, suggesting that epigenetic modifications could play a role in the toxicity of smoking in pregnancy. This study demonstrates the power of pooling studies to detect small effects that can be missed in analyses of smaller, single-cohort studies.

H. H. Burris, MD, MPH

Association between marijuana use and adverse obstetrical and neonatal outcomes

Warshak CR, Regan J, Moore B, et al (Univ of Cincinnati College of Medicine, OH; et al)

J Perinatol 35:991-995, 2015

Objective.—To evaluate associations between marijuana exposure and adverse outcomes excluding women with polysubstance abuse and stratifying for concurrent maternal tobacco use.

Study Design.—We performed a retrospective cohort study evaluating various obstetrical and neonatal outcomes including: preterm delivery, pre-eclampsia, gestational diabetes, cesarean delivery, fetal growth restriction, a composite which included stillbirth or neonatal intensive care unit admission, and perinatal mortality. We stratified study groups according to the maternal tobacco use and performed a logistic regression analysis.

Results.—We included 6468 women, 6107 nonusers and 361 marijuana users. After adjustment for maternal age, race, parity, body mass index and no prenatal care, we found higher rates of small for gestational age (aOR 1.30 (95% CI 1.03 to 1.62)) and neonatal intensive care unit admission (aOR 1.54 (1.14 to 2.07)) in women who were not tobacco users. Other obstetrical outcomes including preterm delivery and fetal anomalies were not increased with maternal marijuana use.

Conclusion.—Maternal marijuana use does not increase the risk of adverse obstetrical outcomes or fetal anomalies, but does increase the risk for small for gestational age and neonatal intensive care unit admission.

▶ As more states legalize sale and use of marijuana, either for medical or recreational purposes, fetal exposure to cannabinoids is certain to become more prevalent. The historical consensus that such exposures have few effects on the developing fetus is based more strongly on the relative lack of data implicating marijuana use in adverse outcomes than on availability of compelling data supporting safety. The few available studies have been confounded by the challenge of separate identification of cannabis effects in the context of exposures to multiple exogenous agents, including tobacco. This important article begins to address that void. After adjustment for maternal age, race, parity, body mass index, and prenatal care, associations between maternal marijuana use and both small size for gestational age (SGA) and neonatal intensive care unit (NICU) admissions were identified. Significantly (and not surprisingly), the rate of tobacco exposure was substantially greater (58%) in marijuana users than in nonusers (20%). Because of that, these authors went on to separately assess the correlates of marijuana use in the subsets of their population who did or did not also use tobacco and found that those associations with marijuana exposure were recapitulated in babies born to women who did not use tobacco (adjusted odds ratios [aOR] for SGA 1.30, 95% confidence interval [CI] 1.03–1.62, and for NICU admission 1.54, 95% CI 1.14–2.07]), but not among those who did use tobacco (aOR for SGA 1.17, 95% CI 0.96–1.41, and for NICU admission aOR 1.29, 95% CI 0.96–1.73). It remains uncertain, however, whether these differences are due to direct effects of marijuana exposure or of confounders not included in the regression model, such as socioeconomic status, education, or nutrition, which also may cosegregate with marijuana use. It is reassuring that maternal marijuana use was not found to be associated with other adverse obstetrical or neonatal outcomes, including preterm birth, antenatal diagnosis of fetal growth delay, gestational diabetes, preeclampsia, abruption, oligohydramnios, nonreassuring fetal condition, induction of labor, cesarean delivery, fetal anomalies, prolonged hospitalization, or neonatal mortality. However, long-term effects on neurodevelopment remain to be explored.

W. E. Benitz, MD

Necrotizing Enterocolitis Is Not Associated With Sequence Variants in Antioxidant Response Genes in Premature Infants

Sampath V, Helbling D, Menden H, et al (Med College of Wisconsin, Milwaukee; et al)

J Pediatr Gastroenterol Nutr 62:420-423, 2016

Reactive oxygen species mediate intestinal injury in necrotizing enterocolitis (NEC), and yet the contribution of antioxidant response (ARE) gene polymorphisms to NEC risk remains unknown. Premature infants recruited in a multicenter study were genotyped for 6 ARE variants. Among 637 infants, 52 had NEC, and 22 developed surgical NEC. Gestational age <28 weeks (P < 0.02) and African American race (*P* = 0.03) were associated with NEC. The *NFE2L2* (rs6721961), *SOD2* (rs4880), *GSTP1* (rs1695), *NQO1* (rs1800566), *GCLC* (rs17883901), and *HMOX1* (rs2071747) variants were not associated with medical or surgical NEC. This study does not support a role for common deleterious ARE variants in NEC.

▶ The suspicion that the necrotizing enterocolitis (NEC) may partially result from genetic sequence variants has been previously questioned largely because of some studies that suggest a slightly higher prevalence of NEC in the identical twins of infants who have previously developed NEC. Based on studies done in animals that suggest that reactive oxygen species may be involved in the pathophysiology of necrotizing enterocolitis, this group evaluated genetic variants of a set of antioxidant genes of the Nrf2-ARE axis.

The samples from the infants used in the study were derived from a prospectively done evaluation of 644 infants born with a gestational age less than or equal to 35 weeks. Genotyping was done using previously developed commercial DNA kits. In this study, necrotizing enterocolitis was defined using the modified Bell staging criteria. However, it was not clear specifically how these stages were compared. For example, if only a drain was placed for suspected necrotizing enterocolitis in the bowel was never visualized by the surgeon, was this considered a case of necrotizing enterocolitis? Nevertheless, the results did not show polymorphisms in antioxidant genes from NEC patients compared to controls. As mentioned by the authors, this study differs from a previous one done by the same group evaluating the nuclear factor Kappa B (NFKB) sites, which appeared to differ in babies with NEC compared with those who did not have NEC. However, the authors did not follow-up on their previous finding because they did find a very high prevalence of that variant in the infants without NEC (65%). So at this time, studies that show a clear genetic variant that predisposes to NEC has not yet been found.

It is the opinion of this reviewer that the search for genetic variants that predispose to NEC should be further pursued, but the likelihood of finding such variants appears to be low. Instead, focusing on modifiable environmental factors that play a role in the pathogenesis of NEC should be priority. Environmental factors could be interacting with the microbes of the infant gastrointestinal tract and very likely producing inflammatory responses, depending on whether the microbes are dysbiotic or commensal. Whether genetic predisposition plays a role in this interaction is still not understood, but at this juncture the studies available do not support this.

J. Neu, MD

4 Labor and Delivery

Partial restoration of the microbiota of cesarean-born infants via vaginal microbial transfer

Dominguez-Bello MG, De Jesus-Laboy KM, Shen N, et al (New York Univ; Univ of Puerto Rico, San Juan; Icahn School of Medicine at Mount Sinai, NY; et al)

Nat Med 22:250-253, 2016

Exposure of newborns to the maternal vaginal microbiota is interrupted with cesarean birthing. Babies delivered by cesarean section (C-section) acquire a microbiota that differs from that of vaginally delivered infants, and C-section delivery has been associated with increased risk for immune and metabolic disorders. Here we conducted a pilot study in which infants delivered by C-section were exposed to maternal vaginal fluids at birth. Similarly to vaginally delivered babies, the gut, oral and skin bacterial communities of these newborns during the first 30 d of life was enriched in vaginal bacteria—which were underrepresented in unexposed C-section–delivered infants—and the microbiome similarity to those of vaginally delivered infants was greater in oral and skin samples than in anal samples. Although the long-term health consequences of restoring the microbiota of C-section–delivered infants remain unclear, our results demonstrate that vaginal microbes can be partially restored at birth in C-section–delivered babies.

► In many parts of the world, cesarean deliveries rates are very high. Clearly, many of these are being done for nonmedical purposes. Because several epidemiologic studies suggest increased odds of developing obesity, autoimmune diseases, and celiac disease in infants born by cesarean delivery,[1] areas where cesarean deliveries are highly prevalent may end up experiencing major public health problems in the future.

Several studies suggest that cesarean versus vaginal delivery affects subsequent microbial colonization in the intestine of the newborn infant. If this is the case, this could also affect the developing immune system, which relies greatly on early intestinal interactions with microbes. One study comparing vaginally to cesarean-delivered baby fecal microbiota[2] using 16SrRNA sequencing showed that vaginally delivered infants acquired bacterial communities resembling their own mother's vaginal microbiota, whereas cesarean-delivered infants were colonized by bacterial communities similar to those found in the mother's skin.

A subsequent study from Canada evaluated fecal microbiota at four months of age[3] in healthy infants who were born by cesarean versus vaginal delivery. Differences were still seen between the 2 modes of delivery at 4 months after birth. In another study from Scandinavia,[4] major differences in microbial diversity were seen up to 2 years after birth in the fecal microbiota. There was a preponderance of *Bacteroidetes* in the infants born by vaginal delivery. This was seen in conjunction with higher levels of anti-inflammatory mediators.

This has raised the question of whether a vaginal swab to introduce maternal vaginal microbes into cesarean-delivered infants' gastrointestinal tracts may be beneficial. The study reported here evaluates a small number of subjects born by cesarean versus vaginal delivery, with 4 of 11 cesarean-delivered babies undergoing a procedure that included swabbing the mouth, face, and body with gauze that had been inoculated with mother's vaginal secretions (including microbes). Rectal swab microbes from the babies who were swabbed after cesarean deliveries showed a rectal swab microbial profile that appeared more similar to the infants born by vaginal delivery than the cesarean-delivered infants who were not swabbed. This suggests that vaginal microbes can be introduced into cesarean-delivered infants. Although this appears to be an exciting finding that should generate larger, well-controlled prospective studies, it is clear that this procedure is still far from the point of being recommended as routine practice. In addition to requiring validation in larger well-controlled trials that show both safety and efficacy, we need to be wary of iatrogenic introduction of pathogens such as HSV, HIV, hepatitis, or Group B *Streptococcus* into infants. Until safety is substantiated with additional studies, routine use of this procedure should be discouraged.

J. Neu, MD

References

1. Cho CE, Norman M. Cesarean section and development of the immune system in the offspring. *Am J Obstet Gynecol.* 2013;208:249-254.
2. Dominguez-Bello MG, Costello EK, Contreras M, et al. Delivery mode shapes the acquisition and structure of the initial microbiota across multiple body habitats in newborns. *Proc Natl Acad Sci U S A.* 2010;107:11971-11975.
3. Azad MB, Konya T, Maughan H, et al. Gut microbiota of healthy Canadian infants: profiles by mode of delivery and infant diet at 4 months. *CMAJ.* 2013; 185:385-394.
4. Jakobsson HE, Abrahamsson TR, Jenmalm MC, et al. Decreased gut microbiota diversity, delayed Bacteroidetes colonisation and reduced Th1 responses in infants delivered by Caesarean section. *Gut.* 2014;63:559-566.

Intra- and interobserver agreement among obstetric experts in court regarding the review of abnormal fetal heart rate tracings and obstetrical management

Sabiani L, Le Dû R, Loundou A, et al (Aix-Marseile Université, France; et al)

Am J Obstet Gynecol 213:856.e1-8, 2015

Objective.—The objective of the study was to evaluate the intra- and interobserver agreement among obstetric experts in court regarding the retrospective review of abnormal fetal heart rate tracings and obstetrical management of patients with abnormal fetal heart rate during labor.

Study Design.—A total of 22 French obstetric experts in court reviewed 30 cases of term deliveries of singleton pregnancies diagnosed with at least 1 hour of abnormal fetal heart rate, including 10 cases with adverse neonatal outcome. The experts reviewed all cases twice within a 3-month interval, with the first review being blinded to neonatal outcome. For each case reviewed, the experts were provided with the obstetric data and copies of the complete fetal heart rate recording and the partogram. The experts were asked to classify the abnormal fetal heart rate tracing and to express whether they agreed with the obstetrical management performed. When they disagreed, the experts were asked whether they concluded that an error had been made and whether they considered the obstetrical management as the cause of cerebral palsy in children if any.

Results.—Compared with blinded review, the experts were significantly more likely to agree with the obstetric management performed ($P < .001$) and with the mode of delivery ($P < .001$) when informed about the neonatal outcome and were less likely to conclude that an error had been made ($P < .001$) or to establish a link with potential cerebral palsy ($P = .003$). The experts' intraobserver agreement for the review of abnormal fetal heart rate tracing and obstetrical management were both mediocre (kappa = 0.46–0.51 and kappa = 0.48–0.53, respectively). The interobserver agreement for the review of abnormal fetal heart rate tracing was low and was not improved by knowledge of the neonatal outcome (kappa = 0.11–0.18). The interobserver agreement for the interpretation of obstetrical management was also low (kappa = 0.08–0.19) but appeared to be improved by knowledge of the neonatal outcome (kappa = 0.15–0.32).

Conclusion.—The intra- and interobserver agreement among obstetric experts in court for the review of abnormal fetal heart rate tracing and the appropriateness of obstetrical care is poor, suggesting a lack of objectivity of obstetrical expertise as currently performed in court.

▶ It is not surprising that there is poor agreement between intra and interobservers in court when interpreting different abnormal fetal monitoring strips and the relationship between interpretation of these strips as signifying neurologic impairment and the subsequent development of cerebral palsy. The use of electronic fetal monitoring (EFM) remains controversial in the obstetrical literature, and we are certain today that interpretations are not always black or white but more frequently "gray." Despite these controversial findings, EFM continues to be used extensively in the intrapartum management of woman and "experts" are often called on in court to testify based on their interpretation of the fetal monitoring strips. In 2008, the National Institute of Child Health and Human Development reported on a workshop on EFM and updated definitions, interpretations and suggested research guidelines.[1] The International Federation of Gynecology and Obstetrics also reported extensive guidelines on intrapartum monitoring.[2] The *Eunice Kennedy Shriver* National Institute of Child Health and Human Development described a 3-tiered fetal heart rate interpretation system was described with Category I being normal, Category III very abnormal (requiring intervention), and Category II having varying necessity for intervention. All of these investigations and meta-analysis with comparisons using intermittent auscultation have shown no significant difference in neonatal outcome.

In addition, there were 116 obstetrical experts contacted, but only 28 (24.1%) actually participated in the study. The use of the Kappa statistic, which measures the agreement between observers, was poor (0.46-0.51), accentuating the disagreements between the obstetrician's interpretations. When neonatal outcome was added to the information, the agreement between physicians improved. Oftentimes in court, when expert witnesses are used, the personality, demeanor, and interaction of the expert with the jury may in fact outweigh the evidence.

This does not mean that there is no place in obstetrical intrapartum management for the use of EFM. Information regarding fetal acidosis, previous neurologic injury and current fetal well-being is still being collected and obstetricians must recognize the limits of the technology when offering opinions in court regarding obstetrical management.

G. I. Martin, MD

References

1. National Institute of Child Health and Human Development Workshop on EFM. *Obstet Gynecol.* 2008;112:3.
2. Visser GR, DeCampo Dfor the FIGO Intrapartum Consensus Panel. FIGO guidelines on intrapartum fetal monitoring: adjunctive technologies. *Int J Gynaecol Obstet.* 2015;131:25-29.

Fetal heart rate abnormalities associated with uterine rupture: a case–control study: A new time-lapse approach using a standardized classification

Desseauve D, Bonifazi-Grenouilleau M, Fritel X, et al (Université de Poitiers, France; Centre Hospitalier Universitaire de Poitiers, France; et al)
Eur J Obstet Gynecol Reprod Biol 197:16-21, 2016

Objective.—The aim of this study was to identify fetal heart rate abnormalities (FHRA) in the two hours preceding uterine rupture during trial of

CTG-Class	FIGO-FHR-class	Baseline heart rate	Variability/reactivity	Deceleration
Normal FHR	*FIGO 1*	•110-150 bpm	•5-25 bpm •Acceleration	•Early uniform decelerations •Uncomplicated variable deceleration with a duration of<60 sec and loss of<60 beats
Intermediate FHR	*FIGO 2*	•100-110 bpm •150-170 bpm •Short bradycardia episode (<100 bpm for ≤ 3 minutes)	•>25 bpm (saltory pattern) •<5 bpm for >40 minutes with absence of acceleration	•Uncomplicated variable deceleartions with a duration <60 sec and loss of >60 beats
		A combinaison of several intermediary observations will result in an abnormal CTG		
Abnormal FHR	*FIGO 3*	•150-170 bpm and reduced variability •>170 bpm •Persistent bradycardia (<100 bpm for >3minutes	•< 5 bpm for >60 minutes •Sinusoidal pattern	•Complicated variable deceleration with a duration of >60 sec •Repeated late uniform deceleratio
Preterminal FHR	*FIGO 4*	***Total lack of variability (<2 bpm) and reactivity with or without deceleration or bradycardia***		

FHR: CardioTocoraphy-class, FIGO : Federation-International-of-Gynecology-and -Obstetric, bpm: beats per minutes

FIGURE 1.—Classification of fetal heart rate according to FIGO, as modified by Amer-Walhin [23]. *Editor's Note*: Please refer to original journal article for full references. (Reprinted from Desseauve D, Bonifazi-Grenouilleau M, Fritel X, et al. Fetal heart rate abnormalities associated with uterine rupture: a case–control study: a new time-lapse approach using a standardized classification. *Eur J Obstet Gynecol Reprod Biol*. 2016;197:16-21, with permission from Elsevier Ireland Ltd.)

labor after a previous C-section compared with successful vaginal birth after cesarean controls.

Study Design.—A multicenter case–control study was conducted from 2006 to 2012. Fetal heart rate tracings of the two-hour period preceding delivery were segmented, anonymized and independently classified by two obstetricians according to a standardized grid based on FIGO guidelines (4 grades: 1 – normal, 2 – intermediate, 3 – abnormal, 4 – preterminal). Each case of uterine rupture was matched to 2 controls.

Survival curves were generated for both groups using the Kaplan–Meier method to analyze the occurrence of each FHR category across time.

Results.—During the study period, 39,773 patients gave birth. 2649 involved women with a previous C-section (6.6%). A total of 33 uterine rupture/scar dehiscence cases occurred (0.08% of all births), of which 22 were included. These were matched to 44 controls.

FIGO grade-3 FHRA were significantly associated with uterine rupture in the hour preceding its diagnosis: odds ratios were 4.1 (95% CI 1.2–14.0), 4.3 (95% CI 1.4–13.0) and 3.7 (95% CI 1.2–11.3), in the 60–40 min, 40–20 min and last 20 min before childbirth, respectively. Agreement between the two reviewers (Cohen's kappa) was 84% (CI 95%: 0.79–0.89).

Conclusion.—In the hour preceding uterine rupture, there are often significant FHRA. This leads us to consider the possibility of an earlier C-section when faced with grade-3 FHRA, before the onset of terminal bradycardia jeopardizing maternal and fetal prognosis (Fig 1).

▶ It is somewhat disturbing that in Europe about a quarter of all deliveries are by cesarean (CD), whereas in the United States, that number is closer to a third, and rising. Although the old adage "once a C-section always a C-section" no longer applies, there has been a general reluctance to expose women to a vaginal birth after a CD (VBAC). A major concern is uterine rupture and the medical and medicolegal implications of this problem. Hypoxic ischemic encephalopathy (HIE) is a major consequence of uterine rupture, and a significant number of babies in the cooling trials that have benefited from this therapy were enrolled after uterine rupture. Be reminded, however, that the uterine scar may give way even if a repeat CD is planned.

This article carefully evaluates fetal heart rate tracings for the 2 hours before the rupture. The study is well designed and controlled. The strips were divided into 20-minute segments, anonymized, and randomly ordered. The selected segments were independently evaluated by 2 senior-grade obstetricians and classified according into 4 grades of increasing severity: normal, intermediate, abnormal, and preterminal (Fig 1). In the event of a disagreement between reviewers, a third-party senior expert analyzed the tracings. They found a significant association between grade 3 fetal heart rate abnormalities during Trial of Labor after C. Section and uterine rupture, in the hour preceding its diagnosis. They concluded, as would any good Monday-morning quarterback knowing the outcomes, that finding significant fetal heart rate abnormalities should be a call to action and an indication for immediate operative delivery for women with previous CD.

A. A. Fanaroff, MD

Modification of the Neonatal Resuscitation Program Algorithm for Resuscitation of Conjoined Twins

Yamada NK, Fuerch JH, Halamek LP (Stanford Univ, Palo Alto, CA)

Am J Perinatol 33:420-424, 2016

There are no national or international guidelines for the resuscitation of conjoined twins. We have described how the U.S. Neonatal Resuscitation Program algorithm can be modified for delivery room resuscitation of omphaloischiopagus conjoined twins. In planning for the delivery and resuscitation of these patients, we considered the challenges of providing cardiopulmonary support to preterm conjoined twins in face-to-face orientation and with shared circulation via a fused liver and single umbilical cord. We also demonstrate how in situ simulation can be used to prepare a large, multidisciplinary team of health care professionals to deliver safe, efficient, and effective care to such patients.

▶ I must say that I was taken aback when I initially saw the title of this article. In the past 40 years, I have encountered but 1 set of conjoined twins, and in the world of protocolized medicine, it seems there is always someone who wants to modify algorithms for each and every exception.

However, as I read the article, I realized that there are some important and key messages contained in it. First, the value of communication cannot be overemphasized. As prenatal diagnosis of anomalous conditions becomes more and more prominent, the challenges of how to deal with unusual and difficult malformations, especially those affecting the airway, have led to novel ways of intervention, such as the EXIT procedure. Interdisciplinary discussion and planning is essential to success in the delivery room. Second, developing an algorithm is great, but it may not be enough, especially if unanticipated complications arise or under the pressure of failing transition. This is the true value of simulation and rehearsal. The authors constructed a 3-dimensional manikin based on fetal magnetic resonance imaging, thus rendering their algorithm feasible and preparing the delivery and resuscitation teams for what to expect and how to react. Well done.

S. M. Donn, MD

Do We Need an Intubation-Skilled Person at All High-Risk Deliveries?

Almudeer A, McMillan D, O'Connell C, et al (Dalhousie Univ, Halifax, Canada)

J Pediatr 171:55-59, 2016

Objective.—To evaluate the significance and predictive value of each of the Neonatal Resuscitation Program (NRP)- listed ante- and intrapartum risk factors for the need of neonatal intubation at birth.

Study Design.—In this population-based study, perinatal data of all infants born at ≥35 weeks gestation in the province of Nova Scotia between 1994 and 2014, were identified and reviewed from the Nova Scotia Atlee Database. The frequency of occurrence of risk factors, incidence of neonatal intubation at birth, and its relationship with the different NRP-listed risk factors, were examined. Variables that were significant ($P < .05$) in univariate analyses were entered into the regression model.

Results.—During the 20-year study period, 176 365 infants ≥35 weeks gestation were born. In presence of any of the listed risk factors, 0.3% of infants received intubation at birth compared with 0.08% in absence of any risk factor ($P < .001$). On logistic regression analysis, only 16 of the NRP-listed risk factors had a significant relationship with intubation at birth ($P < .001$). Delivery in a tertiary care center did not have an impact.

Conclusions.—The presence of an intubation-skilled person at birth may not be indicated in all the NRP-listed ante- and intrapartum risk factors. Stratification of the relative significance of different risk factors may be of importance for the less-resourced health care units providing maternal and newborn care.

▶ The article by Almudeer is provocative and filled with facts and figures. I found the tables particularly interesting. Although the need for intubation in the delivery room is rare, it is nonetheless important that arrangements are in place so that someone skilled in airway management with or without intubation is readily available if not already present at the delivery because seconds count. In their experience, fetal hydrops, fetal major anomaly, cord prolapse, prematurity, chorioamnionitis, and use of general anesthesia were the highest predictors for neonatal endotracheal intubation at birth. But altogether, high-risk predictors identified only 50% of infants who needed intubation.

Wozniak et al[1] validated the currently recommended guideline by the Neonatal Resuscitation Program limiting intubation attempts to less than 30 seconds. The recommendation is supported by stable oxygen saturations and heart rate. Prolonging the intubation more than 30 seconds leads to greater hypoxia and may contribute to increased neonatal morbidity, with no effect on ultimate success rate of intubation. To learn intubation skills, the videolaryngoscope (VL) has proven to be of value. The success rate of endotracheal intubation (ETI) on mannequins was improved, and esophageal intubations decreased while learning ETI using the VL compared with the classic laryngoscope (CL). Once ETI is learned on mannequins using the VL, this skill is transferrable to the CL.[2] When evaluated on infants intubated by residents, the success rate of ETI is 75% with VL and 63% with the video-laryngoscope. Time to successful intubation is longer (57 vs 47 seconds), but the difference is not clinically significant.[3]

Nadler et al[4] argued that time without ventilation is a more physiologically important measure of a resuscitation team's intubation expertise than laryngoscope duration. Because successful attempts took longer than failed attempts, this emphasizes that haste during vocal cord visualization and tube insertion may reduce success rates. Reducing the time without ventilation at either end of the procedure may be achievable with better team coordination and could be just as important to patient well-being as technical precision.

Yang et al[5] reported on a randomized controlled trial comparing laryngeal mask with endotracheal intubation. These authors concluded that laryngeal mask ventilation is an effective alternative to endotracheal intubation during resuscitation of depressed newborns who do not respond to face-mask ventilation. During an emergency, laryngeal mask ventilation may be a preferred technique for medical staff who are unable to acquire or maintain endotracheal intubation skills.

Susan Niermeyer has written an excellent editorial to accompany the article by Almudeer.[6] "There is an acute need to focus on mastery of airway management and effective ventilation during training as performance of endotracheal intubation decreases with revised meconium management, increasing use of continuous positive airway pressure in the delivery room, and minimally invasive surfactant administration. As discussed in the accompanying article, several surveys have shown that pediatric trainees frequently do not master the skill of intubation during residency without deliberate focus on this skill." Furthermore, "Team training with a focus on behavioral skills such as communication, leadership, and situational awareness becomes vital to respond successfully to an unexpected, complex resuscitation. Ventilation remains the key to neonatal resuscitation, with or without endotracheal intubation."

Also don't ignore the circulation—it too needs support.

A. A. Fanaroff, MD

References

1. Wozniak M, Arnell K, Brown M, et al. The 30 second rule: the effects of prolonged intubation attempts on oxygen saturation and heart rate in preterm infants in the delivery room. *Minerva Pediatr.* 2016 [Epub ahead of print].

2. Assaad MA, Lachance C, Moussa A. Learning neonatal intubation using the videolaryngoscope: a randomized trial on mannequins. *Simul Healthc.* 2016;11: 190-193.
3. Moussa A, Luangxay Y, Tremblay S, et al. Videolaryngoscope for teaching neonatal endotracheal intubation: a randomized controlled trial. *Pediatrics.* 2016;137: 1-8.
4. Nadler I, McLanders M, Sanderson P, Liley H. Time without ventilation during intubation in neonates as a patient-centred measure of performance. *Resuscitation.* 2016;105:41-44.
5. Yang C, Zhu X, Lin W, et al. Randomized, controlled trial comparing laryngeal mask versus endotracheal intubation during neonatal resuscitation—a secondary publication. *BMC Pediatr.* 2016;16:17.
6. Niermeyer S. Ventilation remains the key to neonatal resuscitation. *J Pediatr.* 2016;171:8-10.

Efficacy and Safety of Umbilical Cord Milking at Birth: A Systematic Review and Meta-analysis

Al-Wassia H, Shah PS (King Abdulaziz Univ, Jeddah, Saudi Arabia; Mt Sinai Hosp, Toronto, Ontario, Canada)
JAMA Pediatr 169:18-25, 2015

Importance.—Umbilical cord milking (UCM) is suggested to improve neonatal outcomes.

Objectives.—To perform a systematic review and meta-analysis of the efficacy and safety of UCM in full-term and preterm neonates.

Data Sources.—A systematic search of MEDLINE, EMBASE, CINAHL, the Cochrane Database of Clinical Trials, the clinicaltrails.gov database, and the reference list of retrieved articles from 1940 to 2014.

Study Selection.—Randomized clinical trials comparing UCM with other strategies of handling the umbilical cord at birth in full-term and preterm infants. Seven of the 18 initially identified studies were selected.

Data Extraction and Synthesis.—Two reviewers independently extracted data and assessed the risk for bias in included trials using the criteria outlined in the *Cochrane Handbook for Systematic Reviews of Interventions.*

Main Outcomes and Measures.—Neonatal mortality before discharge from the hospital.

Results.—We included 7 randomized clinical trials involving 501 infants. Infants with a gestational age of less than 33 weeks allocated to UCM compared with control conditions showed no difference in the risk for mortality (risk ratio [RR], 0.75 [95% CI, 0.35 to 1.64]; risk difference [RD], −0.02 [95% CI, −0.09 to 0.04]), hypotension requiring volume expanders (RR, 0.71 [95% CI, 0.41 to 1.25]; RD, −0.09 [95% CI, −0.22 to 0.05]), or inotrope support (RR, 0.77 [95% CI, 0.51 to 1.17]; RD, −0.10 [95% CI, −0.25 to 0.05]). Higher initial levels of hemoglobin (mean difference, 2.0 [95% CI, 1.3-2.7] g/dL) and hematocrit (mean difference, 4.5% [95% CI, 1.5%-7.4%]) were identified in the UCM groups. We found a reduced risk for oxygen requirement at 36 weeks (RR, 0.42

[95% CI, 0.21 to 0.83]; RD, −0.14 [95% CI, −0.25 to −0.04]) and for intraventricular hemorrhage of all grades (RR, 0.62 [95% CI, 0.41 to 0.93]; RD, −0.12 [95% CI, −0.22 to −0.02]) in infants assigned to UCM. Among infants with a gestational age of at least 33 weeks, UCM was associated with higher hemoglobin levels in the first 48 hours in 224 infants (mean difference, 1.2 [95% CI, 0.8-1.5] g/dL) and at 6 weeks of life in 170 infants (mean difference, 1.1 [95% CI, 0.7-1.5] g/dL).

Conclusions and Relevance.—Umbilical cord milking was associated with some benefits and no adverse effects in the immediate postnatal period in preterm infants (gestational age, <33 weeks); however, further studies are warranted to assess the effect of UCM on neonatal and long-term outcomes.

▶ In December 2012, the American College of Obstetricians and Gynecologists (ACOG), in association with the American Academy of Pediatrics, released a statement titled "Timing of Umbilical Cord Clamping After Birth."[1] This statement concludes for preterm infants that "Evidence exists to support delayed umbilical cord clamping in preterm infants, when feasible. The single most important clinical benefit for preterm infants is the possibility for a nearly 50% reduction in intraventricular hemorrhage."[1] Since then, a number of publications have reported on the outcomes of delayed cord clamping (DCC) in addition to cord milking. None of the trials have had large sample sizes, so that even the meta-analyses include relatively few infants. It has been encouraging to note that there are definite short-term benefits from the extra blood transfused at birth. Reports are now beginning to filter in on the longer term outcomes, and these too have been positive.

In the review by Al-Wassia and Shah, they included 7 randomized clinical trials of umbilical cord milking (UCM) involving 501 infants. There was no difference in the risk for mortality or hypotension requiring volume expanders between UCM and controls. There were higher initial levels of hemoglobin in the UCM group. Of note, there was a reduced risk for oxygen requirement at 36 weeks and for intraventricular hemorrhage of all grades in infants assigned to UCM. This finding has not held up in other trials where overall intraventricular hemorrhage has been reduced, but not grades II and IV.

Chiruvolu[2] did note a significant decrease in intraventricular hemorrhage compared with a historical control group, but their sample size was small and the incidence of IVH was very high in the control group.

Hemoglobin was higher in the umbilical cord milking group at 6 weeks of life. They concluded that UCM was associated with some benefits and no adverse effects in the immediate postnatal period in preterm infants (gestational age, < 33 weeks); however, further studies are warranted to assess the effect of UCM on neonatal and long-term outcomes UCM group.

Additional benefits of delayed cord clamping have been reported with red cell allo-immunization. Garabedian et al[3] studied 72 pregnancies with red cell allo-immunization. Thirty-six had DCC (30 seconds), and 36 did not. The DCC group had higher hemoglobin at birth (13.4 vs 10.2 g/dL), and indeed none of the infants were anemic at birth. This translated into a longer delay between birth and first transfusion, fewer exchange transfusions, and no increase in severe jaundice.

Ruangkit et al[4] noted that protocol-guided practice of DCC for 30 seconds can be safely performed in both multiple and singleton preterm infants. In addition to higher initial hematocrit, infants in their quality improvement project had lower need for delivery room resuscitation and less metabolic acidosis at birth. The infants with DCC needed less surfactant therapy, medical treatment for patent ductus arteriosus, and red blood cell transfusions after DCC protocol implementation.

As more data are made available, the cases for DCC is strengthened. At this point in time, UCM appears to be equivalent to DCC. Long-term follow-up will determine the optimal methodology.

A. A. Fanaroff, MD

References

1. Committee on Obstetric Practice, American College of Obstetricians and Gynecologists. Committee opinion No. 543: timing of umbilical cord clamping after birth. *Obstet Gynecol.* 2012;120:1522-1526.
2. Chiruvolu A, Tolia VN, Qin H, et al. Effect of delayed cord clamping on very preterm infants. *Am J Obstet Gynecol.* 2015;213:676.e1-7.
3. Garabedian C, Rakza T, Drumez E, et al. Benefits of delayed cord clamping in red blood cell alloimmunization. *Pediatrics.* 2016;137:1-6.
4. Ruangkit C, Moroney V, Viswanathan S, Bhola M. Safety and efficacy of delayed umbilical cord clamping in multiple and singleton premature infants—a quality improvement study. *J Neonatal Perinatal Med.* 2015;8:393-402.

Effect of Delayed Cord Clamping on Neurodevelopment at 4 Years of Age: A Randomized Clinical Trial

Andersson O, Lindquist B, Lindgren M, et al (Uppsala Univ, Sweden; Hosp of Halland, Halmstad, Sweden; Lund Univ, Sweden; et al)
JAMA Pediatr 169:631-638, 2015

Importance.—Prevention of iron deficiency in infancy may promote neurodevelopment. Delayed umbilical cord clamping (CC) prevents iron deficiency at 4 to 6 months of age, but long-term effects after 12 months of age have not been reported.

Objective.—To investigate the effects of delayed CC compared with early CC on neurodevelopment at 4 years of age.

Design, Setting, and Participants.—Follow-up of a randomized clinical trial conducted from April 16, 2008, through May 21, 2010, at a Swedish county hospital. Children who were included in the original study (n = 382) as full-term infants born after a low-risk pregnancy were invited to return for follow-up at 4 years of age. Wechsler Preschool and Primary Scale of Intelligence (WPPSI-III) and Movement Assessment Battery for Children (Movement ABC) scores (collected between April 18, 2012, and July 5, 2013) were assessed by a blinded psychologist. Between

April 11, 2012, and August 13, 2013, parents recorded their child's development using the Ages and Stages Questionnaire, Third Edition (ASQ) and behavior using the Strengths and Difficulties Questionnaire. All data were analyzed by intention to treat.

Interventions.—Randomization to delayed CC (≥180 seconds after delivery) or early CC (≤10 seconds after delivery).

Main Outcomes and Measures.—The main outcome was full-scale IQ as assessed by the WPPSI-III. Secondary objectives were development as assessed by the scales from the WPPSI-III and Movement ABC, development as recorded using the ASQ, and behavior using the Strengths and Difficulties Questionnaire.

Results.—We assessed 263 children (68.8%). No differences were found in WPPSI-III scores between groups. Delayed CC improved the adjusted mean differences (AMDs) in the ASQ personal-social (AMD, 2.8; 95% CI, 0.8-4.7) and fine-motor (AMD, 2.1; 95% CI, 0.2-4.0) domains and the Strengths and Difficulties Questionnaire prosocial subscale (AMD, 0.5; 95% CI, >0.0-0.9). Fewer children in the delayed-CC group had results below the cutoff in the ASQ fine-motor domain (11.0% vs 3.7%; *P* = .02) and the Movement ABC bicycle-trail task (12.9% vs 3.8%; *P* = .02). Boys who received delayed CC had significantly higher AMDs in the WPPSI-III processing-speed quotient (AMD, 4.2; 95% CI, 0.8-7.6; *P* = .02), Movement ABC bicycle-trail task (AMD, 0.8; 95% CI, 0.1-1.5; *P* = .03), and fine-motor (AMD, 4.7; 95% CI, 1.0-8.4; *P* = .01) and personal-social (AMD, 4.9; 95% CI, 1.6-8.3; *P* = .004) domains of the ASQ.

Conclusions and Relevance.—Delayed CC compared with early CC improved scores in the fine-motor and social domains at 4 years of age, especially in boys, indicating that optimizing the time to CC may affect neurodevelopment in a low-risk population of children born in a high-income country.

Trial Registration.—clinicaltrials.gov Identifier: NCT01581489.

▶ In his 1773 "Treatise on the Management of Pregnant and Lying-In Women," Charles White wrote, "The common method of tying and cutting the navel string in the instant the child is born, is likewise one of those errors in practice that has nothing to plead in its favor but custom."[1] Although the origins of this custom are lost in time, it remains deeply ingrained in our culture, despite persistent doubts about its wisdom dating at least to the eighteenth century. Recent decades have seen a gradual evolution in practice, and consensus guidelines now support delayed cord clamping, at least in selected circumstances. The Neonatal Resuscitation Program indicates that delayed cord clamping "for longer than 30 seconds is reasonable for both term and preterm infants who do not require resuscitation at birth.... There is insufficient evidence to recommend an approach to cord clamping for infants who require resuscitation at birth,"[2] and National Institute for Health and Care Excellence guidelines advise: "Do not clamp the cord earlier than 1 minute from the birth of the baby unless there is concern about the integrity of the cord or the baby has a heartbeat below 60 beats/minute that is not getting faster."[3] In practice, delayed cord clamping has been more readily embraced for preterm infants, and adoption for term births has come more slowly, largely because of lingering fears about potential adverse effects and uncertainty about benefits. Other recent studies have provided reassurance that delayed clamping is not associated with severe jaundice, polycythemia, or postpartum hemorrhage. This report provides evidence that even term babies stand to benefit from delayed cord clamping in the form of higher scores for parent-reported social behaviors as well as personal-social and fine-motor development at age 4, although overall neurodevelopment was similar. Notably, these results were obtained in low-risk children in a high-income country (Sweden), extending the scope of potential beneficiaries beyond low- and middle-income countries where early childhood iron deficiency may be more prevalent. As such evidence continues to accumulate, the day when the question is reframed as whether there is sufficient evidence to support the safety of continued use of immediate cord clamping may be approaching.

W. E. Benitz, MD

References

1. White C. *Treatise on the Management of Pregnant and Lying-In Women.* London, UK: Edward and Charles Dilly; 1773:107.
2. Wyckoff MH, Aziz K, Escobedo MB, et al. Part 13: neonatal resuscitation: 2015 American Heart Association guidelines update for cardiopulmonary resuscitation and emergency cardiovascular care. *Circulation.* 2015;132:S543-S560.
3. National Institute for Health and Care Excellence (NICE). Intrapartum care for healthy women and babies (Clinical Guideline 190). 2014. https://www.nice.org.uk/guidance/cg190. Accessed August 29, 2016.

Planned Out-of-Hospital Birth and Birth Outcomes

Snowden JM, Tilden EL, Snyder J, et al (Oregon Health and Science Univ, Portland; et al)
N Engl J Med 373:2642-2653, 2015

Background.—The frequency of planned out-of-hospital birth in the United States has increased in recent years. The value of studies assessing the perinatal risks of planned out-of-hospital birth versus hospital birth has been limited by cases in which transfer to a hospital is required and a birth that was initially planned as an out-of-hospital birth is misclassified as a hospital birth.

Methods.—We performed a population-based, retrospective cohort study of all births that occurred in Oregon during 2012 and 2013 using data from newly revised Oregon birth certificates that allowed for the disaggregation of hospital births into the categories of planned in-hospital births and planned out-of-hospital births that took place in the hospital after a woman's intrapartum transfer to the hospital. We assessed perinatal morbidity and mortality, maternal morbidity, and obstetrical procedures according to the planned birth setting (out of hospital vs. hospital).

Results.—Planned out-of-hospital birth was associated with a higher rate of perinatal death than was planned in-hospital birth (3.9 vs. 1.8 deaths per 1000 deliveries, $P = 0.003$; odds ratio after adjustment for maternal characteristics and medical conditions, 2.43; 95% confidence interval [CI], 1.37 to 4.30; adjusted risk difference, 1.52 deaths per 1000 births; 95% CI, 0.51 to 2.54). The odds for neonatal seizure were higher and the odds for admission to a neonatal intensive care unit lower with planned out-of-hospital births than with planned in-hospital birth. Planned out-of-hospital birth was also strongly associated with unassisted vaginal delivery (93.8%, vs. 71.9% with planned in-hospital births; $P < 0.001$) and with decreased odds for obstetrical procedures.

Conclusions.—Perinatal mortality was higher with planned out-of-hospital birth than with planned in-hospital birth, but the absolute risk of death was low in both settings. (Funded by the Eunice Kennedy Shriver National Institute of Child Health and Human Development.)

▶ Planned home births represent only about 1% of total births in the United States, but the practice has generated enormous controversy regarding its risks, benefits, and appropriateness. Various factors have made it difficult to obtain accurate information regarding outcomes for births at home or in birthing centers. One major difficulty has been that the birth certificate does not document the planned, as well as the actual, place of birth. Oregon, the US state with the highest rate of planned home birth (2.4% in 2012), initiated such documentation on its birth certificate form in 2012. The authors of this article used that data to more accurately determine the outcomes of planned out-of-hospital births in Oregon during 2012–2013.

The authors report that for nonanomalous infants, perinatal deaths were increased by about 1.5 per 1000 and neonatal deaths were increased by about 1 per 1000 live births for planned out-of-hospital birth versus planned hospital births, strikingly consistent with previous work. A previous study of more than 1 million US births attended by midwives found that home delivery carried an increased neonatal mortality of between 0.5/1000 to 1.3/1000 births over delivery in hospital.[1] Additionally, a previous meta-analysis including studies from the United States and other countries reported an increase in nonanomalous neonatal deaths of 1.1/1000 for home delivery compared with hospital birth.[2] These data can be presented in very different ways to expectant families: "the overall neonatal death rate almost tripled" may sound very different from "the absolute increase in neonatal death is around 1 in a thousand," or "the absolute rate of perinatal death in both groups was very low." These statements, although similarly accurate, reflect different points of view that may lead to different recommendations to prospective parents.

Many factors in the United States may contribute to the increase in mortality, including long transport distances. However, likely major contributors are the general separation of home birth providers from the hospital-based health care delivery system, and the highly variable certifications and state regulations for home birth attendants. As the authors of this report say, "Studies from Europe have shown that out-of-hospital birth can be a safe option for women and their babies when the risk of complication is low. The European Union defines uniform standards for the education and training of midwives, whereas the United States takes a piecemeal approach to the training and credentialing of out-of-hospital birth attendants."

Women will continue to choose home birth for a variety of reasons, including control, a family-centered experience, decreased maternal intervention, decreased cost, and others. Future improvements in patient care will not be well served by exclusion. "The goal of providing high-quality care to all newborn infants can best be achieved through continuing efforts by all participating health care providers and institutions to develop and sustain communications and understanding on the basis of professional interaction and mutual respect throughout the health care system."[3]

K. Watterberg, MD

References

1. Malloy MH. Infant outcomes of certified nurse midwife attended home births: United States 2000 to 2004. *Perinatol.* 2010;30:622-627.
2. Wax JR, Lucas FL, Lamont M, Pinette MG, Cartin A, Blackstone J. Maternal and newborn outcomes in planned home birth vs planned hospital births: a metaanalysis. *Am J Obstet Gynecol.* 2010;203:243.e1-8.
3. AAP policy statement: planned home birth. *Pediatrics.* 2013;131:1016-1020.

Planned Out-of-Hospital Birth and Birth Outcomes

Snowden JM, Tilden EL, Snyder J, et al (Oregon Health and Science Univ, Portland; et al)

N Engl J Med 373:2642-2653, 2015

Background.—The frequency of planned out-of-hospital birth in the United States has increased in recent years. The value of studies assessing the perinatal risks of planned out-of-hospital birth versus hospital birth has been limited by cases in which transfer to a hospital is required and a birth that was initially planned as an out-of-hospital birth is misclassified as a hospital birth.

Methods.—We performed a population-based, retrospective cohort study of all births that occurred in Oregon during 2012 and 2013 using data from newly revised Oregon birth certificates that allowed for the disaggregation of hospital births into the categories of planned in-hospital births and planned out-of-hospital births that took place in the hospital after a woman's intrapartum transfer to the hospital. We assessed perinatal morbidity and mortality, maternal morbidity, and obstetrical procedures according to the planned birth setting (out of hospital vs. hospital).

Results.—Planned out-of-hospital birth was associated with a higher rate of perinatal death than was planned in-hospital birth (3.9 vs. 1.8 deaths per 1000 deliveries, $P = 0.003$; odds ratio after adjustment for maternal characteristics and medical conditions, 2.43; 95% confidence interval [CI], 1.37 to 4.30; adjusted risk difference, 1.52 deaths per

1000 births; 95% CI, 0.51 to 2.54). The odds for neonatal seizure were higher and the odds for admission to a neonatal intensive care unit lower with planned out-of-hospital births than with planned in-hospital birth. Planned out-of-hospital birth was also strongly associated with unassisted vaginal delivery (93.8%, vs. 71.9% with planned in-hospital births; $P < 0.001$) and with decreased odds for obstetrical procedures.

Conclusions.—Perinatal mortality was higher with planned out-of-hospital birth than with planned in-hospital birth, but the absolute risk of death was low in both settings. (Funded by the Eunice Kennedy Shriver National Institute of Child Health and Human Development.)

▶ Concerns for overmedicalizing the birth process have led to an increasing trend in favor of parents choosing home birth or birth in a birthing center in preference to delivery in a hospital setting. Prior studies have shown home birth to be associated with higher rates of neonatal complications and death. The study team led by Snowden conducted a population-based, retrospective cohort study of all 79 727 singleton, cephalic presenting, nonanomalous births that occurred in Oregon in 2012 and 2013 using birth certificate data, analyzing by the planned birth setting (in-hospital or out-of-hospital). They also were able to ascertain intrapartum transfers to hospital (16.5%) of planned home births. Similar to previously published reports, the authors found increased neonatal mortality and morbidity and lower rates of obstetrical interventions, despite substantially lower rates of any of multiple maternal pregnancy disorders (eg, diabetes, prior hypertension, preeclampsia, prior cesarean delivery) among the planned out-of-hospital group. In addition, perinatal mortality and cardiorespiratory depression (as reflected by very low 5-minute Apgar scores), neonatal seizures, and maternal blood transfusion all were significantly higher among planned out-of-hospital births, results that persisted after multivariate and propensity score adjustment. In multivariable and propensity-score adjusted analyses, the planned out-of-hospital group also had higher rates of fetal death, perinatal death, and neonatal ventilator support. Adverse neonatal outcomes were worse in several subgroups: maternal parity (nulliparous), age (age ≥35 years), and education (>12 years); both low- and high-risk maternal profiles were associated, significantly or trending toward significantly, with increased neonatal risk. Planned out-of-hospital births also were associated with a higher rate of unassisted vaginal delivery and lower rates of instrumented or surgical deliveries and neonatal intensive care unit admissions. The bottom line offered by these investigators is disappointing: "Perinatal mortality was higher with planned out-of-hospital birth than with planned in-hospital birth, but the absolute risk of death was low in both settings." Really?! The absolute mortality risk associated with planned out-of-hospital birth is 3.9 per 1000 live births compared with 1.8 per 1000 live births for in-hospital planned births—more than double the rate. Furthermore, the adjusted odds ratios (aORs) reflect more than double the risks for fetal death (aOR: 2.3) and perinatal death (aOR: 2.4) and a more than 50% greater risk for infant death (aOR: 1.6) associated with planned home birth—all this without even beginning to assess the long-term implications of the perinatal cardiorespiratory depression and neonatal seizures. Although I have a strong commitment to making the birth process as natural and family-friendly as safely possible and fully appreciate the potential complications of obstetrical interventions, I reject what seems to be a casual brush off of these findings, representing out-of-hospital planned birth as just another low-level risk. Should out-of-hospital birth reach population-wide prevalence, it might fail to reach the level of public health crisis; still, I would argue that it would likely have a detectable adverse effect on the health profile of a generation of children. Furthermore, it's at least worth considering the ethics of subjecting children to nontrivial cumulative risk that is well detailed by these analyses, based mainly on parental preference regarding the birthing experience. These study results highlight the merits of expansion to include long-term investigation of competing maternal and fetal/neonatal/infant outcomes. In the meantime, let's stop pretending that the choice to deliver at home confers just a slightly increased risk to the fetus and newborn and redouble our efforts to work with parents to improve the experience of the safer option—in-hospital birth—for babies and families. For discussion of a number of perspectives, the accompanying article[1] is worth a read, as is Jennifer Holloman's account of her personal experience with a complicated home birth and how it reshaped her thinking (*Boston Globe Magazine*, July 10, 2011).

L. J. Van Marter, MD, MPH

Reference

1. Wilbur MA, Little S, Szymanski LM. Is home birth safe? *N Engl J Med.* 2015;373: 2683-2685.

The impact of ambient operating room temperature on neonatal and maternal hypothermia and associated morbidities: a randomized controlled trial

Duryea EL, Nelson DB, Wyckoff MH, et al (Univ of Texas Southwestern Medical Center, Dallas)

Am J Obstet Gynecol 214:505.e1-7, 2016

Background.—Neonatal hypothermia is common at the time of cesarean delivery and has been associated with a constellation of morbidities in addition to increased neonatal mortality. Additionally, maternal hypothermia is often uncomfortable for the surgical patient and has been associated with intraoperative and postoperative complications. Various methods to decrease the rates of neonatal and maternal hypothermia have been examined and found to have varying levels of success.

Objective.—We sought to determine whether an increase in operating room temperature at cesarean delivery results in a decrease in the rate of neonatal hypothermia and associated morbidities.

Study Design.—In this single-center randomized trial, operating room temperatures were adjusted weekly according to a cluster randomization schedule to either 20°C (67°F), which was the standard at our institution, or 23°C (73°F), which was the maximum temperature allowable per hospital policy. Neonatal hypothermia was defined as core body temperature <36.5°C (97.7°F) per World Health Organization criteria. The primary study outcome was neonatal hypothermia on arrival to the admitting nursery. Measures of neonatal morbidity potentially associated with hypothermia were examined.

Results.—From February through July 2015, 791 women who underwent cesarean deliveries were enrolled, resulting in 410 infants in the 20°C standard management group and 399 in the 23°C study group. The rate of neonatal hypothermia on arrival to the admitting nursery was lower in the study group as compared to the standard management group: 35% vs 50%, $P < .001$. Moderate to severe hypothermia was infrequent when the operating room temperature was 23°C (5%); in contrast such hypothermia occurred in 19% of the standard management group, $P < .001$. Additionally, neonatal temperature in the operating room immediately following delivery and stabilization was also higher in the study group, 37.1 ± 0.6°C vs 36.9 ± 0.6°C, $P < .001$. We found no difference in rates of intubation, ventilator use, hypoglycemia, metabolic acidemia, or intraventricular hemorrhage. Fever (temperature >38.0°C or 100.4°F) on arrival to the admitting unit was uncommon and did not differ between the study groups. Maternal temperature on arrival to the operating room was not different between the 2 groups, however by delivery it was significantly lower in the standard management group, 36.2 ± 0.6°C vs 36.4 ± 0.6°C, $P < .001$. This effect persisted, as maternal temperature on arrival to the postoperative care area was lower in the standard management group, 36.1 ± 0.6°C vs 36.2 ± 0.6°C, $P < .001$, and the rate of hypothermia was higher, 77% vs 69%, $P = .008$.

Conclusion.—A modest increase in operating room temperature at the time of cesarean reduces the rate of neonatal and maternal hypothermia. We did not detect a decrease in neonatal morbidity, but the power to detect a small change in these outcomes was limited.

▶ I often admire studies that put the science behind common sense. Like most neonatologists, I am nearly always amazed at how cold it is in the delivery or operating room and how much effort has to be expended to dry and warm a newborn. "Why don't they just turn up the temperature a little?" has been a nearly 40-year lament. In this single-center, randomized trial, using cluster randomization, Duryea et al showed just that. Increasing the operating room temperature from 20 to 23°C brought about a significant reduction in both maternal and neonatal temperature, the latter upon admission to the admitting nursery. Although the study was underpowered to address specific morbidities associated with hypothermia, at the very least, it enabled more time to be spent on other aspects of transition and resuscitation. For those of you who have had difficulty convincing your obstetrical colleagues to increase the temperature of the operating room, here's the "I told you so" data you need.

S. M. Donn, MD

An economic analysis of immediate delivery and expectant monitoring in women with hypertensive disorders of pregnancy, between 34 and 37 weeks of gestation (HYPITAT-II)

van Baaren G-J, for the HYPITAT-II Study Group (Univ of Amsterdam, the Netherlands; et al)

BJOG 2016 [Epub ahead of print]

Objective.—To assess the economic consequences of immediate delivery compared with expectant monitoring in women with preterm non-severe hypertensive disorders of pregnancy.

Design.—A cost-effectiveness analysis alongside a randomised controlled trial (HYPITAT-II).

Setting.—Obstetric departments of seven academic hospitals and 44 non-academic hospitals in the Netherlands.

Population.—Women diagnosed with non-severe hypertensive disorders of pregnancy between $34^{0/7}$ and $37^{0/7}$ weeks of gestation, randomly allocated to either immediate delivery or expectant monitoring.

Methods.—A trial-based cost-effectiveness analysis was performed from a healthcare perspective until final maternal and neonatal discharge.

Main Outcome Measures.—Health outcomes were expressed as the prevalence of respiratory distress syndrome, defined as the need for supplemental oxygen for >24 hours combined with radiographic findings typical for respiratory distress syndrome. Costs were estimated from a healthcare perspective until maternal and neonatal discharge.

Results.—The average costs of immediate delivery (n = 352) were 10 245 versus 9563 for expectant monitoring (n = 351), with an average difference of 682 (95% confidence interval, 95% CI −618 to 2126). This 7% difference predominantly originated from the neonatal admissions, which were 5672 in the immediate delivery arm and 3929 in the expectant monitoring arm.

Conclusion.—In women with mild hypertensive disorders between $34^{0/7}$ and $37^{0/7}$ weeks of gestation, immediate delivery is more costly than expectant monitoring as a result of differences in neonatal admissions. These findings support expectant monitoring, as the clinical outcomes of the trial demonstrated that expectant monitoring reduced respiratory distress syndrome for a slightly increased risk of maternal complications.

Tweetable Abstract.—Expectant management in preterm hypertensive disorders is less costly compared with immediate delivery.

▶ This study is a secondary analysis of HYPITAT-II, an open-label, controlled trial in which women with nonsevere hypertensive disorders of pregnancy who were between 34 and 37 weeks of gestation were randomly allocated to either induction of labor or cesarean delivery within 24 hours (immediate delivery) or a strategy aimed at prolonging pregnancy until 37 weeks of gestation (expectant monitoring).[1] The primary outcomes of the main trial were a composite of adverse maternal outcome (thromboembolic disease, pulmonary edema, eclampsia, HELLP syndrome, placental abruption, or maternal death) and respiratory distress syndrome (RDS). Immediate delivery significantly increased the risk of neonatal RDS (24 hours of supplemental oxygen + radiographic findings) with a limited reduction of adverse maternal outcomes.[1]

In this article, the investigators report the results of a cost-effectiveness analysis that was performed alongside the HYPITAT-II trial. Overall costs for the expectant monitoring group were lower than those for the immediate delivery group. The higher cost for the immediate delivery group predominately originated in the postpartum period, because of more and longer neonatal stays. Review of the original publication indicated that the median time between randomization and delivery was 5 days longer in the expectant management group and the rate of RDS was 1.7% compared with 5.7% in the immediate delivery cohort, suggesting that the cost benefit of expectant management is due to the delivery of more mature infants.

L. A. Papile, MD

Reference

1. Broekhuijsen K, van Baaren G-J, van Pampus MG, Ganzevoort W, et al. Immediate delivery versus expectant monitoring for hypertensive disorders of pregnancy between 34 and 37 weeks of gestation (HYPITAT-II): an open-label, randomised controlled trial. *Lancet.* 2015;385:2492-2501.

Survival Among Infants Born at 22 or 23 Weeks' Gestation Following Active Prenatal and Postnatal Care

Mehler K, Oberthuer A, Keller T, et al (Univ of Cologne, Germany; et al)
JAMA Pediatr 170:671-677, 2016

Importance.—Rates of survival for infants born at the border of viability are still low and vary considerably among neonatal intensive care units.

Objective.—To determine whether higher survival rates and better short-term outcomes for infants born at 22 or 23 weeks' gestation may be achieved by active prenatal and postnatal care.

Design, Setting, and Participants.—Retrospective study of 106 infants born at 22 or 23 weeks of gestation at a level III neonatal intensive care unit at the University of Cologne Medical Centre in Cologne, Germany, between January 1, 2010, and December 31, 2014. Data analysis was performed in June 2015.

Exposures.—Active prenatal and postnatal care.

Main Outcomes and Measures.—Survival until hospital discharge and survival without neonatal or short-term severe complications (defined as high-grade intraventricular hemorrhage, surgery for abdominal complications, bronchopulmonary dysplasia, or retinopathy of prematurity).

Results.—Of 106 liveborn infants (45 born at 22 weeks and 61 born at 23 weeks and 6 days), 20 (19%) received palliative care (17 born at 22 weeks and 3 born at 23 weeks), and 86 (81%) received active care (28 born at 22 weeks and 58 born at 23 weeks). Of the 86 infants who received active care (mean [SD] maternal age, 32 [6] years), 58 (67%) survived until hospital discharge (17 born at 22 weeks and 41 born at 23 weeks). Eighty-five infants survived without severe complications, with 1 infant born at 22 weeks excluded because of missing data (6 of 27 [22%] born at 22 weeks, and 16 of 58 [28%] born at 23 weeks). Survival was predicted by the Apgar score after 5 minutes (odds ratio, 0.62 [95% CI, 0.46-0.84]) and birth weight (odds ratio, 0.001 [95% CI, 0.00-0.40]).

Conclusions and Relevance.—One in 4 infants born at the border of viability and offered active care survived without severe complications. This finding should be considered for individualized parental approaches and decision making. Active follow-up information is required to determine childhood outcomes.

▶ The key components of "active prenatal and postnatal care"' referred to in the article are (1) antenatal steroid use after parental counseling after 22 weeks of gestation, (2) operative delivery with local anesthesia as the preferred method of delivery, (3) delayed cord clamping, (4) comfort positioning (lateral) of the infant, (5) establishment of spontaneous breathing via a stepwise increase in positive end-expiratory pressure, and (6) less-invasive surfactant application via the use of a thin endotracheal catheter during continuous positive airway pressure—assisted spontaneous breathing. As the authors acknowledge in the discussion, many aspects of their active care approach lack evidence and need to be tested in studies. Nonetheless, they cite their data as adding substance to the assumption that an active prenatal and postnatal approach might improve outcome of extremely premature infants. However, survival per se is only one aspect of outcome; another is survival without neurodevelopmental impairment. The scant follow-up data presented in the article pertain to cognitive outcomes only and are complete for less than half of the survivors. Of the 32 infants who were evaluated, 50% have a developmental delay, which was severe in 28%.

L. A. Papile, MD

5 Infectious Disease and Immunology

Evaluation and Management of Women and Newborns With a Maternal Diagnosis of Chorioamnionitis: Summary of a Workshop

Higgins RD, for the Chorioamnionitis Workshop Participants (Natl Inst of Child Health and Human Development, Bethesda, MD; et al)

Obstet Gynecol 127:426-436, 2016

In January 2015, the *Eunice Kennedy Shriver* National Institute of Child Health and Human Development invited an expert panel to a workshop to address numerous knowledge gaps and to provide evidence-based guidelines for the diagnosis and management of pregnant women with what had been commonly called chorioamnionitis and the neonates born to these women. The panel noted that the term chorioamnionitis has been used to label a heterogeneous array of conditions characterized by infection and inflammation or both with a consequent great variation in clinical practice for mothers and their newborns. Therefore, the panel proposed to replace the term chorioamnionitis with a more general, descriptive term: "intrauterine inflammation or infection or both," abbreviated as "Triple I." The panel proposed a classification for Triple I and recommended approaches to evaluation and management of pregnant women and their newborns with a diagnosis of Triple I. It is particularly important to recognize that an isolated maternal fever is not synonymous with chorioamnionitis. A research agenda was proposed to further refine the definition and management of this complex group of conditions. This article provides a summary of the workshop presentations and discussions.

▶ Over the past 20+ years, those involved in obstetrical research have come to appreciate that many of the pregnancy complications that lead to spontaneous preterm birth (eg, preterm labor, preterm premature rupture of membranes), although separate in their clinical presentation, have their common pathophysiologic origins as inflammatory processes within the uterus. At the same time, the term "chorioamnionitis" has become generalized to the point of losing its clinical utility. Higgins et al present the results of an expert panel workshop convened by the National Institutes of Health in 2015. The panel recommended the replacement of the term chorioamnionitis in clinical parlance with what they believed would be the more descriptive term, "intrauterine inflammation or infection or both." They intended this to be more generally abbreviated as

"Triple I." The panel proposes that this condition is to be diagnosed when maternal fever is present with at least 1 of the following: fetal tachycardia, a maternal white blood cell count >15 000 absent the use of corticosteroids, purulent material leaking across the cervix on speculum exam, and objective laboratory evidence of infection in a sample of amniotic fluid (which would require an amniocentesis). The panel hopes to make the diagnoses more objective and less subject to clinical perception. This is a valid motivation, and the field will not advance if we are not occasionally required to relinquish the comfort of past terminology and the familiarity of the modes of thought that they represent. However, perhaps because of the relative novelty of the effort or perhaps because of the slightly cumbersome nature of the term, I have as of yet to see it yet gain traction in standard clinical vocabulary.

T. F. McElrath, MD, PhD

Low Rate of Perinatal Sepsis in Term Infants of Mothers with Chorioamnionitis

Braun D, Bromberger P, Ho NJ, et al (Kaiser Permanente Southern California, Panorama City, CA; Kaiser Permanente Southern California, San Diego, CA; Kaiser Permanente Southern California, Pasadena, CA)

Am J Perinatol 33:143-150, 2016

Objective.—The risk of infection in infants of mothers with chorioamnionitis (CAM) may be lower than previously reported. This study's objective was to determine the incidence of intrapartum fever (IPF) and culture-positive early-onset bacterial neonatal infection (CPEOI) in the late preterm and term infants of mothers with or without CAM and to assess interhospital variation in neonatal infection management.

Study Design.—This retrospective cohort study included mothers and newborns delivered at ≥35 weeks gestation at Kaiser Permanente Southern California Hospitals in 2010 ($n = 31,112$). Electronic medical and laboratory records from 13 medical centers were examined for maternal temperature, intrapartum, and neonatal antibiotic treatment. Rates for IPF, CAM, and CPEOI were estimated. Rates for starting neonatal antibiotics were calculated.

Results.—The incidence of IPF was 9% and CAM 4%. The overall rate for CPEOI was 0.61/ 1,000 (95% confidence interval [CI] 0.34, 0.89/ 1,000). The rate of CPEOI was 4.0/1,000 (95% CI 0.50, 7.5/1,000) in infants born to mothers with CAM. The rate of beginning antibiotics for infants born to mothers with CAM ranged from 7 to 76% between nurseries.

Conclusion.—The rate of CPEOI in infants born to mothers with CAM is lower than previously reported. There is heterogeneity in initiation of neonatal antibiotics by neonatologists.

► The 1996 Centers for Disease Control and Prevention recommendations for prevention of perinatal group B streptococcal disease[1] did not mention chorioamnionitis (CAM) as a factor to consider in deciding about empiric antimicrobial treatment for infants at risk. Based on new information that had become available in the interim, the 2002 revision[2] singled out CAM as a risk factor that requires a full diagnostic evaluation and empiric antibiotic therapy. That additional information likely included data summarized in a review, of which I was the primary author,[3] in which we noted that nearly 90% of the reported cases in which early-onset neonatal sepsis developed despite intrapartum prophylaxis were associated with maternal CAM. Information that has become available since that review indicates that the conclusion that CAM is a marker of high risk for sepsis was wrong, on at least 2 counts. First, the high conditional probability of prior exposure to maternal CAM among neonates who became infected despite maternal treatment for CAM does not imply the converse, which is a high probability of neonatal sepsis among infants born to women with CAM. Second, the limited data available before 1999 that addressed the latter relationship did not stratify subjects by gestational age, and that has turned out to be quite important.

In this report from the Southern California Kaiser Permanente system, outcomes are reported for the largest cohort of CAM-exposed late-preterm and term neonates (estimated gestational age ≥35 weeks) reported to date. Infants were classified as having been exposed to CAM if the diagnosis appeared in the medical record, reflecting the actual practice of obstetricians, who we depend on to provide that information, and were distinguished from those born to women with intrapartum fever without other signs of CAM. Of 1243 mothers with CAM, 5 had babies with culture-positive early-onset sepsis (all despite intrapartum antibiotic treatment), so the attack rate was only 4 per 1000 births (exact binomial confidence interval 1.3 to 9.4 per 1000), and the number needed to treat to anticipate 1 case of sepsis would be 250. These data support elimination of CAM as a major risk identifier for neonatal sepsis, with 2 important caveats: this only applies to infants ≥35 weeks' gestation, not to less mature infants, and it assumes that mothers with CAM continue to receive intrapartum antibiotic treatment, as was the case for 99% of the affected women in this cohort.

W. E. Benitz, MD

References

1. Prevention of perinatal group B streptococcal disease: a public health perspective. Centers for Disease Control and Prevention. *MMWR Recomm Rep*. 1996;45: 1-24.
2. Schrag S, Gorwitz R, Fultz-Butts K, et al. Prevention of perinatal group B streptococcal disease. Revised guidelines from CDC. *MMWR Recomm Rep*. 2002;51: 1-22.
3. Benitz WE, Gould JB, Druzin ML. Risk factors for early-onset group B streptococcal sepsis: estimation of odds ratios by critical literature review. *Pediatrics*. 1999; 103:e77.

Reconsidering the Current Preterm Premature Rupture of Membranes Antibiotic Prophylactic Protocol

Wolf MF, Miron D, Peleg D, et al (Bar-Ilan Univ, Zefat, Israel; et al)

Am J Perinatol 32:1247-1250, 2015

Objective.—The purpose of our study was to determine whether the current antibiotic regimen for preterm premature rupture of membranes (PPROM) is adequate for covering the current causative agents and sensitivities of chorioamnionitis and early-onset neonatal sepsis.

Study Design.—During a 3-year period, we retrieved the results from placental and amniotic membrane cultures obtained at delivery in cases of maternal fever, chorioamnionitis, and PPROM, and from blood cultures obtained from neonates with early-onset sepsis (EOS) in three participating hospitals. Sensitivity of pathogens to antimicrobial agents was performed using routine microbiologic techniques.

Results.—There were 1,133 positive placental or amniotic cultures, 740 (65.3%) were from gram-negative Enterobacteriaceae. There were 27 neonates diagnosed with EOS with positive blood cultures. Aerobic Enterobacteriaceae accounted for 14 cases (52%) and group B streptococcus for 7 cases (26%). Of the *Escherichia coli* and *Klebsiella* sp., only 38% were sensitive to ampicillin.

Conclusion.—Local pathogens and their antibiotic sensitivity profiles should be explored every few years and an effective antibiotic protocol chosen to cover the main pathogens causing chorioamnionitis and EOS. Consideration should be made for changing ampicillin in women with PPROM to a regimen with better coverage of gram-negative Enterobacteriaceae (Fig 2).

▶ This report of microbial surveillance data from 3 hospitals in Israel from 2011 through 2013 provides a reminder that antepartum or intrapartum antimicrobial prophylaxis may not come without a cost. Taking note of an increase in the number of cases of neonatal sepsis caused by *Enterobacteriaceae* over the interval reviewed, from no cases in 2011 to 4 in 2012 and 10 in 2012, these authors hypothesize that this might have resulted from increasing resistance of local *Escherichia coli* strains to the antibiotics used to prevent neonatal infection in the setting of premature preterm rupture of membranes (PPROM). Review of the antibiotic susceptibilities of *Enterobacteriaceae* isolates from cultures of placenta and amniotic membrane swabs of women deemed at risk for having an infected baby demonstrated that the 62% of the *E coli* isolates and more than 95% of the *Klebsiella* isolates were, in fact, resistant to ampicillin (see Fig 2). The authors conclude that providers need to be aware of evolving patterns of antimicrobial resistance among *Enterobacteriaceae* strains in their communities.

There may be another lesson embedded in this data as well. Sepsis was disproportionately prevalent among preterm infants, accounting for 15 of the 27 cases. Among those 15 preterm infants, *Enterobacteriaceae* caused the sepsis in 12. Only 2 *Enterobacteriaceae* cases occurred in term infants. Six of the preterm infants with sepsis were born to women with preterm premature rupture of

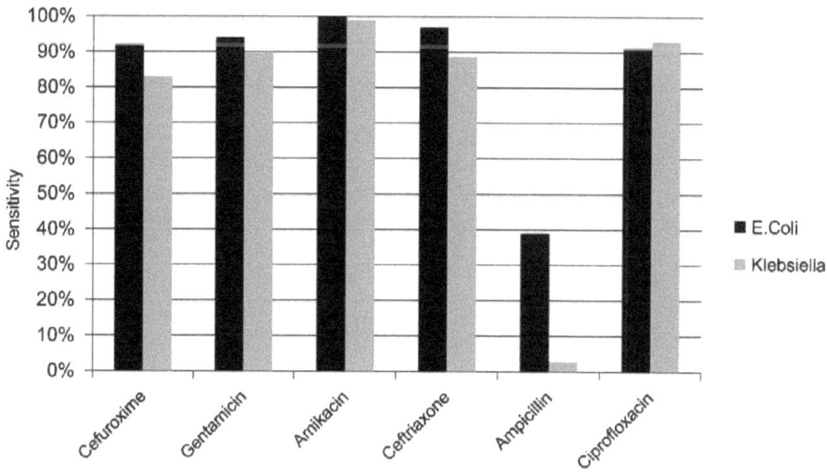

FIGURE 2.—Antibiotic sensitivity profile of *Escherichia coli* and *Klebsiella*. (Reprinted from Wolf MF, Miron D, Peleg D, et al. Reconsidering the current preterm premature rupture of membranes antibiotic prophylactic protocol. *Am J Perinatol*. 2015;32:1247-1250, with permission from Thieme Medical Publishers, Inc.)

membranes (PPROM) and were exposed to antepartum antibiotic prophylaxis for a mean of 6.6 days. Of the 6 neonatal deaths caused by sepsis in this series, 5 were caused by *Enterobacteriaceae* infections in preterm infants. Unfortunately, neither the species and sensitivities of the *Enterobacteriaceae* isolates from neonatal blood cultures nor the identity and sensitivities of the organisms responsible for sepsis after treatment for PPROM were reported. The case could be stronger if those details were available, but these data remind us of the necessity for vigilance for neonatal infection caused by ampicillin-resistant Gram-negative bacilli, particularly in sick preterm infants who have had prolonged antepartum antibiotic exposures. In such infants, initial empiric antibiotic treatment with a third-generation cephalosporin may be preferable to use of ampicillin, at least until culture and sensitivity testing results are available.

W. E. Benitz, MD

Risk of Early-Onset Sepsis following Preterm, Prolonged Rupture of Membranes with or without Chorioamnionitis

Ofman G, Vasco N, Cantey JB (Children's Med Ctr Dallas, TX; Univ of Texas Southwestern Med Ctr, Dallas)

Am J Perinatol 33:339-342, 2016

Objective.—This study aims to determine whether preterm prolonged rupture of membranes (PPROM) increases the risk for early-onset sepsis (EOS) in preterm infants.

Study Design.—Retrospective cohort study of infants 30 to 34 weeks' gestation from 2005 to 2014. Exposure to PPROM (rupture of membranes

≥ 18 hours) or chorioamnionitis (maternal temperature ≥ 38°C during delivery plus notation of chorioamnionitis in the medical record) was collected. The primary outcome was proven or suspected EOS.

Results.—A total of 2,192 infants were included. Overall, 1,750 (80%) were not exposed to PPROM or chorioamnionitis (group 1), 381 (17%) were exposed to PPROM without chorioamnionitis (group 2), and 61 (3%) were exposed to chorioamnionitis ± PPROM (group 3). There was no difference in the incidence of proven or suspected EOS between groups 1 and 2 (5.4 vs. 5.5%, $p = 0.86$). Group 3 had a higher rate of EOS (24.6%) relative to groups 1 and 2 ($p < 0.001$). In multivariate analysis, risk of EOS was 4.1 times higher in infants exposed to chorioamnionitis. PPROM did not increase the risk of EOS in bivariate or multivariate analysis.

Conclusion.—In the absence of chorioamnionitis, PPROM does not increase the risk of proven or clinically suspected EOS in 30 to 34 weeks' gestation infants.

▶ Strategies for prevention of early-onset neonatal sepsis (EOS), particularly cases caused by group B Streptococcus (GBS), have been successful but have also resulted in exposure of a large proportion of parturients and neonates to antibiotic prophylaxis, and many infants also receive postpartum prophylaxis or empiric treatment. Antibiotic stewardship, recognition of adverse effects of antibiotic courses such as increased rates of necrotizing enterocolitis, and the desire to reduce mother-baby separation have drawn attention to opportunities for more selective antibiotic use in the peripartum period. Risk factors identified by epidemiologic studies before 1995 often have been treated as independent factors that compound one another, but more recent data indicate that they are often interrelated and mutually confounded predictors of risk. For example, the remarkable risk associated with GBS bacteriuria during pregnancy may be mediated by the high rate of preterm premature (before onset of labor) rupture of membranes in the reported cases. Similarly, the risk associated with chorioamnionitis reflects the strong relationship between chorioamnionitis and prematurity and the much greater risk of sepsis in preterm infants; chorioamnionitis is not a strong predictor for EOS in late-preterm and term infants. The latter observation provides empirical support for abandonment of empiric antibiotic therapy in well-appearing late-preterm and term infants born to women with clinical signs of chorioamnionitis.

This report provides important data supporting more selective use of empiric antibiotic therapy in moderately preterm infants (30 to 34 weeks' gestation). Unlike reports from the era before adoption of intrapartum prophylaxis for women with prolonged rupture of membranes, these authors did not identify rupture of membranes for ≥18 hours as a risk factor for neonatal sepsis (odds ratio [OR] 1.22; 95% confidence interval [CI] 0.68-2.15), suggesting that the intrapartum intervention largely obviates that risk. These data confirm the strong relationship between chorioamnionitis and EOS (OR 6.30; 95% CI 3.09-10.2) in preterm infants, despite a policy of intrapartum treatment for women with chorioamnionitis. As the authors suggest, it may, therefore, be appropriate to withhold empiric treatment of asymptomatic moderately preterm infants for whom the sole risk factor is prolonged rupture of membranes, provided that intrapartum prophylaxis is sufficient, while continuing that practice for preterm infants whose mothers have chorioamnionitis.

There are 2 important precautions in extrapolation of these data to other settings. First, at-risk infants at that center receive a single dose of penicillin for GBS prophylaxis if not selected for empiric ongoing treatment (and presumably diagnostic evaluation). The proportion of infants for whom cultures were obtained is not reported. The impact of that postpartum prophylaxis is, therefore, difficult to assess, but prior reports suggest that it may prevent 75% of the residual cases not prevented by intrapartum prophylaxis alone. Second, the observed dissociation of risk from preterm prolonged rupture of membranes (PPROM) in the absence of chorioamnionitis must not be confused with the increased risk previously associated with preterm (gestational age < 37 weeks) premature (prior to the onset of labor) rupture of membranes (also commonly abbreviated as PPROM). Although that association might also be mediated by development of chorioamnionitis, that hypothesis is not tested in this report. The latter variety of PPROM continues to merit respect with empiric treatment of babies with that risk factor.

W. E. Benitz, MD

Maternal Immunization With an Investigational Trivalent Group B Streptococcal Vaccine: A Randomized Controlled Trial

Donders GGG, Halperin SA, Devlieger R, et al (Univ Hosps KULeuven, Belgium; IWK Health Centre and Dalhousie Univ, Halifax, Nova Scotia, Canada; GlaxoSmithKline LLC, Cambridge, MA; et al)

Obstet Gynecol 127:213-221, 2016

Objective.—To evaluate the safety and immunogenicity of an investigational trivalent group B streptococcal vaccine in pregnant women and antibody transfer to their newborns.

Methods.—The primary outcome of this observer-blind, randomized study was to estimate placental antibody transfer rates at birth. Secondary outcomes included measurement of serotype-specific antibodies at screening, 30 days postvaccination, at delivery, and 91 days postpartum, infant antibody levels at 3 months of age, the potential effect on routine infant diphtheria vaccination at 1 month after the third infant series dose, and safety in mother and infant participants through at least 5 months postpartum. Sample size was based on 60 participants in the vaccine group giving a probability of observing at least one adverse event of 90% if the actual rate of the event was 3.8%.

Results.—From September 2011 to October 2013, 86 pregnant women were allocated in a 3:2 ratio to receive an investigational group B streptococcal vaccine containing glycoconjugates of serotypes Ia, Ib, and III or placebo. Demographics were similar across groups. Transfer ratios were 66–79% and maternal geometric mean concentrations increased 16-,

23-, and 20-fold by delivery against serotypes Ia, Ib, and III, respectively, Women with no detectable antibodies at inclusion had lower responses than those with detectable antibodies. Three months after birth, infant antibody concentrations were 22–25% of birth levels. Antidiphtheria geometric mean concentrations were similar across groups. In the vaccine and placebo groups, 32 of 51 women (63%) and 26 of 35 women (74%) reported adverse effects, respectively.

Conclusion.—The investigational vaccine was well-tolerated without safety signals in recipients and their infants or interference with routine infant diphtheria vaccination, although further studies on safety and effectiveness are needed. The investigational vaccine was immunogenic for all serotypes, particularly among women with detectable antibody levels at baseline. Antibody transfer to neonates was at similar levels to other maternally administered polysaccharide vaccines.

Clinical Trial Registration.—ClinicalTrials.gov, www.clinicaltrials.gov, NCT01446289.

▶ Reduction of the rate of early-onset neonatal group B streptococcal (GBS) sepsis by nearly an order of magnitude, through use of prenatal screening for colonization and intrapartum antibiotic prophylaxis, ranks among the great public health achievements of the late 20th century. Although unquestionably effective, this strategy is logistically difficult, exposes many new mothers and babies to antibiotics for each case prevented, creates selection pressure antimicrobial resistance, and does little to reduce the rate of late-onset GBS disease. Epidemiological studies done about 40 years ago demonstrated that lack of passively acquired opsonizing antibodies specific for the infecting GBS serotype, prematurity, and maternal vaginal colonization with GBS are major risk factors for development of invasive neonatal disease. Intrapartum risk factors (fever, prolonged rupture of membranes) were associated with early- but not late-onset disease, and maternal colonization was much less closely associated with late-onset disease. Prevention strategies have focused on interrupting vertical transmission through elimination of maternal colonization at delivery. Strategies to reduce neonatal susceptibility through maternal immunization have been much slower in coming to fruition.

As the first phase 2 trial of a GBS vaccine, this work marks a major step forward in pursuit of this second arm of GBS prevention strategies. Prior trials have demonstrated increased specific antibody concentrations in nonpregnant women. This trial extends those observations to pregnant women and addresses 2 additional key questions: are the induced antibodies passively acquired by the fetus, and are antibody responses in nonimmune women sufficient to provide protective immunity? The former is important because elicitation of antibody subclasses that do not cross the placenta will not protect the fetus. The data on placental transfer presented here suggest that may not be an issue. The latter is critical because heavily colonized women who lack specific antibodies—exactly those at greatest risk of having an infected baby—apparently do not lack antibodies as a result of absence of exposure to the organism. As noted in the abstract, subjects who had no detectable antibodies had smaller responses than those who already had detectable antibodies at immunization. At first, this seems to support concern that women whose babies develop invasive GBS disease may have an immunogenetic inability to mount appropriate protective antibody responses to 1 or more GBS serotypes; in such women, immunization is not likely to be a protective strategy. However, the levels of antibodies achieved after immunization in those women closely mirrored that in placebo recipients who had detectable antibody levels at baseline. Although the antibody concentration necessary to protect babies from GBS sepsis is unknown, that similarity provides a basis for hope that even the more modest responses achieved in the previously nonimmune (antibody concentration < lower limit of quantification) women may be sufficient. The proportion of women who did not have detectable antibody for each serotype was remarkably high (76%, 56%, and 64% for serotypes Ia, Ib, and III, respectively), so it remains possible that a few women who had no detectable response to this single dose of vaccine may represent the core of vulnerable mother-infant dyads. It will be of great interest to learn more about the ability of those women to respond to repeated immunization. The authors should be commended for the circumspection reflected in cautioning against generalization of observations in the population at large to the subgroup of concern in their final comment: "Further research is needed to address the needs of women with undetectable antibody concentrations before vaccination."

W. E. Benitz, MD

Maternal Immunization With an Investigational Trivalent Group B Streptococcal Vaccine: A Randomized Controlled Trial

Donders GGG, Halperin SA, Devlieger R, et al (Univ Hosps KULeuven, Belgium; IWK Health Centre and Dalhousie Univ, Halifax, Nova Scotia, Canada; GlaxoSmithKline LLC, Cambridge, MA; et al)
Obstet Gynecol 127:213-221, 2016

Objective.—To evaluate the safety and immunogenicity of an investigational trivalent group B streptococcal vaccine in pregnant women and antibody transfer to their newborns.

Methods.—The primary outcome of this observer-blind, randomized study was to estimate placental antibody transfer rates at birth. Secondary outcomes included measurement of serotype-specific antibodies at screening, 30 days postvaccination, at delivery, and 91 days postpartum, infant antibody levels at 3 months of age, the potential effect on routine infant diphtheria vaccination at 1 month after the third infant series dose, and safety in mother and infant participants through at least 5 months postpartum. Sample size was based on 60 participants in the vaccine group giving a probability of observing at least one adverse event of 90% if the actual rate of the event was 3.8%.

Results.—From September 2011 to October 2013, 86 pregnant women were allocated in a 3:2 ratio to receive an investigational group B streptococcal vaccine containing glycoconjugates of serotypes Ia, Ib, and III or placebo. Demographics were similar across groups. Transfer ratios were 66–79% and maternal geometric mean concentrations increased 16-, 23-, and 20-fold by delivery against serotypes Ia, Ib, and III, respectively, Women with no detectable antibodies at inclusion had lower responses than those with detectable antibodies. Three months after birth, infant antibody concentrations were 22–25% of birth levels. Anti-diphtheria geometric mean concentrations were similar across groups. In the vaccine and placebo groups, 32 of 51 women (63%) and 26 of 35 women (74%) reported adverse effects, respectively.

Conclusion.—The investigational vaccine was well-tolerated without safety signals in recipients and their infants or interference with routine infant diphtheria vaccination, although further studies on safety and effectiveness are needed. The investigational vaccine was immunogenic for all serotypes, particularly among women with detectable antibody levels at baseline. Antibody transfer to neonates was at similar levels to other maternally administered polysaccharide vaccines.

Clinical Trial Registration.—ClinicalTrials.gov, www.clinicaltrials.gov, NCT01446289.

▶ Prevention of the neonatal complications associated with maternal GBS carriage, while having been the subject of standard obstetrical therapy for several decades, has always seemed particularly amenable to vaccine development. In fact, the original 1996 guidelines for group B *Streptococcus* prevention, in a theoretical fashion, noted the potential for vaccine prophylaxis. Donders et al. report the results of a multifaceted trial to evaluate the safety and immunogenicity of an investigational trivalent group B streptococcal vaccine. They found that it was well tolerated and demonstrated appropriately immunogenic properties with adequate placental transfer. Interestingly, however, women with no detectable antibodies at the initiation of the trial had lower subsequent antibody levels, suggesting the vaccine was augmenting nascent immunological responses. Whether this stratification of response would result in a reduced level of protection among women lacking evidence of previous immunological exposure will need to be further evaluated. In addition, the study did not include a large number of premature infants, the population most vulnerable to this infection. Clearly additional trials will be required before this (or a successor) vaccine is routinely available. However, it represents an exciting advance that would clearly benefit mothers and neonates in both developed and developing contexts.

T. F. McElrath, MD, PhD

Targeting IL-17A attenuates neonatal sepsis mortality induced by IL-18

Wynn JL, Wilson CS, Hawiger J, et al (Univ of Florida, Gainesville; Vanderbilt Univ, Nashville, TN, et al)

Proc Natl Acad Sci U S A 113:E2627-E2635, 2016

Interleukin (IL)-18 is an important effector of innate and adaptive immunity, but its expression must also be tightly regulated because it can potentiate lethal systemic inflammation and death. Healthy and septic human neonates demonstrate elevated serum concentrations of IL-18 compared with adults. Thus, we determined the contribution of IL-18 to lethality and its mechanism in a murine model of neonatal sepsis. We find that IL-18–null neonatal mice are highly protected from polymicrobial sepsis, whereas replenishing IL-18 increased lethality to sepsis or endotoxemia. Increased lethality depended on IL-1 receptor 1 (IL-1R1) signaling but not adaptive immunity. In genome-wide analyses of blood mRNA from septic human neonates, expression of the IL-17 receptor emerged as a critical regulatory node. Indeed, IL-18 administration in sepsis increased IL-17A production by murine intestinal γδT cells as well as Ly6G$^+$ myeloid cells, and blocking IL-17A reduced IL-18–potentiated mortality to both neonatal sepsis and endotoxemia. We conclude that IL-17A is a previously unrecognized effector of IL-18–mediated injury in neonatal sepsis and that disruption of the deleterious and tissue-destructive IL-18/IL-1/IL-17A axis represents a novel therapeutic approach to improve outcomes for human neonates with sepsis.

► Multiple studies have consistently established that prematurity is a chronic, hyperinflammatory state compared with adults. Even in the absence of disease, circulating proinflammatory cytokines are increased relative to adults; and, in the face of disease, the inflammatory response is more robust, with preterm infants mounting cytokine levels that far exceed those in adults with similar insults. This unregulated inflammatory response is partially due to an increase in production of proinflammatory mediators, but it is also due to the lack of negative regulators. Understanding this balance and cascading immune networks in preterm neonates will offer insights into future preventative and therapeutic strategies in neonatal disease processes that are exacerbated by immature immune responses and unmitigated inflammation.

In a series of animal and human neonatal experiments, Wynn et al establish interleukin (IL)-18/IL-1/IL-17A as a critical axis in neonatal immune responses to sepsis. IL-18–null mice demonstrated markedly reduced mortality to sepsis compared with wild-type mice. This effect was independent of mature B and T cells and independent of IL-1β but dependent on IL-1R1 signaling. Whole blood transcriptomics in human neonates with and without sepsis confirmed an increase in IL-18 gene expression with sepsis and plasma IL-18 protein elevation among infants with sepsis compared with infants evaluated for sepsis but retrospectively deemed uninfected. In addition, through pathway analysis, IL-17R emerged as a critical node in regulating human neonatal immune responses in sepsis. This IL-18/IL-1/IL-17A linkage was confirmed in a murine model of neonatal sepsis. Interestingly, the major sources of IL-17A transcript were gut and lung, raising an intriguing but plausible mechanism not only to the multisystem effects of sepsis but also an explanation as to why the diagnosis of sepsis is often linked to necrotizing enterocolitis and bronchopulmonary dysplasia.

To date our only tool to combat sepsis is antibiotics, and unfortunately this is often not enough because there remains a high rate of mortality and long-term morbidity with neonatal sepsis. Wynn et al defined a critical and central mediator axis in the immature neonatal immune response system that can be targeted to develop potential adjunctive therapies in neonatal sepsis to increase survival and reduce multisystem morbidity.

C. Martin, MD

Preterm Infants Can Mount Appropriate C-Reactive Protein Responses to Early Onset Sepsis

Shah SD, Talati AJ, Elabiad MT, et al (Univ of Tennessee Health Science Ctr, Memphis)

Am J Perinatol 32:1281-1286, 2015

Objective.—This study aims to evaluate whether infants born at ≤ 32 weeks' gestational age (GA) can mount C-reactive protein (CRP) responses during early onset bacterial sepsis that are comparable to infants born at > 32 weeks' GA.

Methods.—Retrospectively (2003–2012) infants with a positive bacterial culture during the first 72 hours of life were identified and grouped into two categories based on their GA: ≤ 32 weeks (group A) and > 32 weeks (group B).

Results.—Group A included 25 and group B included 122 infants. Both groups responded similarly to sepsis with an increase in CRP ($p = 0.59$). Each group had a significant change in intragroup CRP levels over time ($p < 0.0001$). However, in both groups, the degree of this change was at the same rate over time ($p = 0.74$).

Conclusion.—CRP responses to bacterial sepsis during the first 72 hours of life in infants born at ≤ 32 weeks' GA are comparable to infants born at > 32 weeks' GA (Fig 2).

▶ Since we described the high-sensitivity and negative predictive value of serial C-reactive protein (CPR) measurements in a large case series in 1998, other observational studies have raised concerns that the C-reactive protein response may be less reliable in preterm infants. This report provides some reassurance that the response is similar across gestational ages if cases of positive blood cultures attributable to contamination with skin flora are excluded (Fig 2). Similar to other reports, this analysis grouped all preterm infants ≤32 weeks' gestation into 1 category, leaving the possibility that preterm babies at the extremes of early gestation may still behave differently. Recent studies have suggested selective deficiencies in activation of the innate immune system in such babies, lending plausibility to those concerns, and anecdotal

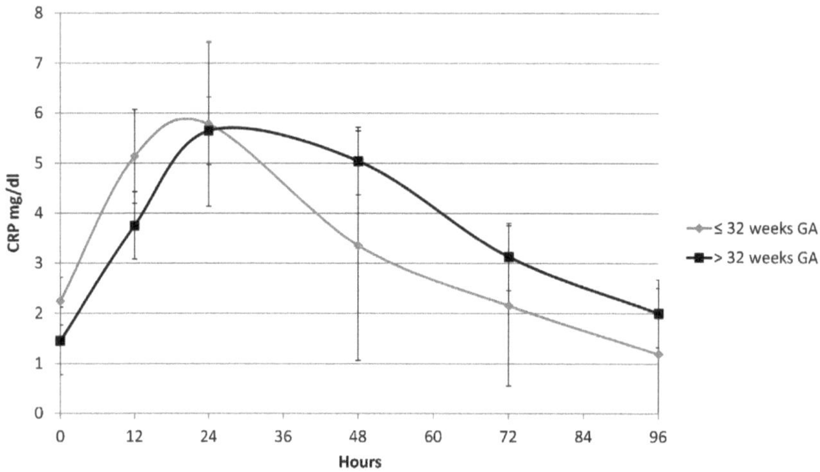

FIGURE 2.—After excluding skin flora, CRP levels of infants in group A (GA ≤ 32 weeks; $n = 15$) and group B (GA > 32 weeks; $n = 76$) at 0, 12, 24, 48, 72, and 96 hours of septic work-up. Values are least square means. Both groups showed significant changes over time ($p < 0.0001$). However, the manner of the response and the change in response rate over time was similar in both the groups, $p = 0.87$, and $p = 0.66$, respectively. CRP, Creactive protein; GA, gestational age. (Reprinted from Shah SD, Talati AJ, Elabiad MT, et al. Preterm infants can mount appropriate c-reactive protein responses to early onset sepsis. *Am J Perinatol.* 2015;32:1281-1286, with permission from Thieme Medical Publishers, Inc.)

evidence suggests that some extremely premature babies do fail to mount an appropriate CRP response despite persistent bacteremia. Although it probably is still true that CRP is "probably the best single test for neonatal sepsis," as stated by Da Silva et al more than 20 years ago,[1] their admonition that "clinicians ... cannot rely on CRP alone to make a decision" about management also remains cogent. In my personal (unpublished) experience, this may be particularly so when dealing with young, extremely immature preterm infants infected with relatively indolent pathogens (such as coagulase-negative *Staphylococci*). Synthesis of the entire clinical situation may support continuation of antimicrobial therapy in the face of normal CRP levels under those circumstances.

W. E. Benitz, MD

Reference

1. Da Silva O, Ohlsson A, Kenyon C. Accuracy of leukocyte indices and C-reactive protein for diagnosis of neonatal sepsis: a critical review. *Pediatr Infect Dis J.* 1995;14:362-366.

Blood Volume Required For Detection of Low Levels and Ultralow Levels of Organisms Responsible for Neonatal Bacteremia by Use of Bactec Peds Plus/F, Plus Aerobic/F Medium, and the BD Bactec FX System: an *In Vitro* Study

Lancaster DP, Friedman DF, Chiotos K, et al (The Children's Hosp of Philadelphia, PA)

J Clin Microbiol 53:3609-3613, 2015

We used an in vitro technique to investigate blood volumes required to detect bacteremia and fungemia with low concentrations of an organism. At 1 to 10 CFU/ml, *Escherichia coli, Staphylococcus epidermidis, Staphylococcus aureus, Listeria monocytogenes, Candida albicans*, and *Candida parapsilosis* isolates were detected in volumes as low as 0.5 ml. Detection of *Streptococcus agalactiae* and detection of bacteremia at<1 CFU/ml were unreliable.

▶ The optimal volume of blood to sample for blood cultures in neonates, especially those who are very low birth weight or extremely low birth weight, remains elusive. Although early studies suggested that neonatal sepsis was characterized by high circulating bacterial colony counts, Kellogg et al[1] found in 1997 that low colony counts are actually quite common in bacteremic infants, with colony counts less than 1 colony-forming unit (CFU)/mL in about 40% of those with positive blood cultures. Their results suggested that neonatal blood cultures had a sensitivity of only about 60%. The minimum necessary inoculum volume was not well delineated, however. Changing culture technologies have made those observations difficult to apply to current practice. For example, these authors note that a pediatric-specific culture system (BACTEC Peds Plus/F) was superior to one designed for use in adults (BACTEC Plus Aerobic/F), so attention to such details of laboratory technique may be critical. The updated simulated culture results presented in this report are, therefore, quite valuable. Although the number of simulated specimens tested for each organism, volume of blood, and level of bacteremia was small (3 for each instance), organisms were recovered from all cultures inoculated with blood at 1 to 10 CFU/mL, including all inocula of only 0.5 mL. At lower bacterial concentrations (<1 CFU/mL), recoveries were poor with inocula of 0.5 mL, better with 1 mL for most organisms, but poor at all volumes up to 3 mL for group B *Streptococcus*, methicillin-resistant *Staphylococcus aureus*, and *Listeria monocytogenes*. Unfortunately, there are very little available data on the prevalence or consequences of low-level bacteremia with these organisms in infants. Accordingly, balancing the risks of failing to diagnose an instance of bacteremia against the costs of using large volumes of blood for cultures seems to favor use of 1 mL inocula into culture bottles optimized for detection of bacteremia in pediatric patients.

W. E. Benitz, MD

Reference

1. Kellogg JA, Ferrentino FL, Goodstein MH, et al. Frequency of low level bacteremia in infants from birth to two months of age. *Pediatr Infect Dis J.* 1997;16: 381-385.

Risk Factors Associated With Laboratory-confirmed Bloodstream Infections in a Tertiary Neonatal Intensive Care Unit

Padula MA, Dewan ML, Shah SS, et al (Children's Hosp of Philadelphia, PA; Cincinnati Children's Hosp Med Ctr, OH; et al)

Pediatr Infect Dis J 33:1027-1032, 2014

Background.—Bloodstream infections (BSI) remain a leading cause of morbidity and mortality among infants admitted to neonatal intensive care units (NICUs). At the time of evaluation for suspected BSI, presenting signs may be nonspecific. We sought to determine the clinical signs and risk factors associated with laboratory-confirmed BSI among infants evaluated for late-onset sepsis in a tertiary NICU.

Methods.—This prospective cohort study included infants >3 days of age admitted to a level 4 NICU from July 2006 to October 2009 for whom a blood culture was drawn for suspected sepsis. Clinicians documented presenting signs at the time of culture. Laboratory-confirmed BSI was defined as per the National Healthcare Safety Network. Multivariate analyses were performed using a logistic regression random effects model.

Results.—Six-hundred and eighty eligible episodes of suspected BSI were recorded in 409 infants. Enteral contrast within the preceding 48 hours was the most significant risk factor for laboratory-confirmed BSI [Odds Ratio: 9.58 (95% confidence interval: 2.03—45.19)] followed by presence of a central venous catheter. Apnea and hypotension were the most strongly associated presenting signs.

Conclusion.—Among infants evaluated in a tertiary NICU, recent exposure to enteral contrast was associated with increased odds of developing BSI. Apnea and hypotension were the most strongly associated clinical signs of infection.

▶ In this study, investigators attempted to establish risk factors associated with culture-proven bacterial sepsis in newborns hospitalized in a neonatal intensive care unit with a unique patient population. Using a prospective cohort study, infants greater than 3 days of age who had blood cultures obtained for suspected sepsis were included. The Centers for Disease Control and Prevention definition of bloodstream infection was used. They enrolled 409 infants (680 episodes) between July 2006 and October 2009. Not surprisingly, hypotension, apnea, and the presence of a central venous catheter were found to be strongly associated with blood stream infections. On the other hand, an unexpected finding was the association of the receipt of enteral contrast material within 48 hours of presentation with sepsis. This was also corroborated by the large number of enteric organisms that were cultured. It is difficult to distinguish whether this finding was the result of the radiologic procedure itself (ie, induction of a bacteremia), the underlying condition that led to the contrast study, or a combination of the two. Nevertheless, this finding is of interest and concern, and it calls for a carefully designed study of the role of prophylactic antibiotic coverage in infants undergoing contrast radiography. As the authors indicate, this problem may be unique to their population, comprising referrals of many "surgical" patients, but I suspect that if we examine our own populations more closely, we will find the same thing.

S. M. Donn, MD

Partial restoration of the microbiota of cesarean-born infants via vaginal microbial transfer

Dominguez-Bello MG, De Jesus-Laboy KM, Shen N, et al (New York Univ; Univ of Puerto Rico, San Juan; Icahn School of Medicine at Mount Sinai, NY; et al)

Nat Med 22:250-253, 2016

Exposure of newborns to the maternal vaginal microbiota is interrupted with cesarean birthing. Babies delivered by cesarean section (C-section) acquire a microbiota that differs from that of vaginally delivered infants, and C-section delivery has been associated with increased risk for immune and metabolic disorders. Here we conducted a pilot study in which infants delivered by C-section were exposed to maternal vaginal fluids at birth. Similarly to vaginally delivered babies, the gut, oral and skin bacterial communities of these newborns during the first 30 d of life was enriched in vaginal bacteria—which were underrepresented in unexposed C-section–delivered infants—and the microbiome similarity to those of vaginally delivered infants was greater in oral and skin samples than in anal samples. Although the long-term health consequences of restoring the microbiota of C-section–delivered infants remain unclear, our results demonstrate that vaginal microbes can be partially restored at birth in C-section–delivered babies.

▶ The composition of the early microbiota of newborn infants is heavily influenced by the mode of delivery. The microbiota of infants born by cesarean delivery (C-section) resembles that of maternal skin, whereas the microbiota of infants delivered vaginally resembles that of the maternal vagina. It has been suggested that these early differences in microbiota heighten the susceptibility of infants delivered by C-section to an increasing number of conditions including obesity, asthma, and autoimmune diseases. "Vaginal seeding," a procedure in which a sterile gauze swab is used to transfer maternal vaginal microbiota on to an infant born by C-section shortly after birth, has gained traction among the lay public, despite no data to support the practice.

In this small interventional study the investigators compared the microbiota of 4 infants delivered by C-section who underwent vaginal seeding to that of 7 infants delivered by C-section who did not undergo vaginal seeding and 7 vaginally delivered infants. Vaginal seeding consisted of swabbing an infant's mouth, face, and then the rest of the body within the first minutes after birth with sterile gauze that had been incubated in their mother's vagina during the hour preceding the C-section. Infants of women who were positive for group B *Streptococcus*, had vaginosis or a vaginal pH >4.5 were excluded. A total of 1519 samples were obtained from anal, oral and skin sites of infants and mothers at 1, 3, 7, 14, 21, and 30 days after birth. The microbiomes of the gauze used for vaginal seeding and vaginal samples obtained on the first postpartum day were similar, indicating that the technique used was effective. Both vaginally delivered and vaginally seeded C-section-delivered babies had a vaginal microbiome-like signal that was absent in unexposed C-section-delivered babies; this pattern persisted throughout the 30-day study period.

As the investigators state in the article, this observational study represents a proof of principle involving a small cohort and with limited follow-up. It would appear that vaginal seeding is feasible; however, its effects on diseases in later life need to be determined before the risk-benefit of the procedure can be ascertained.

L. A. Papile, MD

Neonatal Intensive Care Unit Antibiotic Use

Schulman J, Dimand RJ, Lee HC, et al (California Children's Services, Sacramento; Stanford Univ, CA)

Pediatrics 135:826-833, 2015

Background and Objectives.—Treatment of suspected infection is a mainstay of the daily work in the NICU. We hypothesized that NICU antibiotic prescribing practice variation correlates with rates of proven infection, necrotizing enterocolitis (NEC), mortality, inborn admission, and with NICU surgical volume and average length of stay.

Methods.—In a retrospective cohort study of 52 061 infants in 127 NICUs across California during 2013, we compared sample means and explored linear and nonparametric correlations, stratified by NICU level of care and lowest/highest antibiotic use rate quartiles.

Results.—Overall antibiotic use varied 40-fold, from 2.4% to 97.1% of patient-days; median = 24.5%. At all levels of care, it was independent of proven infection, NEC, surgical volume, or mortality. Fifty percent of intermediate level NICUs were in the highest antibiotic use quartile, yet most of these units reported infection rates of zero. Regional NICUs in the highest antibiotic quartile reported inborn admission rate 218% higher (0.24 vs 0.11, $P = .03$), and length of stay 35% longer (90.2 days vs 66.9 days, $P = .03$) than regional NICUs in the lowest quartile.

Conclusions.—Forty-fold variation in NICU antibiotic prescribing practice across 127 NICUs with similar burdens of proven infection, NEC, surgical volume, and mortality indicates that a considerable portion of antibiotic use lacks clear warrant; in some NICUs, antibiotics are overused. Additional study is needed to establish appropriate use ranges and elucidate the determinants and directionality of relationships between antibiotic and other resource use.

▶ Too many antibiotics for too little proven sepsis in the neonatal intensive care unit (NICU). There are 3 undeniable facts about sepsis in the NICU: (1) neonatal sepsis (early and late onset) is a major cause of morbidity and mortality,[1] (2) identification of infants with possible sepsis is difficult, and (3) most management recommendations from national committees represent expert opinion and are not based on randomized clinical trials.[2] In addition, there are considerable variations in practice within NICUs and among centers participating in networks.[3] In a retrospective study, Schulman et al analyzed variations in antibiotic prescribing among 127 NICUs across California. The data were analyzed according to the level of NICU care (regional, community, and intermediate) and lowest/highest antibiotic use quartiles. Not surprisingly, antibiotic use varied considerably (40-fold). At all level of care, it was independent of proven infection, necrotizing enterocolitis, surgical volume or mortality. Fifty percent of the intermediate care NICUs were in the highest antibiotic use quartile, yet most of their reported infections rates were zero. The study did not detect an association between antibiotic use and late-onset sepsis, necrotizing enterocolitis or mortality.

Although this study clearly indicates practice variations among NICUs, it has several limitations. First, an infection rate of "zero" does not mean that infection was not present. Differences in the rates of maternal antibiotic use and in the technical aspects of performing a blood culture, such as the volume of blood sent for culture, can affect the ability to detect bacteremia. Second, infection at other sites (skin and soft tissue, urinary tract, or central nervous system may not be accompanied by a positive blood culture. Those infections may have contributed to some of the antibiotic usage. Third, use of prophylactic antibiotics (eg, fluconazole) was not identified in this retrospective study. The question remains about how to limit the unnecessary use of antibiotics. For infants with suspected early-onset sepsis, the use of the "sepsis calculators" of Puopolo and Escobar[4] should be effective by determining risk of sepsis based on historical risk factors and clinical signs. The diagnosis of health care–associated infections is more problematic. Although antibiotics will always be used in infants with nonspecific clinical signs suggestive of sepsis, they should be stopped as soon as infection is ruled out (in most cases, by 48 hours) and the infant's condition returns to baseline. In the well-appearing infant, antibiotics should not be continued based on nonspecific indicators of inflammation (eg, acute phase reactants).

R. A. Polin, MD

References

1. Patel RM, Kandefer S, Walsh MC, et al. Causes and timing of death in extremely premature infants from 2000–2011. *N Engl J Med.* 2015;372:331-340.
2. Rysavy BS, Li L, Bell EF, et al. Between hospital variation in treatment and outcomes in extremely preterm infants. *N Engl J Med.* 2015;372:1801-1811.
3. Polin RA, Committee of Fetus and Newborn. Management of neonates with suspected or proven early-onset sepsis. *Pediatrics.* 2012;129:1006-1015.
4. http://www.dor.kaiser.org/external/DORExternal/research/infectionprobabilitycalculator.aspx.

Outcome of Preterm Infants With Postnatal Cytomegalovirus Infection via Breast Milk: A Two-Year Prospective Follow-Up Study

Jim W-T, Chiu N-C, Ho C-S, et al (MacKay Children's Hosp, Taipei, Taiwan; et al)

Medicine 94:e1835, 2015

Approximately 15% of preterm infants may develop postnatal cytomegalovirus (CMV) infection from seropositive mothers via breast milk and are at risk for neurological sequelae in childhood. The aims of this study were to assess the effects and outcomes on growth, neurodevelopmental status, and hearing in very low birth weight (VLBW) premature infants with postnatal CMV infection via breast milk at the corrected age of 12 and 24 months.

The prospective follow-up study population comprised all living preterm children (n = 55) with a birth weight ≤1500 g and gestational age of ≤35 weeks, who had participated in our "postnatal CMV infection via breast milk" studies in 2000 and 2009, respectively. The cohort of children was assessed at 12 and 24 months. Clinical outcomes were documented during hospitalization and after discharge. Long-term outcomes included anthropometry, audiologic tests, gross motor quotient, Infant International Battery, and neurodevelopmental outcomes; all were assessed at postcorrected age in 12 and 24 months during follow-up visits.

Of the 55 infants enrolled in the study (4 noninfected infants were excluded because their parents did not join this follow-up program later), 14 infants postnatally acquired CMV infection through breastfeeding (infected group) and were compared with 41 infants without CMV infection (control group). No significant differences were observed between the groups with regard to baseline characteristics clinical outcomes, anthropometry, or psychomotor and mental development on the Bayley scale of infant development. None of the infants had CMV-related death or permanent sensorineural hearing loss.

Transmission of CMV from seropositive mother via breast milk to preterm infants does not appear at this time to have major adverse effects on clinical outcomes, growth, neurodevelopmental status, and hearing function at 12 and 24 months corrected age.

▶ Preterm infants who acquire postnatal cytomegalovirus (CMV) infection potentially are at an increased risk for developmental delay, cognitive impairment, motor problems, and hearing loss. However, published studies on the neurodevelopmental outcome of preterm infants who acquired postnatal CMV infection from their mother's milk are sparse.

In this observational study, the authors prospectively followed up with a cohort of very low birth weight infants with and without postnatal CMV infection that could be attributed to ingesting infected mother's milk. Postnatal CMV infection was defined as polymerase chain reaction—positive viral DNA in urine and culture-positive urine sample after 3 weeks of age. The infants underwent formal neurodevelopmental evaluation using the Bayley Scales of Infant Development II, Gross Motor Quotient, and Infant International Battery at 1 and 2 years of age. Auditory brainstem responses were measured to assess hearing impairment. Of the 55 infants enrolled in the study, 25% acquired postnatal CMV infection. Baseline characteristics including gestational age, birth weight, and severity of illness score were similar, as were postnatal medical morbidities. At 2 years of age, Mental Developmental Index scores less than 70 were noted in 7% of the non-infected infants and 14% of the CMV-positive infants; 12% and 7% respectively had psychomotor development index score less than 70. Mild peripheral hearing loss was found in 2 infants in each group.

This study adds to the sparse body of literature suggesting that CMV infection acquired postnatally does not increase the risk for neurodevelopmental problems, at least in early childhood. Thus, it would appear that the benefits of feeding preterm infants mother's milk outweigh the risk of acquiring postnatal CMV infection.

L. A. Papile, MD

SENTINEL1: An Observational Study of Respiratory Syncytial Virus Hospitalizations among U.S. Infants Born at 29 to 35 Weeks' Gestational Age Not Receiving Immunoprophylaxis

Anderson EJ, Krilov LR, DeVincenzo JP, et al (Emory Univ School of Medicine, Atlanta, GA; Winthrop Univ Hosp, Mineola, NY; Univ of Tennessee Ctr for Health Sciences, Memphis; et al)

Am J Perinatol 2016 [Epub ahead of print]

Objective.—SENTINEL1 characterized U.S. preterm infants 29 to 35 weeks' gestational age (wGA) < 12 months old hospitalized for laboratory-confirmed respiratory syncytial virus (RSV) disease and not receiving RSV immunoprophylaxis during the 2014 to 2015 RSV season.

Study Design.—This is a noninterventional, observational, cohort study.

Results.—A total of 702 infants were hospitalized with community-acquired RSV disease, of whom an estimated 42% were admitted to the intensive care unit (ICU) and 20% required invasive mechanical ventilation (IMV). Earlier gestational age and younger chronologic age were associated with an increased frequency of RSV-confirmed hospitalization (RSVH), ICU admission, and IMV. Among infants 29 to 32 wGA and < 3 months of age, 68% required ICU admission and 44% required IMV. One death occurred of an infant 29 wGA. Among the 212 infants enrolled for in-depth analysis of health care resource utilization, mean and median RSVH charges were $55,551 and $27,461, respectively, which varied by intensity of care required. Outpatient visits were common, with 63% and 62% of infants requiring visits before and within 1 month following the RSVH, respectively.

Conclusion.—Preterminfants 29 to 35 wGA are at high risk for severe RSV disease, which imposes a substantial health burden, particularly in the first months of life.

▶ Has the American Academy of Pediatrics Committee on Infectious Diseases (COID) missed the boat on respiratory syncytial virus immunoprophylaxis? The results of the SENTINEL 1 study would seem to suggest so. This prospective observational cohort study tracked more than 700 infants of 29 to 35 weeks' gestation, who would have previously received palivizumab but were ineligible according to the 2014 guidelines. The data are not surprising. Nearly half (42%) of the hospitalized infants required admission to an intensive care unit, and half of these required invasive ventilatory support. When stratified by gestational age, there was an inverse relationship, with the more premature infants requiring more intensive care unit admissions and invasive respiratory support. Chronological age showed a similar relationship. Also not a surprise, the costs associated with the hospitalizations were staggering. These data are consistent with those demonstrated earlier. Although true cost-effectiveness may be difficult to calculate, it is clear that the subset of infants 29 to 32 weeks' gestational age are at the highest risk for rehospitalization and need for intensive care and invasive ventilation and are the most costly to support.

Another important factor that has been neglected in arguing cost-effectiveness is how much money we already spend to get these infants through their initial hospitalizations for prematurity. No one in his or her right mind would buy an expensive sports car or luxury sedan without purchasing an automobile insurance policy. Palivizumab seems like a small incremental cost to prevent subsequent respiratory morbidity and its attendant hospitalization and health care resource utilization. The COID must revisit this.

S. M. Donn, MD

6 Cardiovascular System

Randomized, Placebo-Controlled Trial of Dobutamine for Low Superior Vena Cava Flow in Infants

Bravo MC, López-Ortego P, Sánchez L, et al (La Paz Univ Hosp, Madrid, Spain; et al)

J Pediatr 167:572-578, 2015

Objective.—To gather information for a future confirmatory trial of dobutamine (DB) for circulatory impairment (ie, low superior vena cava [SVC] flow).

Study Design.—A total of 127 infants born at <31 weeks gestational age were serially scanned from birth to 96 hours after birth. The infants were randomly assigned to 2 groups and were treated with DB (stepwise dose increase, 5-10-15-20 μg/kg/min) or placebo if they had an SVC flow <41 mL/kg/min within the first 24 hours after birth. The primary outcome measures were the achievement and maintenance of an SVC flow ≥41 mL/kg/min. Secondary outcome measures were the short-term evolution of clinical and biochemical variables, near-infrared spectroscopy, cranial Doppler ultrasound, and clinical outcomes.

Results.—SVC flow increased throughout the first 96 hours for the entire cohort. All of the randomized infants (n = 28) except 2 achieved and maintained an SVC flow ≥41 mL/kg/min after intervention; however, the infants treated with DB (n = 16) showed a higher heart rate and improved base excess compared with those treated with placebo (n = 12). Low SVC flow was associated with low gestational age (P = .02) and poor condition at birth (P = .02). Low SVC flow significantly increased the risk of severe ischemic events (OR, 13; 95% CI, 2.4-69.2; $P < .01$).

Conclusion.—This exploratory trial demonstrates a tendency toward improved short-term clinical and biochemical perfusion variable outcomes in infants with low SVC flow treated with DB.

Trial Registration.—ClinicalTrials.gov (NCT01605279) and the European Clinical Trials Database (EurodraCT 2009-010901-35).

▶ Despite unanswered questions regarding the definitions, clinical relevance, and pathophysiology of hypotension and hypoperfusion in preterm neonates, widespread treatment of these physiologic conditions continues. Several retrospective reports suggest that traditional measures used to address these disorders (most commonly, intravascular volume and dopamine) might not improve outcomes; in fact, some treatments might increase the risk of death or disability. Tremendous strides have been made to optimize diagnostic modalities and elucidate the underlying pathophysiologic mechanisms of hypoperfusion in this challenging population. One of these tools, functional echocardiography was used as the end point of a recent randomized controlled trial conducted in Spain. Specifically, the investigators targeted premature neonates with low superior vena cava (SVC) flow, an end point associated with intraventricular hemorrhage, adverse neurodevelopmental outcome, and death. In this trial, dobutamine was compared with placebo for neonates with low SVC flow, targeting the common underlying pathophysiology of immature myocardial contractility. A total of 127 infants born at < 31 weeks gestational age were serially screened for the first 96 hours of life, and 28 with low SVC flow were randomized. Infants randomized to dobutamine showed greater improvement in base excess, although nearly all infants normalized SVC flow after randomization regardless of treatment group.

The results of this study certainly do not suggest the dobutamine should replace dopamine as the "standard" treatment of cardiovascular dysfunction in preterm neonates. Rather, this study highlights the utility of a long-studied, but infrequently implemented, diagnostic tool: functional echocardiography. Of note, numerous patients in this study were randomized to dobutamine or placebo for low SVC flow, despite treatment with other open-label cardiovascular therapies. The trend toward more rapid normalization of SVC flow among infants randomized to dobutamine is of unclear significance but emphasizes the importance of considering dobutamine as primary therapy for neonates clinically diagnosed with hypotension or hypoperfusion. Although the authors seem enthusiastic about a larger randomized controlled trial, they appropriately highlight the need to consider all available clinical and biochemical variables to ensure randomization of a population of infants who may benefit from the pharmacologic properties of dobutamine. Rigorous criteria for eligibility should be used both for future trials and for the treatment of individual neonates pending results of larger randomized clinical trials.

C. McPherson, PharmD

Early blood pressure, antihypotensive therapy and outcomes at 18–22 months' corrected age in extremely preterm infants

Batton B, for the Eunice Kennedy Shriver National Institute of Child Health & Human Development Neonatal Research Network (Case Western Reserve Univ, Cleveland, OH; et al)

Arch Dis Child Fetal Neonatal Ed 101:F201-F206, 2016

Objective.—To investigate the relationships between early blood pressure (BP) changes, receipt of antihypotensive therapy and 18–22 months' corrected age (CA) outcomes for extremely preterm infants.

Design.—Prospective observational study of infants $23^{0/7}$–$26^{6/7}$ weeks' gestational age (GA). Hourly BP values and antihypotensive therapy exposure in the first 24 h were recorded. Four groups were defined: infants who did or did not receive antihypotensive therapy in whom BP did or did not rise at the expected rate (defined as an increase in the mean arterial BP of ≥5 mm Hg/day). Random-intercept logistic modelling controlling for centre clustering, GA and illness severity was used to investigate the relationship between BP, antihypotensive therapies and infant outcomes.

Setting.—Sixteen academic centres of the *Eunice Kennedy Shriver* National Institute of Child Health and Human Development Neonatal Research Network.

Main Outcome Measures.—Death or neurodevelopmental impairment/developmental delay (NIDD) at 18–22 months' CA.

Results.—Of 367 infants, 203 (55%) received an antihypotensive therapy, 272 (74%) survived to discharge and 331 (90%) had a known outcome at 18–22 months' CA. With logistic regression, there was an increased risk of death/NIDD with antihypotensive therapy versus no treatment (OR 1.836, 95% CI 1.092 to 3.086), but not NIDD alone (OR 1.53, 95% CI 0.708 to 3.307).

Conclusions.—Independent of early BP changes, antihypotensive therapy exposure was associated with an increased risk of death/NIDD at 18–22 months' CA when controlling for risk factors known to affect survival and neurodevelopment.

Clinical Trial Registration Number.—clinicaltrials.gov #NCT00874393.

▶ In this prospective observational study, the investigators evaluated toddler outcomes in a cohort of 367 extremely preterm infants divided into groups defined by early changes in blood pressure (BP) and receipt of antihypotensive therapy. Their objectives were to clarify (1) whether adverse outcomes in infants with concerning BP are related to their not receiving antihypotensive therapy and (2) whether survival and/or intact neurodevelopment in treated infants are related to a rise in BP.

The primary outcome was the incidence of death or neurodevelopmental impairment/developmental delay (NIDD) at 18 to 22 months adjusted age. NIDD was defined as a Bayley Scales of Infant Development III cognitive or motor score <70, cerebral palsy (Gross Motor Function Classification level >2), hearing impairment requiring hearing aids in both ears or blindness (some or no useful vision in either eye). Outcomes were compared among 4 groups: (1) infants who did not receive antihypotensive therapy in whom BP rose >4 mm Hg between 4 and 24 hours of age, (2) infants who did not receive antihypotensive therapy who did not experience a >4 mm Hg rise in BP between 4 and 24 hours of age, (3) infants who received antihypotensive therapy in the first 24 hours in whom BP rose >4 mm Hg between 4 and 24 hours of age, and (4) infants who received antihypertensive therapy in the first 24 hours who did not experience >4 mm Hg rise in BP between 4 and 24 hours of age. Of the 123 infants who received antihypertensive therapy 67% received a fluid bolus, 50% received a blood product, 45% received dopamine, 12% received hydrocortisone, and 9% received dobutamine.

In the untreated group, 58% had a >4-mm rise in BP (91/158) compared with 65% (128/198) in the group receiving therapy. Regression models incorporating gestational age, markers of severity of illness, and changes in BP demonstrated that treatment with any antihypotensive therapy was a significant predictor of death/NIDD but not NIDD alone. Similar regression models incorporating antihypotensive treatment showed that a rise in BP was not significantly associated with either outcome. Thus, it would appear that irrespective of initial BP or changes in BP, antihypertensive therapy, per se, was associated with less good outcome.

Although observational in nature, the study raises concerns about the wisdom of using therapeutic interventions to increase BP shortly after birth in extremely low gestational infants. As the authors state in the conclusions to the article, it is possible that therapeutic interventions for perceived low BP increase the risk of adverse outcomes, at least for some babies.

L. A. Papile, MD

Aspects of pulse oximetry screening for critical congenital heart defects: when, how and why?

Narayen IC, Blom NA, Ewer AK, et al (Leiden Univ Med Ctr, The Netherlands; Birmingham Women's Hosp, UK; et al)

Arch Dis Child Fetal Neonatal Ed 101:F162-F167, 2016

Pulse oximetry (PO) screening for critical congenital heart defects (CCHD) has been studied extensively and is being increasingly implemented worldwide. This review provides an overview of all aspects of PO screening that need to be considered when introducing this methodology. PO screening for CCHD is effective, simple, quick, reliable, cost-effective and does not lead to extra burden for parents and caregivers. Test accuracy can be influenced by targets definition, gestational age, timing of screening and antenatal detection of CCHD. Early screening can lead to more false positive screenings, but has the potential to detect significant pathology earlier. There is no apparent difference in accuracy between screening with post-ductal measurements only, compared with screening using pre-ductal and post-ductal measurements. However, adding pre-ductal measurements identifies cases of CCHD which would have been missed by post-ductal screening. Screening at higher altitudes leads to more false positives. Important non-cardiac pathology is found in 35–74% of false positives in large studies. Screening is feasible in neonatal intensive care units and out-of-hospital births. Training caregivers, simplifying the algorithm and using computer-based interpretation tools can improve the quality of the screening. Caregivers need to consider all aspects of screening to enable them to choose an optimal protocol for implementation of CCHD screening in their specific setting.

▶ Pulse oximetry has rapidly changed the face of the diagnosis of critical congenital heart disease (CCHD). The beauty of the technique is that screening with pulse oximetry can be done quickly, with a high specificity, greater than 94%. This translates into few false positives and unnecessary referral for echocardiography. It is by no means perfect, and there are still a few cases that go undetected, mainly variations of coarctation of the aorta.

Pulse oximetry is now used widely to screen for critical congenital heart disease. An area that needs tweaking of the algorithm is when the screening is done at high altitudes where using the sea level criteria there are a number of false positives.

Jones et al[1] evaluated the impact and efficacy of pulse oximetry screening for CCHD in a level 2 neonatal unit without on-site access to pediatric echocardiography in Middlesex, United Kingdom.

There were 11 233 live births during the study period, with 973 neonatal unit admissions unrelated to pulse oximetry screening. From the remaining

screening population of 10 260 newborns, 23 were admitted on the basis of a screen-positive result; 3 of the 23 patients went on to have urgent echocardiograms, and 2 were found to have critical CHD. In the 21 newborns without critical CHD, an alternative diagnosis was made in 16 cases. These data are in concert with the report from Narayen, which indicated that 80% of the false positives had some other medical diagnosis. Record

linkage with the National Congenital Heart Disease Audit indicated that no newborns born in the hospital during the study period received surgery for critical CHD following negative, and specificity was 99.80, with a false-positive rate of 0.20%. They concluded that "The introduction of pulse oximetry screening to a hospital where pediatric echocardiography services are not available is practical, results in very few referrals to the regional pediatric cardiology center, and detects cases of CHD that would otherwise go undiagnosed."

The review by Naranen et al contains much valuable information and references. The current recommendation to screen after 24 hours of life decreases the false-positive rate but increases the chances of missing an early presentation of CCHD. Overall, this has been a win-win situation and effective—and cost-effective—screening has gained and is gaining traction around the globe, saving the lives of babies born with CCHD.

Narayen et al[2] describe how in the Netherlands, where there are a significant number of home births and very early discharges, they successfully implemented a pulse oximetry screening program. Key factors included training of the nurse midwifes, use of a handheld pulse oximeter, and performing the screening in the first 2 hours of life, before the midwife leaving the home and again 24 hours later. The outcomes were similar to other institutions with few false positives. No cases of CCHD were identified, but none were missed identification of CCHD, and other disorders were diagnosed in the babies who tested positive but did not have CCHD. This demonstrates that in a controlled, well-supervised environment, screening for CCHD can take place in the home. This augurs well for the introduction of screening in resource-limited environments.

A. A. Fanaroff, MD

References

1. Jones AJ, Howarth C, Nicholl R, Mat-Ali E, Knowles R. The impact and efficacy of routine pulse oximetry screening for CHD in a local hospital. *Cardiol Young.* 2016:1-9.
2. Narayen IC, Blom NA, Bourgonje MS, et al. Pulse oximetry screening for critical congenital heart disease after home birth and early discharge. *J Pediatr.* 2016;170: 188-192.e1.

Association Between Early Screening for Patent Ductus Arteriosus and In-Hospital Mortality Among Extremely Preterm Infants

Rozé JC, for the Hemodynamic EPIPAGE 2 Study Group (Nantes Univ Hosp, France; et al)
JAMA 313:2441-2448, 2015

Importance.—There is currently no consensus for the screening and treatment of patent ductus arteriosus (PDA) in extremely preterm infants. Less pharmacological closure and more supportive management have been observed without evidence to support these changes.

Objective.—To evaluate the association between early screening echocardiography for PDA and in-hospital mortality.

Design, Setting, and Participants.—Comparison of screened and not screened preterm infants enrolled in the EPIPAGE 2 national prospective population-based cohort study that included all preterm infants born at less than 29 weeks of gestation and hospitalized in 68 neonatal intensive care units in France from April through December 2011. Two main analyses were performed to adjust for potential selection bias, one using propensity score matching and one using neonatal unit preference for early screening echocardiography as an instrumental variable.

Exposures.—Early screening echocardiography before day 3 of life.

Main Outcomes and Measures.—The primary outcome was death between day 3 and discharge. The secondary outcomes were major neonatal morbidities (pulmonary hemorrhage, severe bronchopulmonary dysplasia, severe cerebral lesions, and necrotizing enterocolitis).

Results.—Among the 1513 preterm infants with data available to determine exposure, 847 were screened for PDA and 666 were not; 605 infants from each group could be paired. Exposed infants were treated for PDA more frequently during their hospitalization than nonexposed infants (55.1%vs 43.1%; odds ratio [OR], 1.62 [95% CI, 1.31 to 2.00]; absolute risk reduction [ARR] in events per 100 infants, −12.0 [95% CI, −17.3 to −6.7). Exposed infants had a lower hospital death rate (14.2% vs 18.5%; OR, 0.73 [95% CI, 0.54 to 0.98]; ARR, 4.3 [95% CI, 0.3 to 8.3]) and a lower rate of pulmonary hemorrhage (5.6% vs 8.9%; OR, 0.60 [95% CI, 0.38 to 0.95]; ARR, 3.3 [95% CI, 0.4 to 6.3]). No differences in rates of necrotizing enterocolitis, severe bronchopulmonary dysplasia, or severe cerebral lesions were observed. In the overall cohort, instrumental variable analysis yielded an adjusted OR for in-hospital mortality of 0.62 [95% CI, 0.37 to 1.04].

Conclusions and Relevance.—In this national population-based cohort of extremely preterm infants, screening echocardiography before day 3 of life was associated with lower in-hospital mortality and likelihood of pulmonary hemorrhage but not with differences in necrotizing enterocolitis, severe bronchopulmonary dysplasia, or severe cerebral lesions. However, results of the instrumental variable analysis leave some ambiguity in the interpretation, and longer-term evaluation is needed to provide clarity.

▶ In the second sentence of the abstract, these authors note that "Less pharmacological closure and more supportive management [of patent ductus arteriosus (PDA) in preterm infants] have been observed without evidence to support these changes." It could also be said that "Routine early pharmacological closure and/or ligation of PDA rather than supportive management continues to be observed, despite considerable evidence that those measures are ineffective." In search of evidence supporting treatment, these authors have undertaken an analysis of data collected on 1513 preterm (< 29 weeks gestation) infants cared for in a national consortium of nurseries in France in 2011. Curiously, screening echocardiography performed at a postnatal age at which patency of the ductus is almost universal (but not reported in this account) was associated with a lower mortality rate (unadjusted odds ratio 0.73, 95% confidence interval 0.54–0.99). This difference was apparent despite echocardiographic evaluation in the 81% of the "nonexposed" subjects at a median age of only 3.5 days (interquartile range 0–98 days vs a median age of 1 day with an IQR of 0–2 days in the "exposed" group), including 16% in whom echocardiography was performed for clinical indications before the third postnatal day. Increased mortality risk was restricted to the subgroup of 390 infants who did not have echocardiographic screening and were not treated for PDA; it is not clear how many of these infants had echocardiography or PDA or whether presence of a PDA was associated with mortality. The differential mortality accrued between approximately 7 and 35 days postnatal age and was predominantly attributable to multiple organ system dysfunction (40% of excess deaths) and respiratory failure (60% of excess deaths). Early screening was also associated with a lower risk of pulmonary hemorrhage, but only 25% of the infants in the "nonexposed" group who died of respiratory failure had pulmonary hemorrhage. This observation is novel, as the only placebo-controlled randomized trial of ibuprofen to report pulmonary hemorrhage as an outcome[1] found no effect of early treatment on the rate of that event. Sophisticated statistical analyses failed to identify potential confounders that might explain this association and no mechanism through which screening might reduce mortality is posited. The instrumental variable analysis, which was the only tested model that included a measure of individual unit preferences, did not demonstrate a statistically significant association, however, and the authors urge caution in interpreting these results. There may be an important signal in these data, but it is not clear just what it means.

W. E. Benitz, MD

Reference

1. Aranda JV, Clyman R, Cox B, et al. A randomized, double-blind, placebo-controlled trial on intravenous ibuprofen L-lysine for the early closure of nonsymptomatic patent ductus arteriosus within 72 hours of birth in extremely low-birth-weight infants. *Am J Perinatol.* 2009;26:235-245.

Paracetamol Accelerates Closure of the Ductus Arteriosus after Premature Birth: A Randomized Trial

Härkin P, Härmä A, Aikio O, et al (Oulu Univ Hosp, Finland)

J Pediatr 2016 [Epub ahead of print]

Objective.—To study the biologic effect of paracetamol, an inhibitor of prostaglandin synthase, on early closure of ductus arteriosus, and to evaluate possible adverse effects associated with the drug.

Study Design.—In a controlled, double-blind, phase I-II trial, very low gestational age (<32 weeks) infants requiring intensive care were randomly assigned to intravenous paracetamol or placebo (0.45% NaCl). A loading dose of 20 mg/kg was given within 24 hours of birth, followed by 7.5 mg/kg every 6 hours for 4 days. Daily cardiac ultrasound examinations of ductal calibers were performed before the first dose, and until 1 day after the last dose. The main outcome was a decrease in the ductal caliber without side effects.

Results.—Of 63 screened infants, 48 were randomized: 23 were assigned to paracetamol and 25 to placebo. Before the intervention, their ductal calibers were similar. During the intervention, the ductus closed faster in the paracetamol group (hazard ratio 0.49, 95% CI 0.25-0.97, $P = .016$). The mean (95% CI) postnatal ages for ductal closure were 177 hours (31.1-324) for the paracetamol-treated vs 338 hours (118-557) for controls ($P = .045$). Paracetamol serum levels were within the therapeutic range, and no adverse effects were evident.

Conclusions.—Prophylactic paracetamol induced early closure of the ductus arteriosus without detectable side effects. Further trials are required to determine whether intravenous paracetamol may safely prevent symptomatic patent ductus arteriosus.

Trial Registration.—ClinicalTrials.gov: NCT01938261; European Clinical Trials Database: EudraCT 2013-008142-33.

▶ Contemporary management of the patent ductus arteriosus (PDA) is a common topic of neonatology debate and lively discussions abound regarding the when, if, and how to treat a PDA and whether outcomes are improved by closure. Paracetamol, a prostaglandin synthetase inhibitor, has been shown in at least 1 previous observational study,[1] to promote PDA closure without some of the adverse effects attributable to the most commonly used treatments: COX inhibitors, ibuprofen, and indomethacin. This double-masked randomized clinical trial of prophylactic paracetamol for closure of the ductus arteriosus enrolled 48 of 63 eligible infants born before 32 weeks of gestation at 1 hospital in Finland. Eligible infants whose parents consented to enrollment were randomized to placebo or paracetamol (the latter as a loading dose followed by smaller doses every 6 hours for 4 days); daily echocardiograms were performed (the first before medication administration). On average, among paracetamol-treated infants, ductus arteriosus closure was quicker than for infants receiving placebo (41 hours vs 78 hours) without any detectable adverse effects. The controversy regarding whether to treat the PDA is not likely to disappear overnight; however, this study at least offers the promise of an alternative to indomethacin, ibuprofen, and surgery that appears to be effective and might be safer.

L. J. Van Marter, MD, MPH

Reference

1. Aikio O, Härkin P, Saarela T, Hallman M. Early paracetamol treatment is associated with lowered risk of persistent ductus arteriosus in very preterm infants. *J Matern Fetal Neonatal Med.* 2014;27:1252-1256.

Neurodevelopmental Outcomes of Premature Infants Treated for Patent Ductus Arteriosus: A Population-Based Cohort Study

Janz-Robinson EM, on behalf of the Neonatal Intensive Care Units Network (Canberra Hosp, Garran, Australian Capital Territory, Australia; et al)

J Pediatr 167:1025-1032, 2015

Objective.—To compare neurodevelopmental outcomes of extremely preterm infants diagnosed with patent ductus arteriosus (PDA) who were treated medically or surgically and those who were not diagnosed with PDA or who did not undergo treatment for PDA.

Study Design.—This retrospective population-based cohort study used data from a geographically defined area in New South Wales and the Australian Capital Territory served by a network of 10 neonatal intensive care units. Patients included all preterm infants born at <29 completed weeks of gestation between 1998 and 2004. Moderate/ severe functional disability at 2-3 years corrected age was defined as developmental delay, cerebral palsy requiring aids, sensorineural or conductive deafness (requiring bilateral hearing aids or cochlear implant), or bilateral blindness (best visual acuity of <6/60).

Results.—Follow-up information at age 2-3 years was available for 1473 infants (74.8%). Compared with infants not diagnosed with a PDA or who did not receive PDA treatment for PDA, those with medically treated PDA (aOR, 1.622; 95% CI, 1.199-2.196) and those with surgically treated PDA (aOR, 2.001; 95% CI, 1.126-3.556) were at significantly greater risk for adverse neurodevelopmental outcomes at age 2-3 years.

Conclusion.—Our results demonstrate that treatment for PDA may be associated with a greater risk of adverse neurodevelopmental outcome at age 2-3 years. This was particularly so among infants born at <25 weeks gestation. These results may support permissive tolerance of PDAs; however, reasons for this association remain to be elucidated through carefully designed prospective trials.

▶ This report on neurodevelopmental outcomes of all infants born before 29 weeks of gestation in New South Wales and Australian Capital Territory in 1998 through 2004 provides an important addition to the literature on the relationship between patent ductus arteriosus (PDA) and long-term outcomes in this vulnerable population. Prior studies amply show that PDA is associated with a variety of adverse outcomes, but data on neurodevelopment have been extensive. The reference group for this study was preterm infants who did not have PDA or who were not treated for PDA, but the authors do not report the number of infants who met the latter criteria. The authors report that "the usual management of a significant symptomatic PDA in the network region included a trial of up to 2 courses of cyclooxygenase inhibitor unless contraindicated, followed by surgical ligation if closure is not achieved," suggesting that most of, if not nearly all, infants in that group did not have a persistent or symptomatic PDA. Infants who did and were then treated with medical or surgical intervention to induce ductal closure, were at substantially greater risk for moderate-to-severe disability (as defined in the abstract), even after correction for potential confounders. The regression analysis can be criticized on several counts, including retention of variables not found to be significantly correlated with the outcome and handling gestational age as a binary variable ($<$vs $\geq$25 weeks of gestation), but the purported association of treated PDA with disability should be a cause for concern. However, the conclusion that "treatment for PDA may be associated with a greater risk of adverse neurodevelopmental outcome" is not exactly correct. What these data suggest is that PDA is associated with worse neurodevelopmental outcomes (as with other adverse outcomes), but the role of the diagnosis cannot be separated from the contribution of treatment. These data also do not address the question of whether PDA has a causal impact on long-term outcomes, which can only be answered by comparison of infants with confirmed PDA who receive treatment to close the ductus with similar infants who are treated expectantly—not with those whose ductuses are inconsequential or close spontaneously. As no group of infants with confirmed PDA who were managed expectantly is described in this report, these data do not "support permissive tolerance of PDAs," but that policy is amply supported by the 53 randomized, controlled trials of PDA treatment (to date) that have uniformly failed to demonstrate a benefit (other than closure of the ductus). What remains open to debate is whether some subset of preterm infants with PDA might benefit from early treatment or if closure of the ductus that remains patent for 2 to 3 weeks or more might be beneficial. It is odd that the burden of proof currently seems to fall on those who question the utility of such treatments rather than those who continue to advocate for them. Certainly, the late Dr. William Silverman would ask, "Where's the evidence?"

W. E. Benitz, MD

Late Diagnosis of Coarctation Despite Prenatal Ultrasound and Postnatal Pulse Oximetry

Lannering K, Bartos M, Mellander M (Queen Silvia Children's Hosp at the Sahlgrenska Univ Hosp, Gothenburg, Sweden)

Pediatrics 136:e406-e412, 2015

Objectives.—To determine what contribution prenatal ultrasound screening and neonatal pulse oximetry screening (POS) make to the timely diagnosis of neonatal coarctation of the aorta (CoA).

Methods.—We identified infants and fetuses diagnosed with isolated CoA in our referral area between 2003 and 2012 who died without surgery, underwent surgical repair before 2 months of age, or were terminated after a prenatal diagnosis. Clinical data were collected from hospital charts.

Results.—Only 3 of the 90 cases were diagnosed prenatally. Two of the 3 were born alive and in 1 case the couple opted for termination of pregnancy. Nineteen of the remaining 87 cases were born in units that used POS (hand and foot) and 4 of 19 screened positive. Of the remaining 83 cases, 46 were discharged undiagnosed (7 after nondiagnostic echocardiography), including 9 with a murmur and weak femoral pulses and 8 with a murmur and normal pulses. One was diagnosed postmortem after dying at home, and 22 of the remaining 45 discharged infants were in circulatory failure on readmission. Five of the patients who were not discharged died without surgery and undiagnosed CoA was the most probable cause of death in 2 of these patients.

Conclusions.—The contribution of prenatal ultrasound screening and postnatal POS to the timely diagnosis of CoA was low. Careful physical examination of all newborns therefore continues to play a fundamental role in detecting this life-threatening cardiac defect, and better screening methods need to be developed.

▶ As screening for critical congenital heart disease using pulse oximetry becomes routine in our nurseries, this report from Sweden provides a pointed reminder that we must not be lulled into a false sense of security about our ability to recognize all cases of significant congenital heart disease. Taking advantage of the data available within their integrated health care system, this population-based survey describes the trajectories of all 90 cases of critical coarctation of the aorta among approximately 360 000 infants born in their region over a 10-year period. It is not surprising that only 3 cases were diagnosed by prenatal echocardiography because this condition is notoriously difficult to recognize while the ductus arteriosus remains open. Pulse oximetry screening (POS) identified only 4 of the 19 infants so tested, reflecting a very low sensitivity (21%, 95% confidence interval 6%–46%) for this condition; 3 of these infants had additional findings identified on routine physical examination, indicating that the incremental yield of POS with respect to this condition is small. These technologies are clearly not reliable tools for ascertainment of infants with this condition.

Of the 83 infants not identified by prenatal echocardiography or POS, 53 had a murmur, weak femoral pulses, or both as the initial clinical sign (Table 1 in original article). Tachypnea was the initial finding in 14 infants. Fourteen infants presented in circulatory collapse, and 11 more experienced circulatory collapse after presenting with another clinical sign. Forty-six infants were discharged before diagnosis. Of the 45 who were readmitted, 22 were already in shock. The authors suggest that more rigorous diagnostic evaluation, including serial echocardiograms until coarctation is excluded after the ductus arteriosus is closed, might have averted some of those shock episodes. Remarkably, only 1 of the infants who were discharged died, at home at age 11 days. The other 5 deaths occurred in infants diagnosed before discharge, including 3 with other significant diagnoses (ELGAN at 26 weeks, congenital diaphragmatic hernia, group B *Streptococcus* sepsis, respectively). Nonetheless, at least 3 of the deaths in this series were potentially preventable. Avoidance of mortality and reduction of the risk for cardiovascular decompensation will have to rely on careful examination of all newborn infants, with particular attention to tachypnea and strength of the femoral pulses, over the first few days after birth. As these authors note, ensuring performance of an additional post-discharge examination of all neonates discharged before 48 hours of age may enable earlier identification of some infants with coarctation and is therefore essential. The contribution of physical examination skills to this process must not be underestimated.

W. E. Benitz, MD

Neurodevelopmental outcomes after neonatal cardiac surgery: Role of cortical isoelectric activity

Seltzer L, Swartz MF, Kwon J, et al (Univ of Rochester Med Ctr, NY; et al)
J Thorac Cardiovasc Surg 151:1137-1144, 2016

Objectives.—Neonates with congenital heart disease are at risk for impaired neurodevelopment after cardiac surgery. We hypothesized that intraoperative EEG activity may provide insight into future neurodevelopmental outcomes.

Methods.—Neonates requiring surgery had continuous intraoperative EEG and hemodynamic monitoring. The level of EEG suppression was classified as either: slow and continuous; moderate burst suppression; severe burst suppression; or isoelectric (no brain activity for >3 minutes). Follow-up neurodevelopmental outcomes were assessed using the Vineland Adaptive Behavior Scale II (Vineland-II).

Results.—Twenty-one neonates requiring cardiac surgery developed a slow and continuous EEG pattern after general anesthesia. Ten neonates (48%) maintained continuous brain electrical activity with moderate burst suppression as the maximum level of EEG suppression. Eleven neonates (52%) developed severe burst suppression that progressed into an isoelectric state during the deep hypothermic period required for circulatory arrest. However, the duration of this state was significantly longer than circulatory arrest times (111.1 ± 50 vs 22.3 ± 17 minutes; $P < .001$). At a mean follow-up at 5.6 ± 1.0 years, compared with neonates with continuous brain electrical activity, neonates who developed an isoelectric state had lower Vineland-II scores in communication. There was an inverse relationship between composite Vineland-II scores and duration of isoelectric activity ($R = -0.75$, $P = .01$). Of neonates who experienced an isoelectric state, durations of >90 minutes were associated with the lowest Vineland-II scores (125.0 ± 2.6 vs 81.1 ± 12.7; $P < .01$).

Conclusions.—The duration of cortical isoelectric states seems related to neurodevelopmental outcomes. Strategies using continuous EEG monitoring to minimize isoelectric states may be useful during complex congenital heart surgery.

▶ Although it is recognized that infants with congenital heart disease who require surgical correction/palliation in the neonatal period are at increased risk for impaired neurodevelopment, the mechanism(s) responsible for the delay remain elusive. In this study, data regarding electroencephalographic (EEG) activity during bypass surgery in the neonatal period and subsequent parental assessment of neurodevelopment at a mean of 5.6 years of age were compared. The children in the report had been enrolled previously in an observational study correlating intraoperative EEG activity and the onset of postoperative seizures.

Of the 26 eligible infants enrolled in the original study, data were available for 21. Evaluation of neurodevelopment was done with the Vineland—II, a parent questionnaire that assesses adaptive skills in multiple domains, including communication, motor function, activities of daily living, social skill, and maladaptive behaviors. Although children who experienced an isoelectric state had lower scores on the Vineland—II than those who did not, the overall mean scores were in the normal range for both groups.

The small sample size precluded performing multivariate analysis for other factors that are known to impact neurodevelopmental outcome including the type of heart lesion, the type of surgical intervention and the need for additional cardiovascular operative procedures. Thus, the authors' suggestion that the duration of isoelectric activity affects neurodevelopmental outcome negatively appears highly speculative.

L. A. Papile, MD

7 Respiratory Disorders

Efficacy and safety of surfactant replacement therapy for preterm neonates with respiratory distress syndrome in low- and middle-income countries: a systematic review

Sankar MJ, Gupta N, Jain K, et al (All India Inst of Med Sciences, New Delhi)

J Perinatol 36:S35-S47, 2016

Surfactant replacement therapy (SRT) has been shown to reduce mortality and air leaks in preterm neonates from high-income countries (HICs). The safety and efficacy of SRT in low- and middle- income countries (LMICs) have not been systematically evaluated. The major objectives of this review were to assess the (1) efficacy and safety, and (2) feasibility and cost effectiveness of SRT in LMIC settings. We searched the following databases—MEDLINE, CENTRAL, CINAHL, EMBASE and WHOLIS using the search terms 'surfactant' OR 'pulmonary surfactant'. Both experimental and observational studies that enrolled preterm neonates with or at-risk of respiratory distress syndrome (RDS) and required surfactant (animal-derived or synthetic) were included. A total of 38 relevant studies were found; almost all were from level-3 neonatal units. Pooled analysis of two randomized controlled trials (RCTs) and 22 observational studies showed a significant reduction in mortality at the last available time point in neonates who received SRT (relative risk (RR) 0.67; 95% confidence interval (CI) 0.57 to 0.79). There was also a significant reduction in the risk of air leaks (five studies; RR 0.51; 0.29 to 0.90). One RCT and twelve observational studies reported the risk of bronchopulmonary dysplasia (BPD) with contrasting results; while the RCT and most before-after/cohort studies showed a significant reduction or no effect, the majority of the case-control studies demonstrated significantly higher odds of receiving SRT in neonates who developed BPD. Two studies—one RCT and one observational—found no difference in the proportion of neonates developing pulmonary hemorrhage, while another observational study reported a higher incidence in those receiving SRT. The failure rate of the intubate-surfactant-extubate (InSurE) technique requiring mechanical ventilation or referral varied from 34 to 45% in four case-series. No study reported on the cost effectiveness of SRT. Available evidence suggests that SRT is effective, safe and feasible in level-3 neonatal units and has the potential to reduce neonatal mortality and air leaks in low-resource settings as well. However, there is a need to generate more evidence on the cost effectiveness of SRT and its effect on BPD in LMIC settings.

▶ This systematic review by Sankar et al analyzed the efficacy and safety of surfactant replacement therapy in preterm infants with RDS in resource-limited settings. Their conclusions, not surprisingly, were analogous to those in the developed world reported in the 1990s. There was an impressive improvement in survival, a reduction in air leaks, and no effect on the incidence of bronchopulmonary dysplasia (BPD; although the evidence is weaker here).

The issue of cost-effectiveness is more difficult to interpret for a number of reasons. As survival improves, the prevalence of BPD will increase. Will the infrastructure be able to support the increasing numbers of infants with chronic respiratory needs and higher risks for neurologic disability? This will have to be offset by the increased numbers of intact survivors. The impact on families also needs to be quantitatively measured. For instance, the need for a working mother to leave the workforce to care for a child with special needs has to be taken into account.

The countries from which the included studies arose are a varied group, and the methods of medical expenditures and reimbursements are often quite different. It may not be appropriate to extrapolate these findings. Nevertheless, these types of analyses may be helpful in negotiating with ministries of health to assure that our preterm population does not remain a therapeutic orphan.

S. M. Donn, MD

Late Surfactant Administration in Very Preterm Neonates With Prolonged Respiratory Distress and Pulmonary Outcome at 1 Year of Age: A Randomized Clinical Trial

Hascoët J-M, Picaud J-C, Ligi I, et al (Université de Lorraine, Nancy, France; Hôpital de la Croix-Rousse, Lyon, France; Assistance Publique-Hopitaux Marseille, France; et al)

JAMA Pediatr 170:365-372, 2016

Importance.—Although immature neonate survival has improved, there is an increased risk of developing bronchopulmonary dysplasia, leading to significant respiratory morbidity. Measures to reduce bronchopulmonary dysplasia are not always effective or have important adverse effects.

Objective.—To evaluate the effect of late surfactant administration in infants with prolonged respiratory distress on ventilation duration, respiratory outcome at 36 weeks postmenstrual age, and at 1 year postnatal age.

Design, Setting, and Participants.—Double-blind randomized clinical trial at 13 level III French perinatal centers. Participants included 118 neonates at less than 33 weeks gestation who still required mechanical ventilation on day 14 (SD, 2) with fraction of inspired oxygen of more than 0.30. All survivors were eligible for follow-up. We performed an intent-to-treat analysis.

Interventions.—Infants received 200 mg/kg of poractant alfa (surfactant) or air after randomization. At 1 year, after parents interview, infants underwent physical examination by pediatricians not aware of the randomization.

Main Outcomes and Measures.—The duration of ventilation was the primary outcome. The combined outcome of death or bronchopulmonary dysplasia at 36 weeks postmenstrual age and respiratory morbidity at 1 year of age were the main secondary outcome measures.

Results.—Of the 118 infants who participated in the study, 65 (55%) were male. Fraction of inspired oxygen requirements dropped after surfactant, but not air, for up to 24 hours after instillation (0.36 [0.11] vs 0.43 [0.18]; $P < .005$). Severe bronchopulmonary dysplasia/death rates at 36 weeks postmenstrual age were similar (27.1% vs 35.6%; $P = .32$). Less surfactant-treated infants needed rehospitalization for respiratory problems after discharge (28.3% vs 51.1%; $P = .03$); 39.5% vs 50% needed respiratory physical therapy ($P = .35$). No difference was observed for weight (7.8 [1.2] kg vs 7.6 [1.1] kg), height (69 [5] cm vs 69 [3] cm), and head circumference (44.4 [1.7] cm vs 44.2 [1.7] cm) measured at follow-up, nor for neurodevelopment outcome.

Conclusions and Relevance.—Late surfactant administration did not alter the early course of bronchopulmonary dysplasia. However, surfactant-treated infants had reduced respiratory morbidity prior to 1 year of age.

Trial Registration.—clinicaltrials.gov Identifier: NCT01039285.

▶ Surfactant treatments are standard of care for premature infants with a diagnosis of respiratory distress syndrome (RDS) or alternatively for infants shortly after birth with a high risk of RDS. Thus, infants normally are treated from minutes to 12 hours of age. Some infants develop progressive RDS beyond 12 hours of age or may be transferred to neonatal units at 2 or more days of age with untreated RDS. The efficacy of surfactant treatments for these older infants has not been formally studied, but the general clinical experience is that they often respond well to surfactant treatments. Based on metabolic studies in animals, the increase in pool size of surfactant in the airspaces after preterm delivery is a slow process, and thus delayed treatment of these infants is both rational and usually effective. The surfactant deficiency component of the pathophysiology of RDS should resolve by 5 to 7 days.

What then is a late surfactant treatment? Surfactant treatments for infants who had RDS or respiratory failure from other causes and continue to require supplemental oxygen and ventilation at 1 to 3 weeks of age have been discussed for surfactant treatment since the 1990s. Small observational reports and trials have demonstrated transient decreased oxygen requirements with surfactant treatments of ventilator-dependent infants, but the reports were underpowered to demonstrate a decrease in bronchopulmonary dysplasia (BPD) or other benefits. The rationale for the late surfactant treatments is that surfactant can be inadequate in amount or function in chronically ventilated infants, resulting in nonuniform regional ventilation, progressive injury, and inflammation that contribute toward progression to BPD.[1] The transient improvement in oxygenation demonstrates some short-term physiological response to the surfactant, which was again reported in the Hascoët trial. Airway samples from chronically ventilated infants can have decreased surface activity, decreased surfactant specific proteins, and increased inflammatory mediators. However, dysplastic type II cells in the lungs of infants and ventilated preterm baboons developing BPD are present in increased numbers and with increased intracellular surfactant. The surfactant dysfunction is likely to result primarily from abnormal surfactant metabolism and inactivation, which may not be effectively treated with more surfactant in an environment where inflammation and injury continue. This phase of early (1–2 weeks) and continual lung injury may be similar to acute RDS, which has not been successfully treated with surfactant despite multiple trials.

Two randomized and controlled trials of late surfactant for ventilator dependent extremely low birth weight infants were recently published.[2] Both trials enrolled infants with mean gestational ages of 25 to 26 weeks and very low birth weights. The ages of randomization and surfactant treatment were similar at 10 to 14 days. All infants were supported with conventional ventilation or high-frequency oscillation, and the infants in the Ballard trial also received inhaled nitrous oxide as a criterion for trial entry. Both trials used animal lung source surfactants but with different initial doses. The Ballard trial retreated the infants at 1- to 3-day intervals up to 4 times. There were no differences in the death, BPD or death, or BPD outcomes in the larger Ballard trial, which was stopped by the Date Safety Monitoring Board for futility. Despite large and repetitive doses of surfactant, there was no death or BPD benefit, which is a strong demonstration of no short-term effect with a minimal risk of a type I error.

The smaller Hascoët trial had no difference in death outcomes or in the combined death or severe BPD outcome ($P = .32$), but with an absolute decrease in severe BPD from 17% to 8.5% of survivors. This low percent of BPD is not easily evaluated relative to the Ballard results with a moderate and severe BPD rate of 60%. The Hascoët trial did not report the incidence of less severe BPD, which I assume would be high. If reproducible, a 50% decrease in severe BPD would be a significant benefit that could justify a larger trial. However, the resoundingly negative results for BPD in the Ballard trial tempers my enthusiasm. The more provocative finding by Hascoët et al is the decreased respiratory-related hospitalization in the surfactant-treated infants over the first year of life with less use of postdischarge steroids. These potentially important outcomes could result from type II error because of the small number of children followed to 1 year. However, an abstract of the 1-year outcomes for the Ballard trial, presented at the European Congress of Perinatal Medicine in June 2016 in Maastricht, Netherlands, demonstrated less home respiratory support and less of a composite assessment of pulmonary morbidity at 1 year of age. These results of improved late outcomes without substantial acute treatment effects are similar to other trials to decrease BPD. Recombinant superoxide dismutase had no effect on the incidence of BPD but the treated group had less respiratory abnormalities over the first year of life.[3] Another trial comparing high-frequency oscillatory ventilation with conventional ventilation did not decrease BPD, but pulmonary function studies were better at 11 to 14 years for the high-frequency group.[4] Similarly, early use of continuous positive airway pressure (CPAP) did not decrease BPD relative to intubation and surfactant treatment, but the CPAP group had less lung disease at 2 years.[5] This disconnect for intervention without large acute treatment benefits or effects on BPD that result in differences in longer term outcomes is a major challenge for all therapeutic research for BPD.

Does the concept of late surfactant for ventilator-dependent infants have a future? Yes, because there may be a new wrinkle. Yeh et al[6] recently published a trial of mixing the steroid budesonide with surfactant for the early treatment of RDS versus surfactant treatments alone. BPD was decreased substantially. The clear result from the Ballard and Hascoët trials is that late surfactant treatments are safe. Within the context of the Hascoët and Ballard trials where the use of postnatal steroids exceeded 72%, an option to explore is the addition of budesonide to a late surfactant treatment. The surfactant will facilitate the targeting and distribution of the steroid to the distal lung, which may be more effective and safer than systemic steroid treatments.

A. H. Jobe, MD, PhD

References

1. Keller RL, Merrill JD, Black DM, et al. Late administration of surfactant replacement therapy increases surfactant protein-B content: a randomized pilot study. *Pediatr Res.* 2012;72:613-619.
2. Ballard RA, Keller RL, Black DM, et al. TOLSURF Study Group. Randomized trial of late surfactant treatment in ventilated preterm infants receiving inhaled nitric oxide. *J Pediatr.* 2016;168:23-29.e24.
3. Davis JM, Parad RB, Michele T, Allred E, Price A, Rosenfeld WNorth American Recombinant Human CuZnSOD Study Group. Pulmonary outcome at 1 year corrected age in premature infants treated at birth with recombinant human CuZn superoxide dismutase. *Pediatrics.* 2003;111:469-476.
4. Zivanovic S, Peacock J, Alcazar-Paris M, et al. United Kingdom Oscillation Study Group. Late outcomes of a randomized trial of high-frequency oscillation in neonates. *N Engl J Med.* 2014;370:1121-1130.
5. Stevens TP, Finer NN, Carlo WA, et al. SUPPORT Study Group of the Eunice Kennedy Shriver National Institute of Child Health and Human Development Neonatal Research Network. Respiratory outcomes of the surfactant positive pressure and oximetry randomized trial (SUPPORT). *J Pediatr.* 2014;165:240-249.e244.
6. Yeh TF, Chen CM, Wu SY, et al. Intratracheal administration of budesonide/surfactant to prevent bronchopulmonary dysplasia. *Am J Respir Crit Care Med.* 2016;193:86-95.

Randomized Trial of Late Surfactant Treatment in Ventilated Preterm Infants Receiving Inhaled Nitric Oxide

Ballard RA, for the TOLSURF Study Group (UCSF Benioff Children's Hosp; et al)

J Pediatr 168:23-29, 2016

Objective.—To assess whether late surfactant treatment in extremely low gestational age (GA) newborn infants requiring ventilation at

7-14 days, who often have surfactant deficiency and dysfunction, safely improves survival without bronchopulmonary dysplasia (BPD).

Study Design.—Extremely low GA newborn infants (GA ≤28 0/7 weeks) who required mechanical ventilation at 7-14 days were enrolled in a randomized, masked controlled trial at 25 US centers. All infants received inhaled nitric oxide and either surfactant (calfactant/Infasurf) or sham instillation every 1-3 days to a maximum of 5 doses while intubated. The primary outcome was survival at 36 weeks postmenstrual age (PMA) without BPD, as evaluated by physiological oxygen/flow reduction.

Results.—A total of 511 infants were enrolled between January 2010 and September 2013. There were no differences between the treated and control groups in mean birth weight (701 ± 164 g), GA (25.2 ± 1.2 weeks), percentage born at GA <26 weeks (70.6%), race, sex, severity of lung disease at enrollment, or comorbidities of prematurity. Survival without BPD did not differ between the treated and control groups at 36 weeks PMA (31.3% vs 31.7%; relative benefit, 0.98; 95% CI, 0.75-1.28; $P = .89$) or 40 weeks PMA (58.7% vs 54.1%; relative benefit, 1.08; 95% CI, 0.92-1.27; $P = .33$). There were no between-group differences in serious adverse events, comorbidities of prematurity, or severity of lung disease to 36 weeks.

Conclusion.—Late treatment with up to 5 doses of surfactant in ventilated premature infants receiving inhaled nitric oxide was well tolerated, but did not improve survival without BPD at 36 or 40 weeks. Pulmonary and neurodevelopmental assessments are ongoing.

Trial Registration.—ClinicalTrials.gov: NCT01022580.

▶ Surfactant treatments are standard of care for premature infants with a diagnosis of respiratory distress syndrome (RDS) or alternatively for infants shortly after birth with a high risk of RDS. Thus, infants normally are treated from minutes to 12 hours of age. Some infants develop progressive RDS beyond 12 hours of age or may be transferred to neonatal units at 2 or more days of age with untreated RDS. The efficacy of surfactant treatments for these older infants has not been formally studied, but the general clinical experience is that they often respond well to surfactant treatments. Based on metabolic studies in animals, the increase in pool size of surfactant in the airspaces after preterm delivery is a slow process, and thus delayed treatment of these infants is both rational and usually effective. The surfactant deficiency component of the pathophysiology of RDS should resolve by 5 to 7 days.

What, then, is a late surfactant treatment? Surfactant treatments for infants who had RDS or respiratory failure from other causes and continue to require supplemental oxygen and ventilation at 1 to 3 weeks of age have been discussed for surfactant treatment since the 1990s. Small observational reports and trials have demonstrated transient decreased oxygen requirements with surfactant treatments of ventilator-dependent infants, but the reports were underpowered to demonstrate a decrease in bronchopulmonary dysplasia (BPD) or other benefits. The rationale for the late surfactant treatments is that surfactant can be inadequate in amount or function in chronically ventilated infants, resulting in nonuniform regional ventilation, progressive injury, and inflammation that contribute toward progression to BPD.[1] The transient improvement in oxygenation demonstrates some short-term physiological response to the surfactant, which was again reported in the Hascoët trial.[2] Airway samples from chronically ventilated infants can have decreased surface activity, decreased surfactant specific proteins, and increased inflammatory mediators. However, dysplastic type II cells in the lungs of infants and ventilated preterm baboons developing BPD are present in increased numbers and with increased intracellular surfactant. The surfactant dysfunction is likely to result primarily from abnormal surfactant metabolism and inactivation, which may not be effectively treated with more surfactant in an environment where inflammation and injury continue. This phase of early (1–2 weeks) and continual lung injury may be similar to acute RDS, which has not been successfully treated with surfactant despite multiple trials.

Two randomized and controlled trials of late surfactant for ventilator-dependent extremely low birth weight infants were recently published.[2] Both trials enrolled infants with mean gestational ages of 25 to 26 weeks and very low birth weights. The ages of randomization and surfactant treatment were similar at 10 to 14 days. All infants were supported with conventional ventilation or high frequency oscillation, and the infants in the Ballard trial also received inhaled NO as a criterion for trial entry. Both trials used animal lung source surfactants, but with different initial doses. The Ballard trial retreated the infants at 1- to 3-day intervals up to 4 times. There were no differences in the death, BPD or death, or BPD outcomes in the larger Ballard trial, which was stopped by the Date Safety Monitoring Board for futility. Despite large and repetitive doses of surfactant, there was no death or BPD benefit, which is a strong demonstration of no short-term effect with a minimal risk of a type I error.

The smaller Hascoët trial had no difference in death outcomes or in the combined death or severe BPD outcome ($P = .32$), but with an absolute decrease in severe BPD from 17% to 8.5% of survivors. This low percent BPD is not easily evaluated relative to the Ballard results with a moderate and severe BPD rate of 60%. The Hascoët trial did not report the incidence of less severe BPD, which I assume would be high. If reproducible, a 50% decrease in severe BPD would be a very large benefit that could justify a larger trial. However, the resoundingly negative results for BPD in the Ballard trial tempers my enthusiasm. The more provocative finding by Hascoët et al is the decreased respiratory-related hospitalization in the surfactant-treated infants over the first year of life with less use of postdischarge steroids. These potentially important outcomes could result from type II error because of the small number of children followed to 1 year. However, an abstract of the 1-year outcomes for the Ballard trial, presented at the European Congress of Perinatal Medicine in June 2016 in Maastricht, Netherlands, demonstrated less home respiratory support and less of a composite assessment of pulmonary morbidity at 1 year of age. These results of improved late outcomes without substantial acute treatment effects are similar to other trials to decrease BPD. Recombinant superoxide dismutase had no effect on the incidence of BPD, but the treated group had less respiratory abnormalities over the first year of life.[3] Another trial comparing high-frequency oscillatory ventilation with conventional ventilation did not decrease BPD but pulmonary function studies were better at 11 to 14 years for the high frequency group.[4] Similarly, early use of CPAP did not decrease BPD relative to intubation and surfactant treatment, but the CPAP group had less lung disease at 2 years.[5] This disconnect for intervention without large acute treatment benefits or effects on BPD that result in differences in longer term outcomes is a major challenge for all therapeutic research for BPD.

Does the concept of late surfactant for ventilator-dependent babies have a future? Yes, because there may be a new wrinkle. Yeh et al[6] recently published a trial of mixing the steroid budesonide with surfactant for the early treatment of RDS versus surfactant treatments alone. BPD was decreased substantially. The clear result from the Ballard and Hascoët trials is that late surfactant treatments are safe. Within the context of the Hascoët and Ballard trials where the use of postnatal steroids exceeded 72%, an option to explore is the addition of budesonide to a late surfactant treatment. The surfactant will facilitate the targeting and distribution of the steroid to the distal lung, which may be more effective and safer than systemic steroid treatments.

A. H. Jobe, MD, PhD

References

1. Keller RL, Merrill JD, Black DM, et al. Late administration of surfactant replacement therapy increases surfactant protein-B content: a randomized pilot study. *Pediatr Res.* 2012;72:613-619.
2. Hascoet JM, Picaud JC, Ligi I, et al. Late surfactant administration in very preterm neonates with prolonged respiratory distress and pulmonary outcome at 1 year of age: a randomized clinical trial. *JAMA Pediatr.* 2016;170:365-372.
3. Davis JM, Parad RB, Michele T, Allred E, Price A, Rosenfeld WNorth American Recombinant Human CuZn SODSG. Pulmonary outcome at 1 year corrected age in premature infants treated at birth with recombinant human CuZn superoxide dismutase. *Pediatrics.* 2003;111:469-476.
4. Zivanovic S, Peacock J, Alcazar-Paris M, et al. United Kingdom Oscillation Study Group. Late outcomes of a randomized trial of high-frequency oscillation in neonates. *N Engl J Med.* 2014;370:1121-1130.
5. Stevens TP, Finer NN, Carlo WA, et al. SUPPORT Study Group of the Eunice Kennedy Shriver National Institute of Child Health and Human Development Neonatal Research Network. Respiratory outcomes of the surfactant positive pressure and oximetry randomized trial (SUPPORT). *J Pediatr.* 2014;165:240-249.e244.
6. Yeh TF, Chen CM, Wu SY, et al. Intratracheal administration of budesonide/surfactant to prevent bronchopulmonary dysplasia. *Am J Respir Crit Care Med.* 2016;193:86-95.

Surfactant therapy and antibiotics in neonates with meconium aspiration syndrome: a systematic review and meta-analysis

Natarajan CK, Sankar MJ, Jain K, et al (All India Inst of Med Sciences, New Delhi)

J Perinatol 36:S48-S53, 2016

Meconium aspiration syndrome (MAS), a common cause of respiratory failure in neonates, is associated with high mortality and morbidity. The objectives of this review were to evaluate the effects of administration of (a) surfactant—either as lung lavage (SLL) or bolus surfactant (BS) and (b) antibiotics on mortality and severe morbidities in neonates with MAS. We searched the following databases: MEDLINE via PubMed, Cochrane CENTRAL, WHOLIS and CABI using sensitive search strategies. We included eight studies on use of surfactant and three studies on use of antibiotics. Neither SLL nor BS reduced the risk of mortality in neonates with MAS (relative risk (RR) 0.38, 95% confidence interval (CI) 0.09 to 1.57; and RR 0.80, 95% CI 0.39 to 1.66, respectively). Both SLL and BS reduced the duration of hospital stay (mean difference −2.0, 95% CI −3.66 to −0.34; and RR −4.68, 95% CI −7.11 to −2.24 days, respectively) and duration of mechanical ventilation (mean difference −1.31, 95% CI −1.91 to −0.72; and mean difference 5.4, 95% CI −9.76 to −1.03 days). Neonates who received BS needed extracorporeal membrane oxygenation (ECMO) less often than the controls (RR 0.64, 95% CI 0.46 to 0.91). Use of antibiotics for MAS did not result in significant reduction in the risk of mortality, sepsis or duration of hospital stay. Surfactant administration either as SLL or BS for MAS was found to reduce the duration of mechanical ventilation and hospital stay; BS also reduced the need for ECMO. Administration of antibiotics did not show any significant clinical benefits in neonates with MAS and no evidence of sepsis. Given the limited number of studies and small number of neonates enrolled, there is an urgent need to generate more evidence on the efficacy and cost-effectiveness of these two treatment modalities before recommending them in routine clinical practice.

▶ The incidence of meconium aspiration syndrome (MAS) appears to have dropped dramatically since our obstetrical colleagues became much more aggressive in limiting postdate pregnancies. As the frequency has waned, so has our respect for the potential dangers of MAS, well known to senior neonatologists but less so to our newer brethren. This review by Natarajan and colleagues examined the impact of systemic antibiotics and surfactant replacement therapy in infants with MAS. The rationale for the use of antibiotics generally stems from 3 reasons: (1) infection might be the stressor that led to meconium passage; (2) although sterile, meconium is a very good bacterial culture medium; and (3) infants who die from MAS often show signs of both inflammation and infection at postmortem examination. In this analysis, no beneficial effects, including for sepsis and mortality, were found in administering systemic broad-spectrum antibiotics.

On the other hand, surfactant administration, whether by bolus or lavage, seems to have a role in improving outcomes and reducing the need for extracorporeal membrane oxygenation (ECMO), although mortality was not reduced. The rationale, that meconium (and inflammation) inactivate surfactant and/or inhibit its production, seems to be borne out, because ventilatory courses were shorter, but there appear to be differences related to either bolus administration or lung lavage.

As the authors indicate, the numbers are small and the studies are very disparate, so interpretation must be done with caution. Nevertheless, the take-home messages are clear: (1) We should avoid the knee-jerk reflex of routinely initiating antibiotic therapy (unless there are other indications), (2) surfactant replacement therapy should be considered for infants requiring mechanical ventilation, and (3) further study is warranted.

S. M. Donn, MD

The Role of Surfactant Therapy in Nonrespiratory Distress Syndrome Conditions in Neonates

Keiser A, Bhandari V (Yale Univ School of Medicine, New Haven, CT)

Am J Perinatol 33:1-8, 2016

While treatment of respiratory distress syndrome (RDS) with surfactant in premature neonates is well established, evidence for its use in non-RDS conditions, especially in the term neonate, has been less abundant. The last published review on a PubMed search was in 2001. In this review, we comprehensively and critically evaluated the evidence from the literature regarding the use of surfactant in specific non-RDS disorders in neonates. Surfactant administered as a bolus should be considered in the treatment of meconium aspiration syndrome with progressive respiratory failure. While controversial in congenital diaphragmatic hernia, it should be considered in Group B streptococcal pneumonia. As evidence evolves, we anticipate the broader application and more routine use of surfactant therapy for respiratory failure because of causes other than RDS.

▶ This article by Keiser and Bhandari is a review of the use of exogenous surfactant for conditions other than respiratory distress syndrome (RDS) in the newborn. Surfactant has been used to treat RDS since the early 1980s, and there is little doubt as to its efficacy in this segment of the neonatal population, where surfactant deficiency is one of the pathophysiologic mechanisms of disease. Repletion of surfactant improves pulmonary gas exchange and lung mechanics. The authors of this article give a salient review of how other disease states can result in the inhibition of surfactant production or the inhibition of surfactant function, and they review the literature for its use in meconium aspiration syndrome (MAS; both bolus administration and lung lavage are addressed), pulmonary hypoplasia (secondary to both congenital diaphragmatic hernia and oligohydramnios-mediated), pulmonary hemorrhage, and pulmonary edema (secondary to bacteria and viruses; aspiration of amniotic fluid, maternal blood, enteral feedings, and bile acid accumulation from cholestasis of pregnancy), and respiratory distress after cardiopulmonary bypass. They concluded that the evidence supports surfactant replacement therapy in MAS. Other uses do not have a sufficient evidence base for routine use.

The authors did not address 2 additional potential uses of surfactant therapy. The first, using later surfactant therapy to prevent or ameliorate bronchopulmonary dysplasia, was studied in a small pilot trial and showed a potential signal for efficacy.[1] The second, which has also only received superficial attention, is the use of surfactant as a vehicle for delivery of pharmaceuticals directly to the lung. Yeh et al[2] showed a potential benefit of administering an intratracheal surfactant/budesonide mixture and obviated the need for systemic corticosteroids. Perhaps this approach might also work for antimicrobials, anti-inflammatories, and broncho- or vasodilating drugs. I have the feeling we are just scratching the surface.

S. M. Donn, MD

References

1. Laughon M, Bose C, Moya F, et al. A pilot randomized controlled trial of later treatment with a peptide-containing, synthetic surfactant for the prevention of bronchopulmonary dysplasia. *Pediatrics.* 2009;123:89-96.
2. Yeh TF, Chen CM, Wu SY, et al. Intratracheal administration of budesonide/surfactant to prevent bronchopulmonary dysplasia. *Am J Respir Crit Care Med.* 2016;193:86-95.

Comparisons and Limitations of Current Definitions of Bronchopulmonary Dysplasia for the Prematurity and Respiratory Outcomes Program

Poindexter BB, for the Prematurity and Respiratory Outcomes Program (Cincinnati Children's Hosp Med Ctr, OH; et al)
Ann Am Thorac Soc 12:1822-1830, 2015

Rationale.—Bronchopulmonary dysplasia is the most common morbidity of prematurity, but the validity and utility of commonly used definitions have been questioned.

Objectives.—To compare three commonly used definitions of bronchopulmonary dysplasia in a contemporary prospective, multicenter observational cohort of extremely preterm infants.

Methods.—At 36 weeks postmenstrual age, the following definitions of bronchopulmonary dysplasia were applied to surviving infants with and without imputation: need for supplemental oxygen (Shennan definition), National Institutes of Health Workshop definition, and "physiologic" definition after a room-air challenge.

Measurements and Main Results.—Of 765 survivors assessed at 36 weeks, bronchopulmonary dysplasia was diagnosed in 40.8, 58.6, and 32.0% of infants, respectively, with the Shennan, workshop and physiologic definitions. The number of unclassified infants was lowest with the workshop definition (2.1%) and highest with the physiologic definition

(16.1%). After assigning infants discharged home in room air before 36 weeks as no bronchopulmonary dysplasia, the modified Shennan definition compared favorably to the workshop definition, with 2.9% unclassified infants. Newer management strategies with nasal cannula flows up to 4 L/min or more and 0.21 *Fio2* at 36 weeks obscured classification of bronchopulmonary dysplasia status in 12.4% of infants.

Conclusions.—Existing definitions of bronchopulmonary dysplasia differ with respect to ease of data collection and number of unclassifiable cases. Contemporary changes in management of infants, such as use of high-flow nasal cannula, limit application of existing definitions and may result in misclassification. A contemporary definition of bronchopulmonary dysplasia that correlates with respiratory morbidity in childhood is needed.

Clinical trial registered with www.clinicaltrials.gov (NCT01435187).

▶ At a time when the spectrum of morbidities consequent on preterm birth has shown a steady decline, bronchopulmonary dysplasia (BPD) bucks the trend. The incidence of BPD in extremely low birth weight infants (< 1000 g) remains stuck in the 30% to 50% range. One factor that has been proposed to contribute to the problem is the absence of well-accepted diagnostic criteria for BPD. Few pathophysiologic disorders in medicine are defined by how they are treated!

The now successfully completed Prematurity and Respiratory Outcomes Program (PROP) was designed to characterize the natural history of respiratory morbidities in preterm infants of 23-286/7 weeks' gestation and characterize potential biomarkers of such morbidities. In the accompanying article, the PROP investigators compared 3 commonly and historically employed diagnostic criteria for BPD. It became immediately apparent that changes in contemporary practice greatly confound the traditionally used definitions. The greatest challenge is to accommodate the widespread use of nasal cannula flow, often in the absence of supplemental oxygen, into existing criteria. For example, if your patient is in 21% oxygen cannula at 36 weeks' postconceptional age, does that classify him or her as "no BPD" based on the Shennan definition? Furthermore, the inspired oxygen may be considerably diminished depending on the magnitude of cannula flow. For example, if your patient is receiving 24% oxygen in a 1 L/min cannula, would that correspond to > 30% in the absence of flow, and so confound the National Institutes of Health Workshop definition? The third or physiologic definition suffered from the largest number of infants who could not be classified.

A future optimal definition of BPD must somehow relate to longer term respiratory morbidity. This is a problem because long-term wheezing is prominent in a large proportion of preterm infants who meet none of our current BPD definitions. That leaves us with the traditional criterion of need for supplemental oxygen at 36 weeks' postconceptional age until further notice.

R. J. Martin, MD

Early Inhaled Budesonide for the Prevention of Bronchopulmonary Dysplasia

Bassler D, for the NEUROSIS Trial Group (Univ of Zurich, Switzerland; et al)
N Engl J Med 373:1497-1506, 2015

Background.—Systemic glucocorticoids reduce the incidence of bronchopulmonary dysplasia among extremely preterm infants, but they may compromise brain development. The effects of inhaled glucocorticoids on outcomes in these infants are unclear.

Methods.—We randomly assigned 863 infants (gestational age, 23 weeks 0 days to 27 weeks 6 days) to early (within 24 hours after birth) inhaled budesonide or placebo until they no longer required oxygen and positive-pressure support or until they reached a postmenstrual age of 32 weeks 0 days. The primary outcome was death or bronchopulmonary dysplasia, confirmed by means of standardized oxygen-saturation monitoring, at a postmenstrual age of 36 weeks.

Results.—A total of 175 of 437 infants assigned to budesonide for whom adequate data were available (40.0%), as compared with 194 of 419 infants assigned to placebo for whom adequate data were available (46.3%), died or had bronchopulmonary dysplasia (relative risk, stratified according to gestational age, 0.86; 95% confidence interval [CI], 0.75 to 1.00; $P = 0.05$). The incidence of bronchopulmonary dysplasia was 27.8% in the budesonide group versus 38.0% in the placebo group (relative risk, stratified according to gestational age, 0.74; 95% CI, 0.60 to 0.91; $P = 0.004$); death occurred in 16.9% and 13.6% of the patients, respectively (relative risk, stratified according to gestational age, 1.24; 95% CI, 0.91 to 1.69; $P = 0.17$). The proportion of infants who required surgical closure of a patent ductus arteriosus was lower in the budesonide group than in the placebo group (relative risk, stratified according to gestational age, 0.55; 95% CI, 0.36 to 0.83; $P = 0.004$), as was the proportion of infants who required reintubation (relative risk, stratified according to gestational age, 0.58; 95% CI, 0.35 to 0.96; $P = 0.03$). Rates of other neonatal illnesses and adverse events were similar in the two groups.

Conclusions.—Among extremely preterm infants, the incidence of bronchopulmonary dysplasia was lower among those who received early inhaled budesonide than among those who received placebo, but the advantage may have been gained at the expense of increased mortality. (Funded by the European Union and Chiesi Farmaceutici; ClinicalTrials.gov number, NCT01035190.)

▶ Bronchopulmonary dysplasia (BPD), regardless of definition, has challenged clinicians caring for extremely preterm infants for decades. Systemic corticosteroids address several conditions of protracted mechanical ventilation by reducing inflammation, decreasing pulmonary edema and fibrosis, minimizing capillary leakage and bronchospasm, and enhancing surfactant and antioxidant production. However, these benefits are accompanied by adverse effects, specifically, potential impairment of brain growth and risk of adverse neurodevelopmental outcome. Therefore, inhaled corticosteroids have been explored with great enthusiasm and caution given the potential for both benefit and adverse effect. Small studies historically show no impact, positive or negative. This year, the long-awaited Neonatal European Study of Inhaled Steroids (NEUROSIS) was published. The investigators randomly assigned 863 infants born at less than 28 weeks of gestation to inhaled budesonide or placebo within 24 hours of birth and continued until 32 weeks postmenstrual age or cessation of oxygen and positive pressure. The incidence of BPD (defined as positive pressure support, supplemental oxygen > 30%, or failure of the oxygen reduction test at 36 weeks postmenstrual age) was significantly lower in the treatment group (28% vs 38%, $P = .004$); however, the composite endpoint of death or BPD achieved only borderline significance (40% vs 46%, $P = .05$) because of a higher rate of death in the treatment group (17% vs 14%, $P = .17$).

These findings are difficult to untangle. A significant reduction in BPD was certainly plausible, given the adequate power, early initiation, and appropriate dosing of budesonide in this trial (higher than previous studies given poor deposition of inhaled therapies in the premature lung). The numerically higher mortality rate in the treatment group is challenging to explain and novel to this study. This result might well be attributable to chance, although infection, especially pneumonia, has been raised as a concern with inhaled corticosteroids. Regardless, the effect size for the composite endpoint is small, and long-term pulmonary and neurodevelopmental outcomes trump assessments at 36 weeks postmenstrual age. Follow-up of this study at 18 to 22 months is nearly complete. The fate of this therapy awaits those results.

C. McPherson, PharmD

Effect of early low-dose hydrocortisone on survival without bronchopulmonary dysplasia in extremely preterm infants (PREMILOC): a double-blind, placebo-controlled, multicentre, randomised trial

Baud O, for the PREMILOC trial study group (Université Paris Diderot, France; et al)

Lancet 387:1827-1836, 2016

Background.—Bronchopulmonary dysplasia, a major complication of extreme prematurity, has few treatment options. Postnatal steroid use is controversial, but low-dose hydrocortisone might prevent the harmful effects of inflammation on the developing lung. In this study, we aimed to assess whether low-dose hydrocortisone improved survival without bronchopulmonary dysplasia in extremely preterm infants.

Methods.—In this double-blind, placebo-controlled, randomised trial done at 21 French tertiary-care neonatal intensive care units (NICUs), we randomly assigned (1:1), via a secure study website, extremely preterm infants inborn (born in a maternity ward at the same site as the NICU) at less than 28 weeks of gestation to receive either intravenous low-dose hydrocortisone or placebo during the first 10 postnatal days. Infants randomly assigned to the hydrocortisone group received 1 mg/kg of hydrocortisone hemisuccinate per day divided into two doses per day for 7 days, followed by one dose of 0·5 mg/kg per day for 3 days. Randomisation was stratified by gestational age and all infants were enrolled by 24 h after birth. Study investigators, parents, and patients were masked to treatment allocation. The primary outcome was survival without bronchopulmonary dysplasia at 36 weeks of postmenstrual age. We used a sequential analytical design, based on intention to treat, to avoid prolonging the trial after either efficacy or futility had been established. This trial is registered with ClinicalTrial.gov, number NCT00623740.

Findings.—1072 neonates were screened between May 25, 2008, and Jan 31, 2014, of which 523 were randomly assigned (256 hydrocortisone, 267 placebo). 255 infants on hydrocortisone and 266 on placebo were included in analyses after parents withdrew consent for one child in each group. Of the 255 infants assigned to hydrocortisone, 153 (60%) survived without bronchopulmonary dysplasia, compared with 136 (51%) of 266 infants assigned to placebo (odds ratio [OR] adjusted for gestational age group and interim analyses 1·48, 95% CI 1·02–2·16, $p = 0·04$). The number of patients needed to treat to gain one bronchopulmonary dysplasia-free survival was 12 (95% CI 6–200). Sepsis rate was not significantly different in the study population as a whole, but subgroup analyses showed a higher rate only in infants born at 24–25 weeks gestational age who were treated with hydrocortisone (30 [40%] of 83 *vs* 21 [23%] of 90 infants; sub-hazard ratio 1·87, 95% CI 1·09–3·21, $p = 0·02$). Other potential adverse events, including notably gastrointestinal perforation, did not differ significantly between groups.

Interpretation.—In extremely preterm infants, the rate of survival without bronchopulmonary dysplasia at 36 weeks of postmenstrual age was significantly increased by prophylactic low-dose hydrocortisone. This strategy, based on a physiological rationale, could lead to substantial improvements in the management of the most premature neonates.

▶ Bronchopulmonary dysplasia (BPD) remains a common morbidity in premature infants, with lifelong implications for both pulmonary and neurocognitive health. Endogenous adrenal insufficiency commonly occurs in sick premature infants and has been linked to the development of BPD. Therefore, prophylactic hydrocortisone represents a relatively intuitive therapy with the potential to reduce the risk of BPD. However, investigation of this therapy has been wrought with complications. Most notably, a promising randomized, controlled trial in the early 2000s was truncated because of frequent concomitant use of open-label prophylactic indomethacin and the association of this dual treatment with a high rate of spontaneous intestinal perforation. Despite these pitfalls, the physiologic rationale for this pharmacologic intervention remains sound. In response, investigators in France recently published the PREMILOC trial. In this trial, 523 infants born at less than 28 weeks of gestation were randomized within the first 24 postnatal hours to 10 days of low-dose hydrocortisone or placebo. The rate of survival without BPD was significantly improved among infants in the treatment group (60% vs 51%, $P = .04$). Notably, this benefit was driven by females, who conferred a dramatic benefit from therapy compared with males, who demonstrated no difference in outcomes. Similarly to the previous truncated trial, infants exposed to chorioamnionitis also derived a disproportionate benefit from therapy. Increased late-onset sepsis was noted in the subgroup of patients born at 24 to 25 weeks of gestation (40% vs 23%, $P = .02$), but other adverse effects were not different between groups.

The expensive lessons of early dexamethasone remind us that short-term gains do not guarantee long-term benefits. Significant effort has been devoted to hydrocortisone, given strong preclinical data and several human studies suggesting no neurodevelopmental detriment. In fact, smaller trials have suggested potential neurologic benefit at 2 years of age. Unfortunately, recruitment of the present trial was also stopped early because of limited funding. This calls into question the power of this trial to detect benefit or detriment at later follow-up. Similarly, subgroup analyses to inform potentially targeted therapy might be limited. Even so, this trial once again offers caregivers the promise of another postnatal pharmacologic tool to assist in the effort to reduce BPD and improve neurodevelopmental outcome.

C. McPherson, PharmD

Association Between Intermittent Hypoxemia or Bradycardia and Late Death or Disability in Extremely Preterm Infants

Poets CF, for the Canadian Oxygen Trial Investigators (Tuebingen Univ Hosp, Germany; et al)

JAMA 314:595-603, 2015

Importance.—Extremely preterm infants may experience intermittent hypoxemia or bradycardia for many weeks after birth. The prognosis of these events is uncertain.

Objective.—To determine the association between intermittent hypoxemia or bradycardia and late death or disability.

Design, Setting, and Participants.—Post hoc analysis of data from the inception cohort assembled for the Canadian Oxygen Trial in 25 hospitals in Canada, the United States, Argentina, Finland, Germany, and Israel, including 1019 infants with gestational ages of 23 weeks 0 days through 27 weeks 6 days who were born between December 2006 and August 2010 and survived to a postmenstrual age of 36 weeks. Follow-up assessments occurred between October 2008 and August 2012.

Exposures.—Episodes of hypoxemia (pulse oximeter oxygen saturation <80%) or bradycardia (pulse rate <80/min) for 10 seconds or longer. Values were sampled every 10 seconds within 24 hours after birth until at least 36 weeks' postmenstrual age.

Main Outcomes and Measures.—The primary outcome was a composite of death after 36 weeks' postmenstrual age, motor impairment, cognitive or language delay, severe hearing loss, or bilateral blindness at

18 months' corrected age. Secondary outcomes were motor impairment, cognitive or language delay, and severe retinopathy of prematurity.

Results.—Downloaded saturation and pulse rate data were available for a median of 68.3 days (interquartile range, 56.8-86.0 days). Mean percentages of recorded time with hypoxemia for the least and most affected 10% of infants were 0.4%and 13.5%, respectively. Corresponding values for bradycardia were 0.1% and 0.3%. The primary outcome was ascertained for 972 infants and present in 414 (42.6%). Hypoxemic episodes were associated with an estimated increased risk of late death or disability at 18 months of 56.5%in the highest decile of hypoxemic exposure vs 36.9% in the lowest decile (modeled relative risk, 1.53; 95% CI, 1.21-1.94). This association was significant only for prolonged hypoxemic episodes lasting at least 1 minute (relative risk, 1.66; 95% CI, 1.35-2.05 vs for shorter episodes, relative risk, 1.01; 95% CI, 0.77-1.32). Relative risks for all secondary outcomes were similarly increased after prolonged hypoxemia. Bradycardia did not alter the prognostic value of hypoxemia.

Conclusions and Relevance.—Among extremely preterm infants who survived to 36 weeks' postmenstrual age, prolonged hypoxemic episodes during the first 2 to 3 months after birth were associated with adverse 18-month outcomes. If confirmed in future studies, further research on the prevention of such episodes is needed.

▶ Apnea of prematurity remains a subject of scrutiny for several reasons. It prolongs hospitalization and increases costs, it requires therapies such as ventilatory support that predispose to lung injury, it serves as a biologic link between the immature lung and central nervous system, and it results in intermittent hypoxic episodes. Whether these episodes of desaturation are of longer term consequence has been the subject of conjecture. Increasing sophistication of pulse oximeter downloads is now enabling us to determine which patterns of intermittent hypoxia are of prognostic significance.

Several years ago Di Fiore et al[1] reported an association between intermittent hypoxic episodes and retinopathy of prematurity. In addition to confirming this finding, Poets and colleagues have now documented an association between hypoxic episodes and adverse 18-month outcomes comprising late death or disability in a post hoc analysis of the Canadian Oxygen Trial [COT] cohort.

More specifically, this association was confined to longer episodes of intermittent hypoxia defined as an oxygen saturation <80% of at least 1-minute duration. Of interest is the observation that this association was strongest in the infants assigned to a higher (92%–95%) target oxygen saturation, presumably reflecting a steeper fall in oxygen saturation. It is tempting to speculate on the biological basis for the adverse effects of episodic desaturation. Prolonged, as opposed to short, desaturation may serve as an adverse oxidant stress, via the fall in oxygenation or its recovery, or both. In both animal models and adults with sleep apnea, the adverse effects of intermittent hypoxia and resultant oxidant stress are well characterized. This study goes a long way to begin to address this problem in the preterm population.

R. J. Martin, MD

Reference

1. Di Fiore JM, Kaffashi F, Loparo K, et al. The relationship between patterns of intermittent hypoxia and retinopathy of prematurity in preterm infants. *Pediatr Res.* 2012;72:606-612.

Association Between Intermittent Hypoxemia or Bradycardia and Late Death or Disability in Extremely Preterm Infants

Poets CF, for the Canadian Oxygen Trial Investigators (Tuebingen Univ Hosp, Germany; et al)

JAMA 314:595-603, 2015

Importance.—Extremely preterm infants may experience intermittent hypoxemia or bradycardia for many weeks after birth. The prognosis of these events is uncertain.

Objective.—To determine the association between intermittent hypoxemia or bradycardia and late death or disability.

Design, Setting, and Participants.—Post hoc analysis of data from the inception cohort assembled for the Canadian Oxygen Trial in 25 hospitals in Canada, the United States, Argentina, Finland, Germany, and Israel, including 1019 infants with gestational ages of 23 weeks 0 days through 27 weeks 6 days who were born between December 2006 and August 2010 and survived to a postmenstrual age of 36 weeks. Follow-up assessments occurred between October 2008 and August 2012.

Exposures.—Episodes of hypoxemia (pulse oximeter oxygen saturation <80%) or bradycardia (pulse rate <80/min) for 10 seconds or longer. Values were sampled every 10 seconds within 24 hours after birth until at least 36 weeks' postmenstrual age.

Main Outcomes and Measures.—The primary outcome was a composite of death after 36 weeks' postmenstrual age, motor impairment, cognitive or language delay, severe hearing loss, or bilateral blindness at 18 months' corrected age. Secondary outcomes were motor impairment, cognitive or language delay, and severe retinopathy of prematurity.

Results.—Downloaded saturation and pulse rate data were available for a median of 68.3 days (interquartile range, 56.8-86.0 days). Mean percentages of recorded time with hypoxemia for the least and most affected 10% of infants were 0.4%and 13.5%, respectively. Corresponding values for bradycardia were 0.1% and 0.3%. The primary outcome was ascertained for 972 infants and present in 414 (42.6%). Hypoxemic episodes were associated with an estimated increased risk of late death or disability at 18 months of 56.5%in the highest decile of hypoxemic exposure vs 36.9% in the lowest decile (modeled relative risk, 1.53; 95% CI, 1.21-1.94). This association was significant only for prolonged hypoxemic episodes lasting at least 1 minute (relative risk, 1.66; 95% CI, 1.35-2.05 vs for shorter episodes, relative risk, 1.01; 95% CI, 0.77-1.32). Relative risks for all secondary outcomes were similarly increased after prolonged hypoxemia. Bradycardia did not alter the prognostic value of hypoxemia.

Conclusions and Relevance.—Among extremely preterm infants who survived to 36 weeks' postmenstrual age, prolonged hypoxemic episodes during the first 2 to 3 months after birth were associated with adverse 18-month outcomes. If confirmed in future studies, further research on the prevention of such episodes is needed.

▶ An ongoing concern in the neonatal intensive care unit is the neurodevelopmental impact of repeated or severe hypoxemia or bradycardic episodes. In this article, a post hoc analysis was undertaken on the data that was collected in the Canadian Oxygen Trial in 25 hospitals internationally including 1019 infants with gestational ages less than 28 weeks of gestation. The authors analyzed the relationship of episodes of hypoxemia (pulse oximeter oxygen saturation < 80%) or bradycardia (pulse rate < 80/min) for 10 seconds or longer to neurodevelopmental disability at 18 months of age. They reported that hypoxemic episodes were associated with an estimated increased risk of late death or disability at 18 months of 56.5% in the highest decile of hypoxemic exposure versus 36.9% in the lowest decile (modeled relative risk, 1.53; 95% confidence interval [CI], 1.21–1.94). This association was significant only for prolonged hypoxemic episodes lasting at least 1 minute (relative risk, 1.66; 95% CI, 1.35–2.05 vs for shorter episodes, relative risk, 1.01; 95% CI, 0.77–1.32). Relative risks for all secondary outcomes were similarly increased after prolonged hypoxemia. Bradycardia did not alter the prognostic value of hypoxemia. They concluded that among extremely preterm infants who survived to 36 weeks' postmenstrual age, prolonged hypoxemic episodes during the first 2 to 3 months after birth were associated with adverse 18-month outcomes. If confirmed in future studies, further research on the prevention of such prolonged hypoxemic episodes is needed. It will be crucial for such intervention studies to be in a randomized controlled trial setting because whether such associations are causative has not been established with this observational study.

T. E. Inder, MD

Automated control of inspired oxygen in ventilated preterm infants: crossover physiological study

Lal M, Tin W, Sinha S (The James Cook Univ Hosp, Middlesbrough, UK)
Acta Paediatr 104:1084-1089, 2015

Aim.—To evaluate the efficacy of automated control of the fraction of inspired oxygen (FiO_2) in comparison with manual FiO_2 control in maintaining target pulse oxygen saturation (SpO_2) range.

Methods.—Crossover physiological study involving preterm infants requiring mechanical ventilation and supplemental oxygen. Each infant was studied for two consecutive 12 hours in a random sequence. Outcome measures included the proportion of time with SpO_2 within and outside the target range of 90–95%, extreme hypoxaemia (<80%) and hyperoxaemia (≥98%).

Results.—Complete data set was available in 27 infants. The percentage of time (median, IQR) within the target range was higher during automated control 72.8 (58.8–82.6) compared to manual control 59.6 (49.3–73.3), $p = 0.031$. Corresponding reduction in per cent time below the target range was 18.1 (12.7–23.6) versus 25.9 (17.8–30.7), $p = 0.028$, and above the target range 4.8 (3–16) versus 10.1 (6.4-22.5), $p = 0.026$. Median (IQR) per cent time spent with severe hypoxaemia (SpO_2<80%) and severe hyperoxaemia (SpO_2≥98%) was 1.3 (0.1–2.9) versus 3.2 (1.4–6.1), $p = 0.022$ and 0.08 (0.05–0.36) versus 1.7 (0.7–6.8), $p = 0.001$, respectively. Median number of manual adjustments of FiO_2 per 12 hour was 0 and 63, respectively.

Conclusion.—Automated control of FiO_2 significantly improved compliance of oxygen saturation targeting and significantly reduced exposure to hypoxaemia as well as hyperoxaemia.

▶ At a time when there is so much discussion in neonatology about optimizing oxygenation, automated control of supplemental oxygen to meet assigned oxygen saturation targets is very tempting. Several groups of investigators are exploring the efficacy of this technology. In the accompanying article, Lal and colleagues documented significant improvement in achieving a target range of 90% to 95% oxygen saturation with such automated versus normal control of inspired oxygen. This technique is being employed as a clinical tool in some European settings, and in the United States, the Food and Drug Administration is restricting its use to investigative study. It also requires incorporation in an Avea ventilator, which limits its use at this time.

In a parallel study, van Kaam and colleagues also documented a greater percent of in target oxygen saturation with such an automated supplemental oxygen delivery system.[1] In contrast to the Lal study, which only studied preterm infants receiving mechanical ventilation, van Kaam randomized infants on noninvasive as well as invasive respiratory support, again employing Avea ventilatory support with a built-in supplemental oxygen delivery function. Although both studies showed statistically significant benefit, the improvement in percent of time in target was relatively modest (in the 10% to 20% range) at 90% to 95% oxygen saturation targeting.

This is consistent with what has recently been learned from the large multicenter oxygen targeting trials: maintaining preterm infants within a narrow oxygen saturation target is a big challenge.

R. J. Martin, MD

Reference

1. van Kaam AH, Hummler HD, Willinska M, et al. Automated versus manual oxygen control with different saturation targets and modes of respiratory support in preterm infants. *J Pediatr.* 2015;167:545-550.

Automated versus Manual Oxygen Control with Different Saturation Targets and Modes of Respiratory Support in Preterm Infants

van Kaam AH, Hummler HD, Wilinska M, et al (Emma Children's Hosp AMC, Amsterdam, The Netherlands; Univ Med Ctr, Ulm, Germany; The Med Ctr of Postgraduate Education, Warsaw, Poland; et al)

J Pediatr 167:545-550, 2015

Objective.—To determine the efficacy and safety of automated adjustment of the fraction of inspired oxygen (FiO_2) in maintaining arterial oxygen saturation (SpO_2) within a higher (91%-95%) and a lower (89%-93%) target range in preterm infants.

Study Design.—Eighty preterm infants (gestational age [median]: 26 weeks, age [median] 18 days) on noninvasive (n = 50) and invasive (n = 30) respiratory support with supplemental oxygen, were first randomized to one of the SpO_2 target ranges and then treated with automated FiO_2 (A-FiO_2) and manual FiO_2 (M-FiO_2) oxygen control for 24 hours each, in random sequence.

Results.—The percent time within the target range was higher during A-FiO_2 compared with M-FiO_2 control. This effect was more pronounced in the lower SpO_2 target range (62 ± 17% vs 54 ± 16%, $P < .001$) than in the higher SpO_2 target range (62 ± 17% vs 58 ± 15%, $P < .001$). The percent time spent below the target or in hypoxemia (SpO_2 <80%) was consistently reduced during A-FiO_2, independent of the target range. The time spent above the target range or at extreme hyperoxemia (SpO_2 >98%) was only reduced during A-FiO_2 when targeting the lower SpO_2 range (89%-93%). These outcomes did not differ between infants on noninvasive and invasive respiratory support. Manual adjustments were significantly reduced during A-FiO_2 control.

Conclusions.—A-FiO_2 control improved SpO_2 targeting across different SpO_2 ranges and reduced hypoxemia in preterm infants on noninvasive and invasive respiratory support.

Trial Registration.—ISRCTN 56626482 (Fig 1).

▶ Tools at our disposal for respiratory support of sick infants have come a long way since the early days of infant ventilation, as the machines have acquired the ability to dynamically respond to infant signals to adjust the timing, frequency, duration, and amplitude of positive pressure breaths. Given the nominally simple relationship between inspired and arterial oxygen tensions, it is somewhat surprising that automation of fraction of inspired oxygen (FIO_2) adjustments, which would seem like easy pickings, has been much slower to reach the bedside. This report marks another step forward in that process. Using a patented proprietary algorithm that is not yet commercially available in the United States, these investigators showed that automated FIO_2 adjustment is capable of producing pulse oximetry distributions that are, at a minimum, comparable to those achieved by manual adjustments guided by a carefully specified practice guideline. In this sample of preterm infants receiving invasive or noninvasive respiratory support, the automated system increased the proportion of time

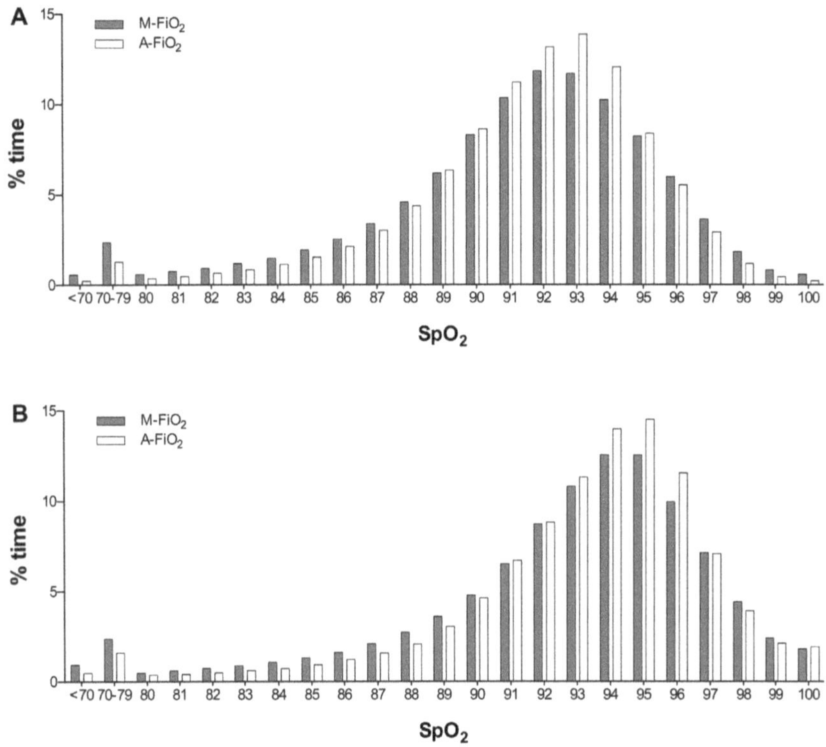

FIGURE 1.—Histograms of SpO_2 measured with pulse oximetry during 24 hours of M-FiO_2 and A-FiO_2 control in the groups of infants assigned to the SpO_2 target range of A, 89%-93% and B, 91%-95%. Data obtained while receiving 21% inspired oxygen are included in the histograms. (Reprinted from van Kaam AH, Hummler HD, Wilinska M, et al. Automated versus manual oxygen control with different saturation targets and modes of respiratory support in preterm infants. *J Pediatr.* 2015;167:545-550, with permission from Elsevier.)

for which the oxygen saturation as measured by pulse oximetry (Spo_2) was in the specified target range, but the gains were modest (increments of 8% and 4% in the low- and high-target range groups), and Spo_2 readings remained outside the target ranges more than one-third of the time. In contrast to prior reports, these gains were primarily achieved through reduction of the time less than the target ranges (Fig 1). Episodes of desaturation to less than 80% for ≥10 seconds that were followed by overcorrection to greater than the target range for at least 60 seconds did not differ between automated and manual control. Prolonged desaturation episodes (>1 minute) were markedly reduced with automated control (episodes of Spo_2 <80% from a median of 15 to 4 per day in the low-target range group and from 13 to 4 in the high-target range group [$P < .001$ for both]; <70% from 1 to 0.5 and 2 to 0.5, respectively [$P < .01$ and $< .001$, respectively]). It is not clear whether the latter will translate into better neurodevelopmental outcomes, despite the association of desaturations lasting more than 1 minute with increased risk of death or severe disability reported elsewhere. Until larger trials determine whether automated control produces better long-term results, the outcome-based case for adoption will remain weak. Virtual elimination of manual adjustments of FIO_2, from a median of 102 (interquartile range, 73–173) to 1 (0–3) per day in the low-target range group ($P < .001$) and from 109 (79–156) to 1 (0-3) ($P < .001$), which will free nursing time and attention for other tasks, may provide a compelling economic argument for adoption of this technology. The data provided in the Figure suggest that it is at least safe to do so.

W. E. Benitz, MD

Diode laser spectroscopy for noninvasive monitoring of oxygen in the lungs of newborn infants

Svanberg EK, Lundin P, Larsson M, et al (Lund Univ, Malmö, Sweden; Lund Univ, Sweden)

Pediatr Res 79:621-628, 2016

Background.—Newborn infants may have pulmonary disorders with abnormal gas distribution, e.g., respiratory distress syndrome. Pulmonary radiography is the clinical routine for diagnosis. Our aim was to investigate a novel noninvasive optical technique for rapid nonradiographic bedside detection of oxygen gas in the lungs of full-term newborn infants.

Methods.—Laser spectroscopy was used to measure contents of oxygen gas (at 760 nm) and of water vapor (at 937 nm) in the lungs of 29 healthy newborn full-term infants (birth weight 2,900–3,900 g). The skin above the lungs was illuminated using two low-power diode lasers and diffusely emerging light was detected with a photodiode.

Results.—Of the total 390 lung measurements performed, clear detection of oxygen gas was recorded in 60%, defined by a signal-to-noise ratio of >3. In all the 29 infants, oxygen was detected. Probe and detector positions for optimal pulmonary gas detection were determined. There were no differences in signal quality with respect to gender, body side or body weight.

Conclusion.—The ability to measure pulmonary oxygen content in healthy full-term neonates with this technique suggests that with further development, the method might be implemented in clinical practice for lung monitoring in neonatal intensive care.

▶ I wasn't quite sure whether to title this commentary "Building a Better Mousetrap" or "Buck Rogers meets Joseph Priestly." These investigators examined the potential use of low-intensity diode laser spectroscopy to determine the presence of oxygen in the lungs of newborns. Their ultimate goal appears to be replacing ionizing radiation as a diagnostic tool in the neonatal intensive care unit. Although the study certainly demonstrated the ability of the device to detect oxygen in the lungs, I do not yet see this as an "imaging" technique that will be able to distinguish the subtle differences between conditions such as respiratory distress syndrome and transient tachypnea of the newborn. As an adjunct to radiography, it might help to examine ventilation/perfusion mismatching or regional atelectasis. From a technical standpoint, application of the leads and use of the probe, as well as interobserver variability may limit its practical usefulness. Maybe "Not Ready for Prime Time Player" is the best description.

S. M. Donn, MD

Endotracheal Intubation in Neonates: A Prospective Study of Adverse Safety Events in 162 Infants

Hatch LD, Grubb PH, Lea AS, et al (Vanderbilt Univ Med Ctr, TN; Monroe Carell Jr Children's Hosp at Vanderbilt, Nashville, TN; et al)

J Pediatr 168:62-66, 2016

Objective.—To determine the rate of adverse events associated with endotracheal intubation in newborns and modifiable factors contributing to these events.

Study Design.—We conducted a prospective, observational study in a 100-bed, academic, level IV neonatal intensive care unit from September 2013 through June 2014. We collected data on intubations using standardized data collection instruments with validation by medical record review. Intubations in the delivery or operating rooms were excluded. The primary outcome was an intubation with any adverse event. Adverse events were defined and tracked prospectively as nonsevere or severe. We measured clinical variables including number of attempts to successful intubation and intubation urgency (elective, urgent, or emergent). We used logistic regression models to estimate the association of these variables with adverse events.

Results.—During the study period, 304 intubations occurred in 178 infants. Data were available for 273 intubations (90%) in 162 patients. Adverse events occurred in 107 (39%) intubations with nonsevere and severe events in 96 (35%) and 24 (8.8%) intubations, respectively. Increasing number of intubation attempts (OR 2.1, 95% CI, 1.6-2.6) and emergent intubations (OR 4.7, 95% CI, 1.7-13) were predictors of adverse events. The primary cause of emergent intubations was unplanned extubation (62%).

Conclusions.—Adverse events are common in the neonatal intensive care unit, occurring in 4 of 10 intubations. The odds of an adverse event doubled with increasing number of attempts and quadrupled in the emergent setting. Quality improvement efforts to address these factors are needed to improve patient safety.

► In this prospective observational study, conducted over a 9-month period, the effects of 273 endotracheal intubations performed in 162 patients were documented. Adverse events occurred in 39% of cases, with nearly 9% classified as severe. Predictors of adverse events included increasing number of attempts (doubling the odds) and emergent intubations (quadrupling the odds). Adverse events classified as nonsevere included esophageal intubations, oral or airway bleeding, difficult bag/mask ventilation, mainstem bronchus intubation, emesis, and chest wall rigidity. Some of these could certainly be considered severe.

I suspect that the results of this study are commonplace in today's neonatal intensive care unit. Twenty-five or so years ago, most neonatologists and pediatricians learned how to intubate and gained experience with meconium-stained babies. These newborns are seldom intubated nowadays, and pediatric residents spend much less time in neonatology training. Couple this with the changing demographics of the preterm population, and the recipe for disaster has been written. It is unfortunate for many reasons. For the baby, it is indeed a patient safety issue. For the trainee, it's a variant of not being able to get a job because of a lack of experience. For care providers, they are often placed in an uncomfortable position of "policing" the procedure and being the "bad guy" who terminates the attempt.

The authors suggest, rightly so, that the incidence of adverse events is probably higher than believed. The severity may also be higher than reported in this study because measures of central nervous system physiology (such as intracranial pressure or near-infrared spectroscopy) were not included.

The increasing popularity of noninvasive respiratory support may, on the one hand, decrease the prevalence of the problem, but on the other hand, the incidence may rise because intubations will occur is sicker babies who fail continuous positive airway pressure.

It is clear that as a discipline, we have a problem. It will require careful thought and adequate resources to solve.

S. M. Donn, MD

Premedication Use Before Nonemergent Intubation in the Newborn Infant

Muniraman HK, Yaari J, Hand I (SUNY Downstate School of Medicine, Brooklyn)

Am J Perinatol 32:821-824, 2015

Objective.—In 2010, an American Academy of Pediatrics (AAP) clinical report recommended that except for emergent situations, premedication should be used for all endotracheal intubations in newborns. The purpose of this study is to ascertain the current practice of premedication before elective intubation.

Study Design.—An online, survey-based questionnaire on the practice of premedication before nonemergent intubations was distributed via e-mail to neonatologists who are members of the Perinatal Section of the AAP.

Results.—Although 72% of respondents believed premedication should be used in nonemergent intubations, only 34% of the respondents report frequently premedicating before intubation with significant variation among the neonatal units (46% among level 4 units and 27% in level 3 and 2 units) p = 0.000. About 44% of respondents report having a written protocol or guideline on premedication which significantly correlated with the use of premedication (62% in level 4, 33% in level 3, and 16% in level 2 units), p = 0.000.

Conclusion.—Despite a recent AAP clinical report recommending the use of premedication before nonemergent endotracheal intubation, only one-third of neonatologists report frequent use of premedication and less than half of the institutions have a written protocol on premedication.

▶ It has been nearly 10 years since we published the results of a national survey reporting very similar findings to those of Muniraman and colleagues: that neonatologists infrequently premedicate newborns for elective endotracheal intubation.[1] Subsequent to our publication, the American Academy of Pediatrics Committee on the Fetus and Newborn issued a strong recommendation to premedicate in nonemergent situations.[2] Our group also demonstrated that having a protocol for such increases the frequency of premedication.[3]

The present survey sadly reports that almost nothing has changed in the past 10 years. This is a travesty. There is little doubt that intubation is a potentially harmful procedure, resulting in bradycardia, desaturation, and increased intracranial pressure, and is a very uncomfortable and possibly painful procedure. This practice would be unacceptable in a population that could verbalize pain and discomfort. Why are we allowing it to continue in newborns?

We see a lot of "repeat surveys" and often disregard them as "nothing new." This survey, despite the limitations of survey methodology, shows us that human behavior is difficult to change. Despite the fact that a majority of neonatologists believe that medication should be given, it isn't. "Do as we say, not as we do" is apparently ineffective.

S. M. Donn, MD

References

1. Sarkar S, Schumacher RE, Baumgart S, Donn SM. Are newborns receiving premedication before elective intubation? *J Perinatol.* 2006;26:286-289.
2. Kumar P, Denson SE, Mancuso TJCommittee on Fetus and Newborn, Section on Anesthesiology and Pain Medicine. Premedication for nonemergency endotracheal intubation in the neonate. *Pediatrics.* 2010;125:608-615.
3. VanLooy JW, Schumacher RE, Bhatt-Mehta V. Efficacy of a premedication algorithm for nonemergent intubation in a neonatal intensive care unit. *Ann Pharmacother.* 2008;42:947-955.

Endotracheal Suction for Nonvigorous Neonates Born through Meconium Stained Amniotic Fluid: A Randomized Controlled Trial

Chettri S, Adhisivam B, Bhat BV, et al (Jawaharlal Inst of Postgraduate Med Education and Res (JIPMER), Pondicherry, India)

J Pediatr 166:1208-1213, 2015

Objective.—To assess whether endotracheal suctioning of nonvigorous infants born through meconium stained amniotic fluid (MSAF) reduces the risk and complications of meconium aspiration syndrome (MAS).

Study Design.—Term, nonvigorous babies born through MSAF were randomized to endotracheal suction and nosuction groups (n = 61 in each). Risk of MAS, complications of MAS and endotracheal suction, mortality, duration of neonatal intensive care unit stay, and neurodevelopmental outcome at 9 months were assessed.

Results.—Maternal age, consistency of meconium, mode of delivery, birth weight, sex, and Apgar scores were similar in the groups. In total, 39 (32%) neonates developed MAS and 18 (14.8%) of them died. There were no significant differences in MAS, its severity and complications, mortality, and neurodevelopmental outcome for the 2 groups. One infant had a complication of endotracheal suctioning, which was mild and transient.

Conclusions.—The current practice of routine endotracheal suctioning for nonvigorous neonates born through MSAF should be further evaluated.

Trial Registration.—Clinical Trial Registry of India: CTRI/2013/03/003469.

▶ Chettri et al. performed an randomized controlled trial to assess the effect of endotracheal intubation and suctioning in a population of nonvigorous, meconium-stained infants. The trial took place at their institution in India. This is the first trial published to date that has assessed the potential benefits of the procedure in nonvigorous patients in a prospective randomized, controlled trial.

The standard of care for more than 40 years has been to intubate and suction nonvigorous meconium-stained infants. This has continued to be recommended even during the more than 15 years since it has been known that this procedure is not of benefit among vigorous infants. The retrospective and cohort data of the mid-1970s supported routine suctioning and intubation of all meconium-stained infants (the publications of Gregory et al[1]; Ting and Brady,[2] and Burke-Strickland and Edwards[3]). The American Heart Association website identifies an additional 7 observational studies indicating improved outcomes among all tracheally suctioned meconium-stained infants. These 10 studies noted better outcomes, including a considerably lower rate in the occurrence of meconium aspiration syndrome (MAS) among tracheally suctioned infants born through meconium stained amniotic fluid. None of these reports, however, were specifically limited to nonvigorous infants, nor did they examine lack of vigor as part of subgroup analysis. Because depressed infants are at greater risk for developing MAS, routine intubation and suctioning in the latter population has continued to be advocated despite the lack of supportive evidence in prospective randomized, controlled trials. Many clinicians and researchers believe that most aspiration of meconium occurs in utero before birth and would not be prevented by postnatal intubation/suctioning. Nevertheless, the data from the aforementioned publications are compelling in the face of appropriately sized RCTs providing contrary information.

Chettri and colleagues used the 40-year-old retrospective data of Ting and Brady to plan their sample size. However, the rate of MAS among babies born through MSAF has dropped substantially since the mid-1970s. The authors should have used more current data to determine their sample size. Indeed, the published rate of MAS in India (where the trial took place) is considerably lower than what the authors used to determine sample size. Other data, perhaps from the National Perinatal-Neonatal Data Base of India (which has been available for more than 10–15 years) could have been used. As a result, the Chettri trial was clearly too small in size and underpowered, a deficiency the authors acknowledge.

The demographic characteristics of the population appeared to support the study population consisted of truly "nonvigorous" infants—a high rate of Category III fetal heart rate tracings, low cord pH's, low Apgar scores, need for resuscitation, among other concerns.

A major criticism concerns the tracheal suction procedure in those infants randomized to suction. The authors report that negative pressure was produced by the "medflo wall suction device" at 80–100 mm Hg. However, we do not know whether there was any type of meconium suction aspirator interspaced between suction tubing and the endotracheal tube. Numerous such devices specifically for retrieval of meconium are available to connect between the endotracheal tube and the tubing coming from wall or portable suction. There is wide variability among devices in the quantity of meconium-stained fluid that can be retrieved. This is a critical piece of information not provided in the article. In the United States, the Neotech meconium aspirator is most commonly used. Moreover, it has been demonstrated that greater quantities of meconium may be retrieved when higher levels of negative pressure are used.[4]

There was a trend toward "other respiratory disorders" being more common in one of the groups ($P = .35$), but it is unknown in which group. It is unclear why the mean duration of "NICU stay" was so short (2.7–3.4 days) despite there being a considerable proportion of each group either mechanically ventilated, dying, having shock, or manifesting seizures. One would have expected a longer mean duration of "NICU stay" even had the majority of infants "recovered" in the first day or two following birth. We have no data concerning the causes of death in the 20% of infants that died, other than the 2 that died from sepsis. We do not know at what age infants died during the neonatal hospitalization.

The data in this report may not be able to be extrapolated to developed countries. In India, the rate of MAS in infants born through MSAF has been reported as 3 times or more common than in developed countries. The rate of MAS in the Chettri trial (31%–33%) was particularly high. No data were presented regarding use of high-frequency ventilation, surfactant, inhalational nitric oxide, or extracorporeal membrane oxygenation (ECMO). Most likely, none of these therapies were available. The persistent pulmonary hypertension of the newborn rate (3% and 7%) is exceptionally low, presumably because of the lack of echocardiogram data. The death rate seemed excessive (11%–12% during hospitalization and 19%–21% of all known infants by 9 months of age, excluding those lost to follow-up).

Chettri and colleagues final conclusion was that further evaluation is needed concerning endotracheal suctioning for nonvigorous neonates born through MSAF.

Of note, the latest recommendation concerning management of nonvigorous infants born through MSAF will appear in the seventh edition of the Neonatal Resuscitation Program (NRP) textbook, to be published in 2016. A preliminary version of the recommendation was recently published.[5] The authors of the latter publication considered the Chettri article to be of "low-quality evidence, downgraded for risk of bias and imprecision." In the 2016 NRP, there will be a major change in that routine intubation of nonvigorous infants born through MSAF is no longer "suggested" because of insufficient evidence to continue recommending the practice. As part of this new recommendation is the suggestion that appropriate interventions should be initiated as indicated for individual infants. This "may include intubation and suction if the airway is obstructed." In contrast, however, on the American Heart Association website concerning this topic, reportedly the agreed-on terminology for the recommendation was "We suggest that routine tracheal intubation for suctioning of meconium in nonvigorous infants should not be considered as a standard of care, but may be considered a reasonable alternative to no tracheal intubation if a meconium plug is suspected. There was concern that the legal profession could misinterpret the term standard of care." The authors of the document in *Pediatrics* and the upcoming NRP textbook acknowledge that a definitive clinical trial is still needed. This reviewer is not aware of any such large randomized controlled trials that are either being planned or are underway. If no such trial(s) are performed, hopefully large neonatal databases will be assessed over the next 5 years or so to evaluate whether the decision to change the recommendation was appropriate.

T. E. Wiswell, MD

References

1. Gregory, et al. *J Pediatr.* 1974;85:848-855.
2. Ting P, Brady JP. Tracheal suction in meconium aspiration. *Am J Obstet Gynecol.* 1975;122:767-771.
3. Burke-Strickland M, Edwards NB. Meconium aspiration in the newborn. *Minn Med.* 1973;56:1031-1035.
4. Bent RC, Wiswell TE, Chang A. Removing meconium from infant tracheae. What works best? *Am J Dis Child.* 1992;146:1085-1089.
5. *Pediatrics.* 2015;136:S196-S218.

Unplanned Extubation and Subsequent Trial of Noninvasive Ventilation in the Neonatal Intensive Care Unit

Nesbitt G, Guy KJ, König K (Mercy Hosp for Women, Melbourne, Victoria, Australia)

Am J Perinatol 32:1059-1063, 2015

Objective.—Unplanned extubation (UE) occurs as an infrequent complication of mechanical ventilation in the neonatal intensive care unit (NICU). Following UE, a trial of noninvasive ventilation (NIV) may be considered if a neonate is showing adequate respiratory effort. This study investigated the success and failure rate of NIV management of neonates experiencing UE.

Study Design.—Retrospective single-center study of neonates experiencing UE in the NICU over a 9-year period. Reintubation within 12 hours of a trial of NIV following UE was defined as treatment failure. Short-term respiratory outcomes were analyzed for all infants plus the incidence of bronchopulmonary dysplasia for preterm infants born less than 32 weeks' gestation.

Results.—A total of 43 patients were included. Of those, 30 infants were trialed on NIV following UE. Baseline demographics were similar between both the groups except for the oxygen requirement before UE. The NIV was successful in 20 and failed in 10 infants. Infants who failed a trial of the NIV were reintubated between 0.45 and 5.25 hours following UE. Respiratory outcomes in very preterm infants did not differ between groups.

Conclusion.—A trial of NIV may be considered as a treatment option in preterm and term newborns experiencing UE in the NICU.

▶ This retrospective observation examined the responsiveness to noninvasive respiratory support in a group of preterm infants who had inadvertent or "unplanned" extubations. It was a retrospective, single-center experience and thus subjected to enormous selection bias that was further complicated by a very small sample size compiled over a relatively long (9-year) observation period. What can be learned from this report? Some infants self-extubate, some can be supported by noninvasive means, those who succeeded probably should have been electively extubated, and if we examine enough variables and do not apply a Bonferroni correction, something just might be statistically significant. Or not.

How does this stuff get published?

S. M. Donn, MD

Effect of Meconium-Stained Amniotic Fluid on Perinatal Complications in Low-Risk Pregnancies at Term

Hiersch L, Krispin E, Aviram A, et al (Tel Aviv Univ, Israel)

Am J Perinatol 33:378-384, 2016

Objective.—This study aims to determine the impact of meconium-stained amniotic fluid (MSAF) in low-risk pregnancies at term on pregnancy outcome.

Study Design.—A retrospective cohort study of women with MSAF during labor who delivered in a tertiary hospital at 37 to 41^{+6} weeks of gestation (2007–2013). Exclusion criteria included: multiple gestations, noncephalic presentation, fetal structural/chromosomal anomalies, hypertensive disorders, diabetes, oligohydramnios, or small for gestational age. Pregnancy outcome of women with MSAF ($N = 4{,}893$) was compared with a control group of women without MSAF ($N = 39{,}651$). Neonatal respiratory morbidity was defined as the presence of any of the following: respiratory distress syndrome, transient tachypnea of the newborn, meconium aspiration syndrome, or need for ventilatory support.

Results.—Overall, 10.9% of low-risk pregnancies at term were diagnosed with MSAF. Compared with the controls, women with MSAF had higher rates of nulliparity, gestational age at delivery ≥41 weeks, induction of labor, nonreassuring fetal heart rate, and operative deliveries. In multivariate analysis MSAF was associated with operative delivery (odds ratio [OR], 1.82; 95% confidence interval [CI], 1.63–2.09; $p < 0.001$), cesarean section (OR, 1.48; 95% CI, 1.31–1.69; $p < 0.001$), respiratory morbidity (OR, 4.74; 95% CI, 3.87–5.82; $p < 0.001$), and increased risk for short-term neonatal morbidity.

Conclusions.—MSAF is associated with a higher rate of adverse perinatal outcome even in low-risk pregnancies at term.

▶ This large cohort study attempted to address the effect of meconium passage in utero with perinatal complications in pregnancies deemed to be low-risk between 37 and 42 weeks of gestation. Meconium-stained amniotic fluid was found to be associated with a higher incidence of perinatal morbidities, including operative delivery/cesarean delivery, neonatal respiratory morbidity, and an increased risk of other short-term neonatal morbidity (including seizures, hypoxic-ischemic encephalopathy, and hypoglycemia).

The authors acknowledge the weaknesses of the study, including its retrospective nature, lack of information regarding the timing of meconium passage, and other important confounders, such as maternal obesity and smoking. Exclusions included chronic maternal disease, uncertain gestational age dating, anomalies, nonvertex presentations, maternal diabetes, oligohydramnios, growth restriction, and suspected chorioamnionitis. Thus, presumably the study examined only the passage of meconium on outcomes.

A larger weakness of the study can be attributed to the choice of definitions used to characterize neonatal morbidities. The investigators defined hypoxic-ischemic encephalopathy, for instance, on the basis of an umbilical arterial pH < 7.1 or an

Apgar score < 7 at 5 minutes and a neonatal seizure occurring in the first 24 hours of life. These are rather soft and might have resulted in an overstatement of these problems. Bonferroni correction was not applied to statistical analyses either.

The database was limited to 37 to 42 weeks' gestation. What might have been more meaningful is an analysis of whether the morbidities increased with advancing gestational age. We have certainly seen the incidence of deliveries beyond 42 weeks drop dramatically, and perhaps not going beyond 40 weeks is equally impactful.

S. M. Donn, MD

High-flow nasal cannulae are associated with increased diaphragm activation compared with nasal continuous positive airway pressure in preterm infants

Nasef N, El-Gouhary E, Schurr P, et al (Sunnybrook Health Sciences Centre, Toronto, Ontario, Canada; et al)

Acta Paediatr 104:e337-e343, 2015

Aim.—High-flow nasal cannulae (HFNC) are increasingly used for respiratory management of preterm infants. However, their ability to provide support compared to nasal continuous positive airway pressure (CPAP) has been questioned. We compared the effect of HFNC versus nasal CPAP on diaphragm electrical activity (EAdi) in preterm infants.

Methods.—Preterm infants ≤1500 g were randomised in a crossover design to receive 2 hours of either Infant Flow® CPAP (IF-CPAP) at 5–6 cmH_2O or HFNC with the flow rate adjusted to achieve an equivalent pharyngeal pressure. A feeding catheter with miniaturised sensors was inserted for continuous EAdi measurement.

Results.—The study comprised ten infants. Physiologic parameters and oxygen requirements were not different between the two modes. However, seven infants demonstrated a higher EAdi peak and six showed a higher EAdi tonic on HFNC, even though the mean group data showed no difference between HFNC and IF-CPAP. Neural inspiratory time was significantly longer with HFNC than IF-CPAP (0.55 ± 0.11 versus 0.48 ± 0.06 seconds, $p = 0.018$).

Conclusion.—In this cohort of preterm infants, the majority exhibited greater diaphragm activation, as assessed by neural breathing patterns, when supported with HFNC than IFCPAP, suggesting that nasal CPAP may provide more effective respiratory support.

▶ Publication of a handful of short-term observations in a small number of preterm infants in 2001 was followed by rapid and widespread adoption of high-flow nasal cannula (HFNC) therapy as an alternative to continuous positive airway pressure (CPAP) in infants and children with respiratory failure. Understanding of how HFNC works and evidence to guide its use have been slow to develop but are gradually accruing. Several beneficial effects of HFNC have been proposed, including washout of the nasopharyngeal dead space and maintenance of functional residual capacity through delivery of distending airway pressure. Despite the small number of subjects studied and marginal statistical significance, this study suggests that the former may be more important than the latter, at least with HFNC as implemented by these investigators. The important implication is that HFNC may be well suited to support infants whose chest wall mechanics are sufficient to maintain functional residual capacity (FRC) but who do not have the strength or stamina to maintain normocapnia, or in whom modest hypercapnia predisposes to apnea episodes because reduction in dead space can be expected to improve carbon dioxide removal. If support of FRC is required or if the objective is modification of pulmonary blood flow (as in infants with left-to-right shunts), the more predictable increases in airway distending pressure achieved with CPAP devices may be preferable. As familiarity with these options grows, the question should not be simply which is better but which is better for management of different specific pathophysiologies, and how they are best applied in those circumstances.

W. E. Benitz, MD

Impact of Prophylactic Continuous Positive Airway Pressure on Transient Tachypnea of the Newborn and Neonatal Intensive Care Admission in Newborns Delivered by Elective Cesarean Section

Celebi MY, Alan S, Kahvecioglu D, et al (Ankara Univ School of Medicine, Turkey; Hitit Univ Corum Training and Res Hosp, Corum, Turkey)
Am J Perinatol 33:99-106, 2016

Objective.—This study aims to evaluate the effect of the prophylactic continuous positive airway pressure (CPAP) administration in the delivery room to newborns who were delivered by elective cesarean section (CS).

Study Design.—Inborn infants with gestational age between $34^{0/7}$ to $38^{6/7}$ and born by elective CS were prospectively randomized to receive either prophylactic CPAP for 20 minutes via face mask or standardized care without CPAP in the delivery room. Primary outcomes were the incidence of transient tachypnea of the newborn (TTN) and neonatal intensive care unit (NICU) admission due to respiratory distress.

Results.—A total of 259 infants with a mean gestational age of 37.7 ± 0.8 weeks and birth weight of 3,244 ± 477 g were included. A total of 134 infants received prophylactic CPAP and 125 received control standard care. The rate of NICU admission was significantly lower in prophylactic CPAP group ($p = 0.045$). Although the rate of TTN was lower in the prophylactic CPAP group, the difference was not statistically significant ($p = 0.059$). The rate of NICU admission due to respiratory distress was significantly higher in late-preterm cohort than early-term cohort ($p < 0.0001$).

Conclusion.—Prophylactic CPAP administration decreases the rate of NICU admission without any side effect in late-preterm and early-term infants delivered by elective CS.

▶ In this study, a group of Turkish investigators hypothesized that prophylactic continuous positive airway pressure (CPAP) after elective cesarean delivery would be beneficial in reducing the severity of transient tachypnea of the newborn (TTNB). They randomized 259 infants between 34 and 39 weeks to treatment or control arms in the delivery room. The treatment group received CPAP (5–6 cm H_2O) and 24% to 30% oxygen by mask, whereas the control arm did not. Outcome measures were the incidence of TTNB and admission to the neonatal intensive care unit (NICU).

Sample size calculations were made based on the predicted incidence of TTNB of 4.2%. A total of 825 infants were eligible, but only 259 (31%) were enrolled. Differences in the incidence of TTNB between groups failed to reach statistical significance, but there were fewer NICU admissions attributable to TTNB (3% vs 8.8%, $P = .045$).

The authors focused on the latter finding as the success of the trial. However, (1) the study was not masked, and bias cannot be excluded; (2) the study does not appear to have been powered for this outcome parameter; and (3) admission criteria appear to be both soft and subjective. Morbidity related to CPAP was not addressed.

The number needed to treat for both outcome measures was very high, 18 for NICU admission and 25 for TTNB. I don't think I'm ready to try this.

S. M. Donn, MD

A randomised controlled trial of flow driver and bubble continuous positive airway pressure in preterm infants in a resource-limited setting

Mazmanyan P, Mellor K, Doré CJ, et al (Scientific Res Centre of Maternal and Child Health, Yerev, Armenia; BirthLink, London, UK; Med Res Council Clinical Trials Unit at Univ College London, UK; et al)

Arch Dis Child Fetal Neonatal Ed 101:F16-F20, 2016

Objectives.—The variable-flow flow driver (FD; EME) and continuous-flow bubble (Fisher-Paykel) continuous positive airway pressure (CPAP) systems are widely used. As these differ in cost and technical requirements, determining comparative efficacy is important particularly where resources are limited.

Design.—We performed a randomised, controlled, equivalence trial of CPAP systems. We specified the margin of equivalence as 2 days. We analysed binary variables by logistical regression adjusted for gestation, and log transformed continuous variables by multiple linear regression adjusted for gestation, sex and antenatal steroids.

Setting.—A neonatal unit with no blood gas analyser or surfactant availability and limited X-ray and laboratory facilities.

Patients.—Neonates <37 weeks of gestation.
Interventions.—We provided CPAP at delivery followed by randomisation to FD or bubble (B).
Outcomes.—Primary outcome included total days receiving CPAP; secondary outcomes included days receiving CPAP, supplemental oxygen, ventilation, death, pneumothorax and nasal excoriation.
Results.—We randomised 125 infants (B 66, FD 59). Differences in infant outcomes on B and FD were not statistically significant. The median (range) for CPAP days for survivors was B 0.8 (0.04 to 17.5), FD 0.5 (0.04 to 5.3). B:FD (95% CI) ratios were CPAP days 1.3 (0.9 to 2.1), CPAP plus supplementary oxygen days 1.2 (0.7 to 1.9). B:FD (95% CI) ORs were death 2.3 (0.2 to 28), ventilation 2.1 (0.5 to 9), nasal excoriation 1.2 (0.2 to 8) and pneumothorax 2.4 (0.2 to 26).
Conclusions.—In a resource-limited setting we found B CPAP equivalent to FD CPAP in the total number of days receiving CPAP within a margin of 2 days.
Trial Registration Number.—ISRCTN22578364.

▶ Mazmanyan and colleagues performed a randomized controlled trial of variable flow and constant flow CPAP in babies less than 37 weeks' gestation in an Armenian hospital. Eligible infants were randomized to treatment with either bubble continuous positive airway pressure (CPAP; Fisher-Paykel) or flow-driven CPAP (EME) in an equivalency trial that used a 2-day margin of equivalence. In this setting, there was neither surfactant therapy nor blood gas analyses and only limited radiographic assessment. Investigators randomized 125 infants and found the 2 CPAP devices to be equivalent with respect to total days of CPAP, supplemental oxygen, need for ventilation, survival, pneumothorax, and nasal excoriation. They concluded that the 2 CPAP generators were equivalent and that bubble CPAP is a relatively simple and inexpensive technology that can be successfully applied in this setting.

This type of clinical trial is essential in resource-limited settings. Although the study did not address cost-effectiveness, it is clear that the bubble CPAP device is less expensive and thus easier to implement. Moreover, this study was performed without funding and produced results relevant to the setting in which the trial was conducted. The question remains as to whether these results will be exportable to other resource-limited or developing countries. Importantly, however, the methodology is exportable for addressing device issues elsewhere. For this, I congratulate the investigators.

S. M. Donn, MD

Conventional Mechanical Ventilation Versus High-frequency Oscillatory Ventilation for Congenital Diaphragmatic Hernia: A Randomized Clinical Trial (The VICI-trial)

Snoek KG, on behalf of the CDH EURO Consortium (Erasmus Med Centre-Sophia Children's Hosp, Rotterdam, The Netherlands; et al)

Ann Surg 263:867-874, 2016

Objectives.—To determine the optimal initial ventilation mode in congenital diaphragmatic hernia.

Background.—Congenital diaphragmatic hernia is a life-threatening anomaly with significant mortality and morbidity. The maldeveloped lungs have a high susceptibility for oxygen and ventilation damage resulting in a high incidence of bronchopulmonary dysplasia (BPD) and chronic respiratory morbidity.

Methods.—An international, multicenter study (NTR 1310), the VICI-trial was performed in prenatally diagnosed congenital diaphragmatic hernia infants (n = 171) born between November 2008 and December 2013, who were randomized for initial ventilation strategy.

Results.—Ninety-one (53.2%) patients initially received conventional mechanical ventilation and 80 (46.8%) high-frequency oscillation. Forty-one patients (45.1%) randomized to conventional mechanical ventilation died/ had BPD compared with 43 patients (53.8%) in the high-frequency oscillation group. An odds ratio of 0.62 [95% confidence interval (95% CI) 0.25–1.55] ($P = 0.31$) for death/BPD for conventional mechanical ventilation vs high-frequency oscillation was demonstrated, after adjustment for center, head-lung ratio, side of the defect, and liver position. Patients initially ventilated by conventional mechanical ventilation were ventilated for fewer days ($P = 0.03$), less often needed extracorporeal membrane oxygenation support ($P = 0.007$), inhaled nitric oxide ($P = 0.045$), sildenafil ($P = 0.004$), had a shorter duration of vasoactive drugs ($P = 0.02$), and less often failed treatment ($P = 0.01$) as compared with infants initially ventilated by high-frequency oscillation.

Conclusions.—Our results show no statistically significant difference in the combined outcome of mortality or BPD between the 2 ventilation groups in prenatally diagnosed congenital diaphragmatic hernia infants. Other outcomes, including shorter ventilation time and lesser need of extracorporeal membrane oxygenation, favored conventional ventilation.

▶ Successful management of the infant with a congenital diaphragmatic hernia (CDH) remains an elusive challenge. This study attempted to define the optimal initial ventilation strategy and compared conventional mechanical ventilation (CMV) and high-frequency oscillatory ventilation (HFOV) in an international randomized clinical trial. Infants with a prenatal diagnosis of CDH who were > 34 weeks of gestation were eligible for randomization providing they did not have an exclusionary criterion likely to confound the results. The authors concluded that there were no differences in the primary outcome (death or

BPD) and that secondary outcomes such as duration of ventilation and less need for extracorporeal membrane oxygenation (ECMO) favored infants randomized to CMV.

Although I applaud the effort of the VICI trial group to address this issue through a well-planned randomized controlled trial, there are both methodological and ethical issues that must be addressed before we accept its findings and conclusions.

The management of infants was standardized by using the CDH EURO consortium protocol, but it appears that multiple devices for both CMV and HFOV were used. Moreover, designing a trial that dictates the initial ventilator settings rather than allowing individual settings based on individual pathophysiology is likely to result in few patients receiving what they actually need. In the CMV group, the initial peak inspiratory pressure was limited to 20 to 25 cm H_2O and positive end expiratory pressure was surprisingly initiated at only 3 to 5 cm H_2O. Despite using triggered ventilation, control rates were set at 40 to 60 beats/min, which discourages spontaneous breathing. In the HFOV group, a mean airway pressure of 13 to 17 cm H_2O was used with a rate that was relatively high (10–12 Hz) and an amplitude of 30 to 50 cm H_2O. Thus, the strategy essentially assigned much higher pressures to the HFOV group.

Conducting the trial in centers not able to provide ECMO to subjects failing either CMV or HFOV could certainly have altered mortality rates and encouraged crossover. The use of sildenafil to treat elevated pulmonary pressure is an off-label application with unproven efficacy and unknown safety.[1]

Finally, the trial did not reach its intended enrollment. It was terminated early because of slower than anticipated enrollment, lack of resources, and "a lack of research infrastructure in 1 high-volume center."

This study demonstrates the difficulties in studying a multifactorial disease process, but it also shows that great care must be taken to design comparable study arms. The hypothesis going in was that a considerable proportion of infants with CDH sustain ventilator-induced lung injury, which compounds the problems of pulmonary hypoplasia and pulmonary hypertension. If the goal is to reduce barotrauma and volutrauma, perhaps the strategy adopted here was wrong. A better high-frequency option (although not used in Europe) might be high-frequency jet ventilation, which has been used with increasing success in some US centers.[2]

S. M. Donn, MD

References

1. Bhatt-Mehta V, Donn SM. Sildenafil for pulmonary hypertension complicating bronchopulmonary dysplasia. *Expert Rev Clin Pharmacol*. 2014;7:393-395.
2. Zhang Q, Macartney J, Sampaio L, O'Brien K. High frequency jet ventilation during initial management, stabilization, and transport of newborn infants with congenital diaphragmatic hernia: a case series. *Crit Care Res Pract*. 2013;2013:937871.

Effects of Multiple Ventilation Courses and Duration of Mechanical Ventilation on Respiratory Outcomes in Extremely Low-Birth-Weight Infants

Jensen EA, DeMauro SB, Kornhauser M, et al (The Children's Hosp of Philadelphia and The Univ of Pennsylvania School of Medicine; Alere Inc, Waltham, MA; et al)

JAMA Pediatr 169:1011-1017, 2015

Importance.—Extubation failure is common in extremely preterm infants. The current paucity of data on the adverse long-term respiratory outcomes associated with reinitiation of mechanical ventilation prevents assessment of the risks and benefits of a trial of extubation in this population.

Objective.—To evaluate whether exposure to multiple courses of mechanical ventilation increases the risk of adverse respiratory outcomes before and after adjustment for the cumulative duration of mechanical ventilation.

Design, Setting, and Participants.—We performed a retrospective cohort study of extremely low-birth-weight (ELBW; birth weight <1000 g) infants born from January 1, 2006, through December 31, 2012, who were receiving mechanical ventilation. Analysis was conducted between November 2014 and February 2015. Data were obtained from the Alere Neonatal Database.

Exposures.—The primary study exposures were the cumulative duration of mechanical ventilation and the number of ventilation courses.

Main Outcomes and Measures.—The primary outcome was bronchopulmonary dysplasia (BPD) among survivors. Secondary outcomes were death, use of supplemental oxygen at discharge, and tracheostomy.

Results.—We identified 3343 ELBW infants, of whom 2867 (85.8%) survived to discharge. Among the survivors, 1695 (59.1%) were diagnosed as having BPD, 856 (29.9%) received supplemental oxygen at discharge, and 31 (1.1%) underwent tracheostomy. Exposure to a greater number of mechanical ventilation courses was associated with a progressive increase in the risk of BPD and use of supplemental oxygen at discharge. Compared with a single ventilation course, the adjusted odds ratios for BPD ranged from 1.88 (95% CI, 1.54-2.31) among infants with 2 ventilation courses to 3.81 (95% CI, 2.88-5.04) among those with 4 or more courses. After adjustment for the cumulative duration of mechanical ventilation, the odds of BPD were only increased among infants exposed to 4 or more ventilation courses (adjusted odds ratio, 1.44; 95% CI, 1.04-2.01). The number of ventilation courses was not associated with increased risk of supplemental oxygen use at discharge after adjustment for the length of ventilation. A greater number of ventilation courses did not increase the risk of tracheostomy.

Conclusions and Relevance.—Among ELBW infants, a longer cumulative duration of mechanical ventilation largely accounts for the increased risk of chronic respiratory morbidity associated with reinitiation of mechanical ventilation. These results support attempts of extubation in ELBW infants receiving mechanical ventilation on low ventilator settings, even when success is not guaranteed.

▶ Jensen and colleagues examined the effects of multiple ventilation courses and the duration of mechanical ventilation on the incidence of bronchopulmonary dysplasia (BPD) in surviving extremely low-birth-weight infants. They found that the risk of BPD increased with a longer cumulative duration of mechanical ventilation but did not increase appreciably with repetitive courses of mechanical ventilation until after 4 courses.

Although this was a retrospective cohort study, subject to the usual selection biases, and was dependent on the accuracy of data input in an electronic medical record system, I found the results both encouraging and validating. Years ago, as I was making sign-out rounds in the neonatal intensive care unit, a colleague presented a 900-g baby who was being ventilated with room air at a rate of 20 and pressures of 10/3. I asked why the baby was still on the ventilator and was surprised at his response, "To grow." Although mechanical ventilation has certainly improved since those days, with triggering, synchronization, and pressure support, we are still left with a high imposed work of breathing from narrow lumen endotracheal tubes and increased dead space ratios in this population. As the present study affirms, nothing ventured, nothing gained.

Failed extubations may be the neonatal equivalent of a surgeon finding a negative appendix when operating for appendicitis. Although we can argue that reintubation is uncomfortable, probably invasive, and has physiologic consequences, remaining intubated and on mechanical ventilation unnecessarily also has significant risks and costs.

We all espouse the axiom that discharge planning begins at admission. So should we believe that weaning and preparation for extubation begin with intubation. If you need evidence, it is here.

S. M. Donn, MD

Extubating Extremely Preterm Infants: Predictors of Success and Outcomes following Failure

Manley BJ, Doyle LW, Owen LS, et al (The Royal Women's Hosp, Parkville, Victoria, Australia)
J Pediatr 173:45-49, 2016

Objectives.—To identify variables that predict extubation success in extremely preterm infants born <28 weeks gestational age (GA), and to compare outcomes between those who had successful or failed extubation.

Study Design.—A secondary analysis of data from a randomized trial of postextubation respiratory support that included 174 extremely preterm infants. "Extubation success" was defined as not requiring reintubation within 7 days, and "extubation failure" the converse. Predictive variables that were different between groups were included in a multivariable logistic regression model.

Results.—Sixty-eight percent of infants were successfully extubated. Compared with those infants who had extubation failure, they had a higher GA and birth weight, were extubated earlier, were more often exposed to prolonged ruptured membranes, more often avoided intubation in the delivery room, had a higher pre-extubation pH, and had lower mean pre-extubation fraction of inspired oxygen and partial pressure of carbon dioxide (PCO_2). Only GA and PCO_2 remained significant in the multivariable analysis (area under a receiver operating characteristic curve = 0.81). Extubation failure was associated with death, bronchopulmonary dysplasia, severe retinopathy of prematurity, patent ductus arteriosus ligation, and longer durations of respiratory support, oxygen supplementation, and hospitalization. When adjusted for allocated treatment in the randomized trial, GA, and birth weight z-score, extubation failure remained associated with death before discharge and prolonged respiratory support and hospitalization.

Conclusions.—In extremely preterm infants, higher GA and lower pre-extubation PCO_2 predicted extubation success. Infants in whom extubation failed were more likely to die and have prolonged respiratory support and hospitalization.

Trial Registration.—Australian New Zealand Clinical Trials Network: ACTRN12610000166077.

▶ Widespread appreciation among neonatologists of the risks of mechanical ventilation of extremely preterm infants, including bronchopulmonary dysplasia and neurodevelopmental disability among survivors, has led to increased use of noninvasive methods of respiratory support and to efforts, among those intubated, to taper off mechanical ventilation to extubation as soon as possible. The challenge of providing respiratory support to extremely preterm infants presents a catch-22 situation in which those who are most at risk of ventilator-induced lung injury are also those least likely to succeed without it. In this publication, investigators of the Australia New Zealand Clinical Trials Network explore factors related to success or failure of extubation of extremely preterm infants receiving mechanical ventilation. Lower FiO_2 and a number of individual factors unrelated to ventilator settings were associated with extubation success. In multivariable analyses, extubation success was associated only with more advanced gestational age and lower pre-extubation PCO_2. Infants who failed extubation were at increased risk of death and serious morbid sequelae of prematurity including bronchopulmonary dysplasia, retinopathy of prematurity, patent ductus arteriosus ligation, and more prolonged respiratory support and hospitalization. Of note, those successfully extubated were, on average, first extubated on postnatal day 2 whereas those infants whose extubations were unsuccessful were, on average, first extubated on day 5. These findings might be explained by confounding by indication in which 1 or more complications leading to failed extubation (eg, hemodynamically significant patent ductus arteriosus, infection) also leads to mortality or morbidity. Another possibility is that the decision to ventilate longer before attempting extubation might be a contributing factor to extubation failure. In a still illuminating now 10-year-old study, Thomson and colleagues[1] found that lambs randomized to surfactant and early extubation (24 h) versus later (5 days) had more favorable pulmonary cytokine profiles, pulmonary histology, and in vitro measures of lung compliance, putting them at a pulmonary advantage. The current study might prove most useful in providing objective criteria that strengthen neonatologists' resolve to proceed with a trial of extubation at the earliest rational time point, thereby minimizing the risk of prolonged mechanical ventilation and its associated sequelae.

L. J. Van Marter, MD, MPH

Reference

1. Thomson M, Yoder BA, Winter VT, Giavedoni L, Chang LY, Coalson JJ. Delayed extubation to nasal continuous positive airway pressure in the immature baboon model of bronchopulmonary dysplasia: lung clinical and pathological findings. *Pediatrics*. 2006;118:2038-2050.

Respiratory Outcomes of the Surfactant Positive Pressure and Oximetry Randomized Trial (SUPPORT)

Stevens TP, on behalf of the SUPPORT Study Group of the *Eunice Kennedy Shriver* National Institute of Child Health and Human Development Neonatal Research Network (Univ of Rochester Med Ctr and Golisano Children's Hosp, Rochester, NY; et al)

J Pediatr 2014 [Epub ahead of print]

Objective.—To explore the early childhood pulmonary outcomes of infants who participated in the National Institute of Child Health and Human Development's Surfactant Positive Airway Pressure and Pulse Oximetry Randomized Trial (SUPPORT), using a factorial design that randomized extremely preterm infants to lower vs higher oxygen saturation targets and delivery room continuous positive airway pressure (CPAP) vs intubation/surfactant.

Study Design.—The Breathing Outcomes Study, a prospective secondary study to the Surfactant Positive Airway Pressure and Pulse Oximetry Randomized Trial, assessed respiratory morbidity at 6-month intervals from hospital discharge to 18-22 months corrected age (CA). Two prespecified primary outcomes—wheezing more than twice per week during the worst 2-week period and cough longer than 3 days without a cold—were compared for each randomized intervention.

Results.—One or more interviews were completed for 918 of the 922 eligible infants. The incidences of wheezing and cough were 47.9% and 31.0%, respectively, and did not differ between the study arms of either randomized intervention. Infants randomized to lower vs higher oxygen saturation targets had a similar risk of death or respiratory morbidity (except for croup and treatment with oxygen or diuretics at home). Infants randomized to CPAP vs intubation/surfactant had fewer episodes of wheezing without a cold (28.9% vs 36.5%; $P < .05$), respiratory illnesses diagnosed by a doctor (47.7% vs 55.2%; $P < .05$), and physician or emergency room visits for breathing problems (68.0% vs 72.9%; $P < .05$) by 18-22 months CA.

Conclusion.—Treatment with early CPAP rather than intubation/surfactant is associated with less respiratory morbidity by 18-22 months CA. Longitudinal assessment of pulmonary morbidity is necessary to fully evaluate the potential benefits of respiratory interventions for neonates.

▶ The SUPPORT trial[1,2] evaluated the effects of both oxygen saturation targets and early continuous positive airway pressure (CPAP) versus intubation and surfactant treatment among extremely preterm infants and found no significant difference in the composite outcome death or bronchopulmonary dysplasia (BPD) among infants randomized to the 2 target ranges for oxygen saturation and CPAP versus intubation/surfactant. On the other hand, the early outcomes showed that, when compared with the group who were intubated and received surfactant, infants randomized to receive CPAP were more likely to be alive and free from mechanical ventilation (MV) at age 7 days, had fewer MV days, and were less likely to be intubated or receive glucocorticoids for BPD. The current study evaluated breathing outcomes among a subset of the original cohort: 922 of the original 1316 infants met inclusion criteria and 918 were followed until age 18 to 22 months and their parents were interviewed. In this analysis, treatment with early CPAP, rather than intubation/surfactant, was associated with fewer episodes of spontaneous wheezing (in the absence of respiratory infection), fewer physician-diagnosed respiratory infections, and fewer visits to a physician or emergency department for breathing problems. Despite the failure to detect a benefit of CPAP over intubation/surfactant in the early primary pulmonary and 18- to 22-month neurodevelopmental[3] outcomes, the absence of adverse effects, and modest but persistent signs of improved pulmonary health underscore the validity of CPAP as an optional first-line therapy for pulmonary failure in extremely preterm newborns.

L. J. Van Marter, MD, MPH

References

1. SUPPORT Study Group of the Eunice Kennedy Shriver NICHD Neonatal Research Network, Carlo WA, Finer NN, Walsh MC, et al. Target ranges of oxygen saturation in extremely preterm infants. *N Engl J Med.* 2010;362:1959-1969.
2. SUPPORT Study Group of the Eunice Kennedy Shriver NICHD Neonatal Research Network, Finer NN, Carlo WA, Walsh MC, et al. Early CPAP versus surfactant in extremely preterm infants. *N Engl J Med.* 2010;362:1970-1979.
3. Vaucher YE, Peralta-Carcelen M, Finer NN, et al. Neurodevelopmental outcomes in the early CPAP and pulse oximetry trial. *N Engl J Med.* 2012;367:2495-2504.

Functional evidence for continued alveolarisation in former preterms at school age

Yammine S, Schmidt A, Sutter O, et al (Univ Children's Hosp of Basel (UKBB), Switzerland; Univ Children's Hosp Bern, Switzerland; et al)

Eur Respir J 47:147-155, 2016

Prematurity is the most common disruptor of lung development. The aim of our study was to examine the function of the more vulnerable peripheral airways in former preterm children by multiple-breath washout (MBW) measurements.

86 school-aged children, born between 24 and 35 weeks of gestation and 49 term-born children performed nitrogen MBW. Lung clearance index (LCI), and slope III-derived Scond and Sacin were assessed as markers for global, convection-dependent and diffusion–convection-dependent ventilation inhomogeneity, respectively.

We analysed the data of 77 former preterm (mean (range) age 9.5 (7.2–12.8) years) and 46 term-born children (mean age 9.9 (6.0–15.9) years). LCI and Sacin did not differ between preterm and term-born children. Scond was significantly elevated in preterm compared to term-born participants (mean difference z-score 1.74, 95% CI 1.17–2.30; $p < 0.001$), with 54% of former preterm children showing elevated Scond. In multivariable regression analysis Scond was significantly related only to gestational age ($R^2 = 0.37$).

Normal Sacin provides evidence for a functionally normal alveolar compartment, while elevated Scond indicates impaired function of more proximal conducting airways. Together, our findings support the concept of continued alveolarisation, albeit with "dysanaptic" lung growth in former preterm children.

▶ In 2012 Dr Alan Jobe wrote, "The concept that BPD [bronchopulmonary dysplasia] at the anatomic level is decreased or arrested alveolarization and pulmonary microvascular development is based on excellent animal models and limited anatomic evaluations of infants who have died of BPD. There are no recent anatomic studies of lungs of infants who have died of BPD. There is essentially no information about the anatomical abnormalities in the lungs of infants that recover from BPD.... the diagnosis of BPD provides no information about the pulmonary function of the infant, other than the need for supplemental oxygen. In 2012, the realization is that we know very little about this disease and its variants."[1] Little has changed in the ensuing four years. We still don't know much about the nature and natural history of this "new BPD" in human infants, what we learned from "old BPD" is largely just inapplicable, and we collectively remain insufficiently attuned to those circumstances.

This important study begins to address one of the key unanswered questions: How does BPD influence long-term pulmonary outcomes? The answer seems to be "Not much, if at all." In this comparison of detailed tests of pulmonary function in former preterm infants to control children born at term, few differences were evident. Notably, their data (Sacin measurements) suggest normal function of the acinar compartment—the primary locus of disease in the new BPD. Scond determinations, which were elevated in more than half of the preterm subjects, provided evidence of nonuniform distribution of ventilation in the distal conducting airways in the preterm cohort. Remarkably, after adjustment for gestational age, there was no difference between infants with or without BPD, and there was no association between Scond and the hallmark risk factors for BPD, days of exposure to oxygen, intubation, or respiratory support. More preterm infants than expected had reductions in forced expiratory volume in 1 second or forced expiratory flow at 25% to 75%, providing further evidence of distal airway obstruction in this group, but these measurements were not different between those with and those without BPD. These data suggest that prematurity itself is a risk factor for small airways dysfunction in childhood, but that diagnosis of BPD is not predictive of irreversible alveolar dysfunction or of small airways disease. Accordingly, we must question the utility of empiric treatments—diuretics, bronchodilators, inhaled steroids, etc—for infants with BPD, particularly in the convalescent period preceding and following discharge from the neonatal intensive care unit. It is not clear just what those treatments might be able to prevent.

W. E. Benitz, MD

Reference

1. Jobe AH. What is BPD in 2012 and what will BPD become? *Early Hum Dev.* 2012;88:S27-S28.

Lung ultrasound decreased radiation exposure in preterm infants in a neonatal intensive care unit

Escourrou G, De Luca D (South Paris Univ Hosps, Paris, France)

Acta Paediatr 105:e237-e239, 2016

Background.—Lung ultrasound findings are available for typical neonatal respiratory conditions, and the procedure shows better diagnostic accuracy than chest radiographs for some critical care adult conditions. The technique is quick, free of radiation, and available for bedside use by clinicians. It potentially should reduce the radiation exposure of neonates, but evidence is lacking.

Methods.—A retrospective analysis of hospital administration data was performed to evaluate the impact of lung ultrasound on the use of chest radiographs and on radiation exposure levels. Lung ultrasound was used as the first-line imaging technique for all infants admitted to the neonatal intensive care unit (NICU) in respiratory distress, with chest radiographs done as a second-line procedure in cases with uncertain findings, for infants suspected to have a rare condition, or in those requiring control over central lines. The study population consisted of preterm infants with a gestational age of 24 to 36 weeks between 2012 and 2014. Data on mortality, NICU stay length, incidence of bronchopulmonary dysplasia, and grade III-IV intraventricular hemorrhage were collected along with average number of chest radiographs per infant and mean radiation dose per infant. Chest radiograph entrance surface doses used were 28, 30, and 32 μGy for infants weighing less than 1500 g, 1500-2500 g, and more than 2500 g, respectively.

Results.—Eighty-one percent of the 402 preterm infants admitted to the NICU in 2012 had at least one chest radiograph, but by 2014, this had fallen to 69.7% of 565 preterm infants in the NICU. In 2012, a total of 1976 chest radiographs were preformed, whereas in 2014, 1476 were done. Mean number of chest radiographs per infant declined from 4.9 in 2012 to 2.6 in 2014, which lowered the mean radiation dose per infant from 183 μGy in 2012 to 68 μGy in 2014. The change in mortality from 6.8% in 2012 to 4.5% in 2014 was not significant.

Conclusions.—Lung ultrasound has a steep learning curve and is easy to perform and interpret. Its use is relatively uncommon principally because it takes time to convince people of the usefulness of the technique, train them, and then expand the technique in accordance with a dedicated formal protocol. Lung ultrasound has proved useful as a means for diagnosing hyaline membrane disease, transient tachypnea of the neonate, and meconium aspiration and to guide the administration of surfactant. This study shows it can significantly reduce the radiation exposure for preterm infants in the NICU.

▶ This short article describes the experience of a single center that used lung ultrasonography as a diagnostic technique and demonstrated an impressive reduction in the number of x-rays and amount of radiation exposure to infants in its neonatal intensive care unit.

Although I am a great fan of nonionizing imaging techniques, I viewed this publication as a feasibility study. These investigators, as well as others, have demonstrated several patterns suggestive of neonatal pulmonary pathology, but before we all jump on the bandwagon, it will take a fair amount of research and correlation before there are enough trained individuals and diagnostic accuracy in each center to accept this in place of our current gold standard, the plain film radiograph.

Still, we should strive to reduce radiation exposures to our patients. Do we routinely need a lateral view to accompany an anteroposterior one? Can we "batch" x-rays, for instance, to combine a single exposure to assess endotracheal tube and umbilical catheter positions? And I've been very disappointed that transillumination[1] has become a lost art. Today's 24-week baby receives a much larger radiation exposure than the 28-week baby of a decade ago. Will this come back to bite us in a few years?

S. M. Donn, MD

Reference

1. Donn SM. Historical perspective: neonatal transillumination. *Neoreviews*. 2005;6: e1-e3.

Lung ultrasound decreased radiation exposure in preterm infants in a neonatal intensive care unit

Escourrou G, De Luca D (South Paris Univ Hosps, Paris, France)

Acta Paediatr 105:e237-e239, 2016

Lung ultrasound is a relatively new technique with a well-defined semiology, and lung ultrasound findings have been described for typical neonatal respiratory conditions, such as meconium aspiration syndrome, hyaline membrane disease, transient tachypnoea of the neonate and pneumothorax. Moreover, lung ultrasound also shows better diagnostic accuracy than chest X-rays for some critical conditions in adult critical care. Finally, it has the advantage of being a quick and radiation-free bedside technique that may be directly performed by clinicians. Thus, lung ultrasound has also the potential to reduce radiation exposure in neonates, but no data are available on this topic (Figs 1 and 2).

▶ Lung ultrasound (LUS) has increased in popularity over the past decade because it is simple, provides instant answers, and avoids irradiation. Lung ultrasound readily differentiates between surfactant deficient respiratory distress syndrome (RDS) and transient tachypnea of the newborn (TTNB) and can be used to recognize pulmonary edema, pleural effusion, and air leaks; in addition, the lung ultrasound score is predictive of the need for surfactant.[1,2] In meconium aspiration syndrome (MAS), LUS images corresponded well with x-ray findings. Piastra et al[3] concluded that LUS is a useful and promising tool in the diagnosis and management of MAS, providing real-time bedside imaging, with the additional potential benefit of limiting radiation exposure in sick neonates. The "Choosing Wisely" report identified 5 therapies or tests that could not be justified on the basis of efficacy, safety, or cost. One of the recommendations was to avoid routine daily chest radiographs without an indication for intubated infants.[4] This may increase the demand for LUS.

Escourrou and DeLuca, in this brief communication, demonstrate how with the introduction of LUS (Fig 2), no x-rays are performed on 30% of their admissions; for those that do require x-rays, the number needed has diminished, together with the exposure to irradiation (Fig 1).

Brusa et al[5] assessed the reliability of lung sonography in neonates between physician interpreters with different degrees of experience. Four experienced observers, blinded to the clinical situation, studied the first ultrasound clips from infants admitted with respiratory distress in the first 24 hours of life. They reported that there was excellent differentiation between RDS and TTNB. There was high interobserver agreement even between interpreters with varying levels of experience.

Vergine[6] studied 59 infants, 23 with RDS and 30 with TTNB, reported on the accuracy of LUS in differentiating these 2 conditions. LUS showed a sensitivity of 95.6% and specificity of 94.4%, with a positive predictive value (PPV) of 91.6% and a negative predictive value of 97.1% for RDS; for TTNB, sensitivity was 93.3% and specificity 96.5%, with a positive predictive value of 96.5% and a negative predictive value of 93.4%.

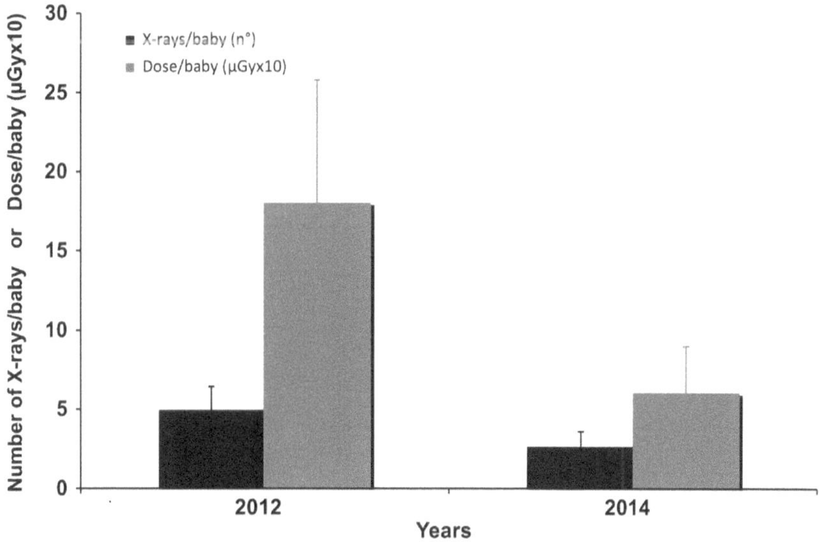

FIGURE 1.—Effect of lung ultrasound introduction in the NICU care of preterm neonates. Mean number of chest X-rays per baby (black columns) and mean dose per baby (grey columns). T-bars represent standard deviations. 2012 and 2014 were the years before and after the introduction of the formal lung ultrasound programme. (Reprinted from Escourrou G, De Luca D. Lung ultrasound decreased radiation exposure in preterm infants in a neonatal intensive care unit. *Acta Paediatr.* 2016;105:e237-e239, with permission from Foundation Acta Pædiatrica.)

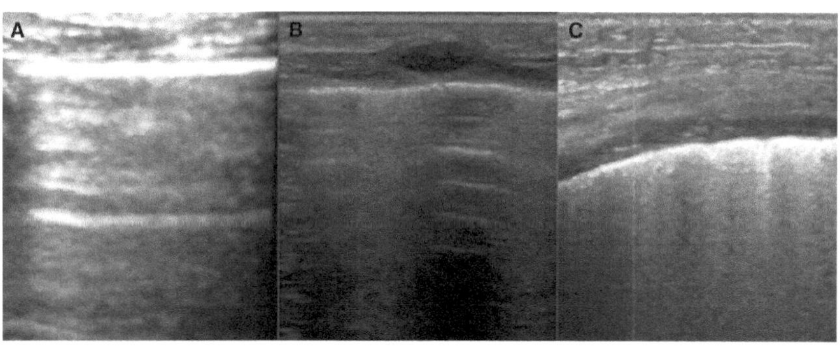

FIGURE 2.—Some typical lung ultrasound findings. Panel A shows a normal lung: typical A-lines pattern (horizontal line, reflecting to the pleura, representing a well aerated lung). Panel B shows an interstitial pattern with typical B-lines (vertical comet tales originating from the pleura) and a double lung point (A-lines and B-lines on the same scan), typical of transient tachypnoea of the neonate (1). Panel C shows an alveolar pattern with confluent B-lines creating a white lung, more typical of hyaline membrane disease (1). All images were obtained by transversal scan, with a micro-linear high-frequency (15 MHz) golf probe, placed between two ribs on the anterior and lateral chest. Black asterisks indicate A-lines. B-lines, the double lung point, the pleura and the white lung pattern are indicated either directly or with arrows. (Reprinted from Escourrou G, De Luca D. Lung ultrasound decreased radiation exposure in preterm infants in a neonatal intensive care unit. *Acta Paediatr.* 2016;105:e237-e239, with permission from Foundation Acta Pædiatrica.)

Most of the reports on LUS in the neonate have come from the pioneers in this field in Udine, Italy, and more recently France. In these clinicians' hands, this has become an excellent clinical tool. With some training and practice, I believe that LUS will be used with increased frequency at many other centers.

A. A. Fanaroff, MD

References

1. Cattarossi L. Lung ultrasound: its role in neonatology and pediatrics. *Early Hum Dev.* 2013;89:S17-S19.
2. Brat R, Yousef N, Klifa R, Reynaud S, et al. Lung ultrasonography score to evaluate oxygenation and surfactant need in neonates treated with continuous positive airway pressure. *JAMA Pediatr.* 2015;169:e151797.
3. Piastra M, Yousef N, Brat R, Manzoni P, Mokhtari M, De Luca D. Lung ultrasound findings in meconium aspiration syndrome. *Early Hum Dev.* 2014;90: S41-S43.
4. Ho T, Dukhovny D, Zupancic JA, Goldmann DA, Horbar JD, Pursley DM. Choosing wisely in newborn medicine: five opportunities to increase value. *Pediatrics.* 2015;136:e482-e489.
5. Brusa G, Savoia M, Vergine M, Bon A, Copetti R, Cattarossi L. Neonatal lung sonography: interobserver agreement between physician interpreters with varying levels of experience. *J Ultrasound Med.* 2015;34:1549-1554.
6. Vergine M, Copetti R, Brusa G, Cattarossi L. Lung ultrasound accuracy in respiratory distress syndrome and transient tachypnea of the newborn. *Neonatology.* 2014;106:87-93.

Car Seat Screening for Low Birth Weight Term Neonates

Davis NL (Univ of Maryland School of Medicine, Baltimore)
Pediatrics 136:89-96, 2015

Background and Objective.—Car seat tolerance screening (CSTS) is a common predischarge assessment of neonates. Almost half of nurseries and NICUs have low birth weight (LBW, <2.5 kg) as an inclusion criterion, regardless of birth gestational age (GA). Little is known about the epidemiology of CSTS in this cohort. The objective of this study was to identify incidence and risk factors for CSTS failure in term LBW infants.

Methods.—This was a retrospective medical record review of 220 full-term LBW infants qualifying for CSTS over a 4-year period between January 2010 to December 2013. We described CSTS results and performed bivariate analyses to evaluate for predictors of failure.

Results.—Overall failure incidence was 4.8%. There were no differences between those who passed and those who failed based on birth weight, birth GA, race, gender, Apgar scores, respiratory support requirements, magnesium exposure, corrected GA, or weight at the time of CSTS. Maternal urine toxicology positive for opiates was found to be a significant predictor of CSTS failure. Of the 9 subjects who failed, 2 had a specific diagnosis identified (Prader–Willi syndrome and long QT syndrome) after a failed CSTS prompted closer examination and workup before discharge.

Conclusions.—We found a similar incidence of failure for full-term LBW infants as has been previously reported for preterm infants. The infants who failed were more likely to have mothers who tested positive for opiates before delivery. Epidemiologic data are provided to help guide future CSTS policies and protocol development for this group.

▶ Current recommendations from the American Academy of Pediatrics include testing for cardiorespiratory instability in the infant's car seat before discharge of all infants born before 37 weeks' gestation, and suggests consideration in term infants with other conditions placing them at risk for obstructive apnea, bradycardia, or oxygen desaturation. This report describes extension to another group, term infants with low birth weights (LBW). Car seat test failure is reported in 4.8% of their subjects, but the actual rate of failure in otherwise well-appearing LBW term infants is difficult to ascertain. Of the total of 220 subjects, 101 received all of their care in the full-term nursery, and 7 of them failed their car seat test. It is not apparent how many of the 119 infants admitted to the neonatal intensive care unit would have qualified for car seat testing based on other indications, but at least 1 was referred transferred from another facility for evaluation of desaturation episodes. Two infants had significant pathologic syndromes (Prader-Willi and long QT) identified by evaluations prompted by failure of the car seat test; however, that is not the intended purpose of such testing, and it is not clear whether the now mandatory pulse oximetry screening for cyanotic congenital heart disease would have made the car seat test results redundant. In the Conclusions section of the text, the authors state, "Because very little is published on the topic, it is difficult to make evidence-based recommendations related to testing [LBW term infants]. More evidence is needed to support routine testing of all LBW infants, narrowed testing to a specific demographic group, or completely eliminating this test. Right now, it is unclear which of these options is best." Until car seat observations in otherwise well preterm and LBW term infants are demonstrated to have predictive value for unexpected deaths while in the car, this procedure should be relegated to the category of useless interventions and not extended to additional patient groups.

W. E. Benitz, MD

Surgical intervention strategies for pediatric congenital cystic lesions of the lungs: A 20-year single-institution experience

Furukawa T, Kimura O, Sakai K, et al (Kyoto Prefectural Univ of Medicine, Japan)

J Pediatr Surg 50:2025-2027, 2015

Background.—The aim of this study was to assess surgical intervention strategies for congenital cystic lesions of the lungs (CCL), focusing on the safety of lung resection.

Materials and Methods.—The clinical features of 27 children (CCAM, n = 16; bronchial atresia, n = 4; bronchogenic cyst, n = 3; pulmonary sequestration, n = 3; lobar emphysema, n = 1) who were treated at our institution between 1995 and 2014 were analyzed.

Results.—Of the 27 patients, 14 were asymptomatic, and 13 were symptomatic. The youngest symptomatic patient presented with pneumonia at 9 months of age. The mean age at surgery was 4 months in the asymptomatic group and 4.1 years in the symptomatic group. The mean operating time was 167 minutes in the asymptomatic group and 275 minutes in the symptomatic group ($P < 0.001$). The mean amount of intraoperative bleeding was 15 g in the asymptomatic group and 83.4 g in the symptomatic group ($P < 0.05$). All of the prenatally diagnosed patients underwent surgery within six months of birth. Three patients had remnant cystic lesions, all of which involved cystic lesions located over the lobulation anomalies of the lung.

Conclusions.—To minimize surgical invasiveness, surgery for CCL should be performed during the asymptomatic period or within six months after birth.

▶ Seriously? This article presented the results of a single-center experience over a 20-year period in which 27 patients—about 1 per year—were treated for congenital cystic lesions of the lung. What did we learn? Asymptomatic babies do better than symptomatic babies.

I find it hard to understand why series like this are published. Certainly, both diagnostic and therapeutic technologies have advanced significantly in this time frame, especially fetal diagnosis and treatment.

Conclusions from reports like this are fraught with hazard and should not be taken to heart.

S. M. Donn, MD

Risk-stratification of severity for infants with CDH: Prenatal versus postnatal predictors of outcome

Akinkuotu AC, Cruz SM, Abbas PI, et al (Texas Children's Fetal Ctr, Houston)
J Pediatr Surg 51:44-48, 2016

Purpose.—The purpose of this study was to compare the predication accuracy of a newly described postnatally-based clinical prediction model to fetal imaging-based predictors of mortality for infants with CDH.

Methods.—We performed a retrospective review of all CDH patients treated at a comprehensive fetal care center from January 2004 to January 2014. Prenatal data reviewed included lung-to-head ratio (LHR), observed/ expected-total fetal lung volume (O/E-TFLV), and percent liver herniation (%LH). Based on the postnatal prediction model, neonates were categorized as low, intermediate, and high risk of death. The primary outcome was 6-month mortality.

Results.—Of 176 CDH patients, 58 had a major cardiac anomaly, and 28 had a genetic anomaly. Patients with O/ETFLV <35% and %LH >20% were at increased risk for mortality (44% and 36%, respectively). There was a significant difference in mortality between low, intermediate, and high-risk groups (4% vs. 22% vs. 51%; $p < 0.001$). On multivariate regression, the O/E-TFLV and postnatal-based mortality risk score were the two independent predictors of 6-month mortality.

Conclusion.—The CDH Study Group postnatal predictive model provides good discrimination among three risk groups in our patient cohort. The prenatal MRI-based O/E-TFLV is the strongest prenatal predictor of 6-month mortality in infants with CDH and will help guide prenatal counseling and discussions regarding fetal intervention and perinatal management.

► Congenital diaphragmatic hernia (CDH) accounts for approximately 8% of all congenital defects. Forty percent of infants born with CDH have additional anomalies that increase mortality risk substantially. The CDH study group has recently published an expanded clinical scoring system applicable at the bedside for predicting mortality risk postnatally.[1] This model scores +1 for very low birth weight (< 1500 g), +1 for low 5-minute APGAR score < 7, +2 for missing Apgar score, +2 for severe pulmonary hypertension on echocardiogram, +2 for major cardiac anomaly (other than a patent ductus arteriosus or patent foramen ovale), and +1 for chromosomal anomaly. Patients were than stratified into low (score of 0, mortality risk of 10%), intermediate (score of 1–2, mortality risk of 25%), and high (score ≥3, mortality risk of 50%) risk. Drawing from outcome data in 2202 infants in the CDH Registry, this model was found to discriminate mortality risk within the first days of admission to the neonatal intensive care unit, which can be helpful in predicting the severity of the neonatal course as well as mortality risk.

For the majority of families who face a prenatal diagnosis of CDH, however, survival prediction before delivery is of paramount importance because decisions about termination of pregnancy or assessment for fetal surgical intervention in cases with severe lung hypoplasia must be addressed expeditiously. The retrospective study by Akinkuotu et al reviews various ultrasound and magnetic resonance imaging measurements of fetal lung volume reported in a cohort of 176 CDH infants treated at Texas Children's Hospital over a 10-year period ending in 2014. A multivariate regression analysis identified observed/expected-total fetal lung volume (O/E-TFLV) < 35% (adjusted odds ratio [OR]: 15.9; 95% confidence interval [CI] 1.35–188) and postnatal based CDH mortality risk score (adjusted OR: 2.35; 95% CI 1.11–4.97) as independent predictors of CDH mortality at 6 months of life. The O/E-TFLV < 35% was also the strongest independent predictor of extracorporeal membrane oxygenation (ECMO) use. The rate of liver herniation > 20% into the chest, another risk factor associated with severe pulmonary hypoplasia,[2,3] was higher in the CDH nonsurvivor group, but was not an independent predictor of mortality in this retrospective cohort.

Counseling parents who are facing the delivery of a baby diagnosed prenatally to have a CDH is a difficult task, as none of the predictors of mortality in this condition is absolute. Fetal echocardiogram and chromosomal analysis are essential to know whether one is dealing with more than an isolated diaphragmatic defect, given the high rate of associated anomalies. Prenatal discussions range from anticipated straightforward surgical repair to probable need for prolonged ventilator support, inhaled nitric oxide, and ECMO. In cases of suspected severe pulmonary hypoplasia, evaluation for fetal surgical intervention (tracheal plugging), although still considered experimental, should also be reviewed. These are weighty and, frankly, scary subjects to relay to expectant parents, but necessary to optimize the infant's chances for survival.

E. K. Stork, MD

References

1. Brindle ME, Cook EF, Tibboel D, Lally PA, Lally KPon behalf of the Congenital Diaphragmatic Hernia Study Group. A clinical prediction rule for the severity of congenital diaphragmatic hernias in newborn. *Pediatrics*. 2014;134:e413-e419.
2. Ruano R, Lazar DA, Cass DL, et al. Fetal lung volume and quantification of liver herniation by magnetic resonance imaging in isolated congenital diaphragmatic hernia. *Ultrasound Obstet Gynecol*. 2014;43:662-669.
3. Zamora IJ, Olutoye OO, Cass DL, et al. Prenatal MRI fetal lung volumes and percent liver herniation predict pulmonary morbidity in congenital diaphragmatic hernia [CDH]. *J Pediatr Surg*. 2014;49:688-693.

8 Central Nervous System and Special Senses

Detection and Management of Delirium in the Neonatal Unit: A Case Series

Groves A, Traube C, Silver G (Weill Cornell Med College, NY)

Pediatrics 137:e20153369, 2016

Delirium is increasingly recognized as a common syndrome in critically ill children, but in our experience, it is rarely considered in the NICU. Delirium is independently associated with prolonged length of stay and adverse longterm outcomes in children. We report the cases of 3 infants cared for in our NICU at corrected gestational ages of 4, 11, and 17 weeks who presented with classic symptoms of delirium. All 3 children had complex medical problems and were receiving multiple analgesic and sedative medications. All 3 children exhibited agitation that was unresponsive to increasing doses of medications, and they all appeared to improve after treatment with quetiapine, allowing weaning of other medications. It is possible that with increased vigilance, delirium will be increasingly recognized in newborns, thus allowing tailored intervention. Further research is needed to investigate the prevalence and associated risk factors for developing delirium in the NICU and to explore possible treatment options.

▶ Delirium, a global brain dysfunction, is defined as an acute and fluctuating change in awareness and cognition that can occur as a result of illness or with the use of some medications, particularly anxiolytics and opioids. Children treated in intensive care units who are heavily sedated and on ventilators are particularly vulnerable; one study places the rate at more than 20%.[1] The authors of this case series suggest that the syndrome also occurs in medically fragile infants cared for in newborn intensive care units, particularly those who continue to be agitated and to breathe against the ventilator despite escalating doses of sedative/hypnotic and anxiolytic medication.

Each of the 3 infants in the above report was receiving daily doses of an anxiolytic medication and an opioid. The diagnosis of delirium was entertained when it became apparent that the infants' agitation and restlessness were not responsive to an escalation in medication dosing. The diagnosis of delirium was made using the Cornell Assessment of Pediatric Delirium, a clinical tool that has been validated in children.[2] The infants were treated with quetiapine, an atypical antipsychotic drug that has been used off label for the treatment of intensive care delirium in adult and pediatric populations. Potential adverse events associated with the medication include QTc prolongation and anticholinergic and hypotensive effects.

There is increasing evidence that benzodiazepine use, especially when given continuously, is associated with an increased risk of delirium.[3] In addition, there is growing concern regarding the adverse effect of benzodiazepines on the developing brain.[4] Thus, it would seem prudent to avoid using medications that are associated with an increased risk of delirium rather that promoting the treatment of a potentially avoidable problem.

L. A. Papile, MD

References

1. Silver G, Traube C, Gerber LM, et al. Pediatric delirium and associated risk factors: a single-center prospective observational study. *Pediatr Crit Care Med.* 2015;16:303-309.
2. Traube C, Silver G, Kearney J, Patel A, et al. Cornell assessment of pediatric delirium: a valid, rapid, observational tool for screening delirium in the PICU. *Crit Care Med.* 2014;42:656-663.
3. Zaal IJ, Devlin JW, Hazelbag M, Klouwenberg K, et al. Benzodiazepine-associated delirium in critically ill adults. *Intensive Care Med.* 2015;41:2130-2137.
4. McPherson C, Grunau RE. Neonatal pain control and neurologic effects of anesthetics and sedatives in preterm infants. *Clin Perinatol.* 2014;41:209-227.

Postnatal Steroids and Febrile Seizure Susceptibility in Preterm Children

Tu Y-F, Wang L-W, Wang S-T, et al (National Cheng Kung Univ, Tainan, Taiwan; Chi Mei Med Ctr, Tainan, Taiwan; et al)

Pediatrics 137:e20153404, 2016

Objective.—To investigate risk factors, seizure characteristics, and outcomes of febrile seizure (FS) in children born very preterm.

Methods.—This study used a prospective registry data set of 844 preterm infants (birth weight <1500 g and gestational age <32 weeks) admitted to NICUs from 2001 to 2009 in southern Taiwan. We investigated the prevalence, risks, seizure patterns, and outcomes of FS in children aged 5 years.

Results.—Among 575 children (follow-up rate, 85.8%) followed up for 5 years, 35 (6.1%) developed FS. The FS and non-FS groups were comparable regarding their mean gestational age, birth weight, 5-minute Apgar score <6, and prenatal and postnatal complications. No difference was observed in the use of prenatal corticosteroids between the 2 groups. The FS group had a significantly higher rate of postnatal corticosteroid treatment than the non-FS group, even after adjusting for confounding factors (odds ratio, 5.4 [95% confidence interval, 1.9–15.8]; $P = .006$). No differences were observed in IQs or subsequent epilepsy rates between the 2 groups. Although no difference was observed in the age of FS onset or neurodevelopmental outcomes between the 2 groups, children with FS who received postnatal corticosteroid treatment had a significantly lower mean body temperature during the first FS attack compared with those who did not receive postnatal corticosteroid treatment (38.6 ± 0.4°C vs 39.2 ± 0.6°C; $P = .034$).

Conclusions.—Children born very preterm have a higher rate of FS, and postnatal corticosteroid treatment was associated with FS susceptibility in these children.

▶ In this prospective observational study, investigators attempted to characterize later febrile seizures in a population of preterm infants weighing less than 1500 g at birth and less than 32 weeks' gestation. Infants were followed at 6 months, 1, 2, and 5 years of age.

There were 844 infants; 7 were excluded for congenital anomalies, 165 died (a very high 20% mortality rate), and more than 14% of survivors were lost to follow-up, which may have biased the results. The authors looked at 20 demographic and prenatal, perinatal, and postnatal complications. An association was found between subsequent febrile seizures (without electroencephalographic confirmation) and receipt of steroids in the neonatal intensive care unit, $P = .006$. However, the investigators failed to correct for multiple comparisons, and application of the Bonferroni correction required a P value of $< .0025$ to achieve significance. Among children with febrile seizures, the temperature at onset was about 0.6°C lower in those who received steroids.

Although several speculative mechanisms were proposed by the authors, it is unlikely the study had adequate statistical power to even confirm the association. On the other hand, if the association turns out to be valid, it is yet another thing we will have to consider when we reach for the steroids. There is so little we know.

S. M. Donn, MD

Postnatal Steroids and Febrile Seizure Susceptibility in Preterm Children

Tu Y-F, Wang L-W, Wang S-T, et al (Natl Cheng Kung Univ, Tainan, Taiwan; Chi Mei Med Ctr, Tainan, Taiwan; et al)

Pediatrics 137:e20153404, 2016

Objective.—To investigate risk factors, seizure characteristics, and outcomes of febrile seizure (FS) in children born very preterm.

Methods.—This study used a prospective registry data set of 844 preterm infants (birth weight <1500 g and gestational age <32 weeks) admitted to NICUs from 2001 to 2009 in southern Taiwan. We investigated the prevalence, risks, seizure patterns, and outcomes of FS in children aged 5 years.

Results.—Among 575 children (follow-up rate, 85.8%) followed up for 5 years, 35 (6.1%) developed FS. The FS and non-FS groups were comparable regarding their mean gestational age, birth weight, 5-minute Apgar score <6, and prenatal and postnatal complications. No difference was observed in the use of prenatal corticosteroids between the 2 groups. The FS group had a significantly higher rate of postnatal corticosteroid treatment than the non-FS group, even after adjusting for confounding factors (odds ratio, 5.4 [95% confidence interval, 1.9–15.8]; $P = .006$). No differences were observed in IQs or subsequent epilepsy rates between the 2 groups. Although no difference was observed in the age of FS onset or neurodevelopmental outcomes between the 2 groups, children with FS who received postnatal corticosteroid treatment had a significantly lower mean body temperature during the first FS attack compared with those who did not receive postnatal corticosteroid treatment (38.6 ± 0.4°C vs 39.2 ± 0.6°C; $P = .034$).

Conclusions.—Children born very preterm have a higher rate of FS, and postnatal corticosteroid treatment was associated with FS susceptibility in these children.

▶ The dataset used in this observational study included not only demographic factors and medical complications of 844 very preterm/very low birth weight infants and their mothers during the prenatal, perinatal, and postnatal period but also detailed neurodevelopmental assessments at 6, 12, and 24 months and 5 years of age. Information regarding seizures and medication use was obtained from parental report. Medical records were further reviewed in cases in which a history of seizures was reported.

Despite the plethora of data available for analysis, there were only 35 children with identifiable febrile seizure who were born very preterm/very low birth weight. This small sample size might have confounded the posthoc findings of the study. Thus, although the study raises yet another concern about the adverse consequences of postnatal corticosteroid therapy use in very preterm/very low birth weight infants, a long-term follow-up study with a larger sample is needed to validate or refute the above observation.

L. A. Papile, MD

Pregnancy risk factors in autism: a pilot study with artificial neural networks

Grossi E, Veggo F, Narzisi A, et al (Villa Santa Maria Inst, Tavernerio, Italy; IRCCS Stella Maris Foundation, Calambrone, Italy; Univ of Bergamo, Italy; et al)

Pediatr Res 79:339-347, 2016

Background.—Autism is a multifactorial condition in which a single risk factor can unlikely provide comprehensive explanation for the disease origin. Moreover, due to the complexity of risk factors interplay, traditional statistics is often unable to explain the core of the problem due to the strong inherent nonlinearity of relationships. The aim of this study was to assess the frequency of 27 potential risk factors related to pregnancy and peri-postnatal period.

Methods.—The mothers of 45 autistic children and of 68 typical developing children completed a careful interview. Twenty-four siblings of 19 autistic children formed an internal control group.

Results.—A higher prevalence of potential risk factors was observed in 22 and 15 factors in external control and internal control groups, respectively. For six of them, the difference in prevalence was statistically significant. Specialized artificial neural networks (ANNs) discriminated between autism and control subjects with 80.19% global accuracy when the dataset was preprocessed with TWIST (training with input selection and testing) system selecting 16 out of 27 variables. Logistic regression applied to 27 variables gave unsatisfactory results with global accuracy of 46%.

Conclusion.—Pregnancy factors play an important role in autism development. ANNs are able to build up a predictive model, which could represent the basis for a diagnostic screening tool.

▶ We are only beginning to scratch the surface of the pathophysiological underpinnings of autism spectrum disorders. Although reported rates of autism are increasing, there is uncertainty whether this reflects a true increase in the disorder, improved recognition, or both. In any case, we have much to learn about the pathogenesis of autism. Genetics, health, and environmental factors have been found to play roles, with the prior research studies mainly focusing on infancy and early childhood health and exposures. The current study takes a step further back in time, exploring pregnancy risk factors in a maternal interview based comparison of 45 autistic and 68 typically developing children using advanced epidemiological analyses via artificial neural networks (ANNs). Inspired by the functioning and learning of the human brain, ANNs are computerized systems that employ multilayer connectionist models that dynamically find connections between various data sets and are used to reveal previously unrecognized or weak relationships between the input and output variables, by overcoming some of the statistical challenges that impair traditional logistic regression modeling. They have been used to study other multifactorial disorders such as Alzheimer disease. Despite the modest sample size of the current study, the investigators found evidence of associations among several pregnancy, perinatal, and neonatal factors and autism, including paint/solvent occupational exposures during pregnancy, number of stressful events during pregnancy, pregnancy complications, perinatal complications, no breastfeeding, and early antibiotic therapy. In addition, the ANNs performance, specifically 80% predictive accuracy on the receiver-operating characteristic curve, substantially outperformed the sensitivity and specificity estimates generated by standard logistic regression. Pretty cool! How exciting to contemplate the potential of this powerful new analytic approach to the study of other vexing multifactorial disorders, such as bronchopulmonary dysplasia and necrotizing enterocolitis.

L. J. Van Marter, MD, MPH

The Association of Maternal Obesity and Diabetes With Autism and Other Developmental Disabilities

Li M, Fallin MD, Riley A, et al (Johns Hopkins Bloomberg School of Public Health, Baltimore, MD; et al)

Pediatrics 137:e20152206, 2016

Background.—Obesity and diabetes are highly prevalent among pregnant women in the United States. No study has examined the independent and combined effects of maternal prepregnancy obesity and maternal diabetes on the risk of autism spectrum disorder (ASD) in parallel with other developmental disorders (DDs).

Methods.—This study is based on 2734 children (including 102 ASD cases), a subset of the Boston Birth Cohort who completed at least 1 postnatal study visit at Boston Medical Center between 1998 and 2014. Child ASD and other DDs were based on physician diagnoses as documented in electronic medical records. Risks of ASD and other DDs were compared among 6 groups defined by maternal prepregnancy obesity and diabetes status by using Cox proportional hazard regression controlling for potential confounders.

Results.—When examined individually, maternal prepregnancy obesity and pregestational diabetes (PGDM) were each associated with risk of ASD. When examined in combination, only mothers with obesity and PGDM (hazard ratio 3.91, 95% confidence interval 1.76–8.68) and those with obesity and gestational diabetes (hazard ratio 3.04, 95% confidence interval 1.21–7.63) had a significantly increased risk of offspring ASD. Intellectual disabilities (IDs), but not other DDs, showed a similar pattern of increased risk associated with combined obesity and PGDM. This pattern of risk was mostly accounted for by cases with co-occurring ASD and ID.

Conclusions.—Maternal prepregnancy obesity and maternal diabetes in combination were associated with increased risk for ASD and ID. ASD with ID may be etiologically distinct from ASD without ID.

▶ This study of 2734 children in the Boston Birth Cohort (1998–2014), including 102 cases of children with autism spectrum disorder (ASD), explored prenatal antecedents of ASD. The investigators found associations between both diabetes (pregestational as well as gestational) and obesity and ASD, individually and in combination, with the greatest risk occurring among those with both prepregnancy obesity and diabetes. ASD accompanied by intellectual impairment was limited to those with both prepregnancy diabetes mellitus and obesity. This study is intriguing from the perspective of underlying unexplained pathophysiological mechanisms. We are well aware that maternal obesity is a risk factor for obstetrical complications; however, this factor alone is unlikely to explain the observed association. Both diabetes and obesity are pro-inflammatory states associated with circulating cytokines that can cause fetal brain injury. Further, diabetes is associated with intrauterine (fetal) hyperglycemia and, sometimes, neonatal hyperinsulinemia and hypoglycemia. Better understanding of the mechanisms linking a pregnant woman's obesity and diabetes with later ASD in her child must await further investigation, yet it is clear from this and prior investigations that obesity and diabetes are important pregnancy and perinatal risks and that infants born to mothers with these conditions must be followed closely to ensure they are making appropriate neurodevelopmental progress.

L. J. Van Marter, MD, MPH

Serial cranial ultrasonography or early MRI for detecting preterm brain injury?

Plaisier A, Raets MMA, Ecury-Goossen GM, et al (Erasmus Med Ctr—Sophia, Rotterdam, The Netherlands; et al)

Arch Dis Child Fetal Neonatal Ed 100:F293-F300, 2015

Objective.—To investigate detection ability and feasibility of serial cranial ultrasonography (CUS) and early MRI in preterm brain injury.

Design.—Prospective cohort study.

Setting.—Level III neonatal intensive care unit.

Patients.—307 infants, born below 29 weeks of gestation.

Methods.—Serial CUS and MRI were performed according to standard clinical protocol. In case of instability, MRI was postponed or cancelled. Brain images were assessed by independent experts and compared between modalities.

Main Outcome Measures.—Presence of preterm brain injury on either CUS or MRI and discrepant imaging findings on CUS and MRI.

Results.—Serial CUS was performed in all infants; early MRI was often postponed (n=59) or cancelled (n=126). Injury was found in 146 infants (47.6%). Clinical characteristics differed significantly between groups that were subdivided according to timing of MRI. 61 discrepant imaging findings were found. MRI was superior in identifying cerebellar haemorrhage; CUS in detection of acute intraventricular haemorrhage, perforator stroke and cerebral sinovenous thrombosis.

Conclusions.—Advanced serial CUS seems highly effective in diagnosing preterm brain injury, but may miss cerebellar abnormalities. Although MRI does identify these lesions, feasibility is limited. Improved safety, better availability and tailored procedures are essential for MRI to increase its value in clinical care.

▶ In this study, the investigators compared the detection ability and clinical feasibility of routine MRI scan with serial cranial ultrasonongraphy (CUS) until discharge in infants born at less than 29 weeks of gestational age. CUS was obtained at days 0, 1, 2, 7 and weekly thereafter. MRI scan was done at 30 weeks of corrected gestational age or later if an infant was clinically unstable. MRI scan was not performed in 126 of the 307 infants, as 57 died before 30 weeks of corrected gestational age, 55 were transferred to another facility before 30 weeks of corrected gestational age, and 14 encountered technical difficulties. The MRI scan could not be done at 30 weeks of corrected gestational age for 73 infants because they were too unstable to be moved to the MRI suite; of these, only 59 were available for a scan at a later date. MRI was a better imaging technique for the detection of germinal matrix hemorrhage (80% vs 36%) and posterior fossa abnormalities (100% vs 27%), whereas CUS outperformed MRI in the detection of intraventricular hemorrhage (85% vs 52%) and cerebral sinovenous thrombosis (100% vs 22%). Because the number of infants with white matter injury was low, comparison of the 2 techniques was not practical. Although MRI was superior to detect posterior fossa abnormalities, its clinical use was limited; approximately 28% of the infants were not scanned because of transfer to another facility or clinical instability. Thus it seems that CUS is a more feasible imaging modality than MRI to detect and monitor preterm brain injury.

L. A. Papile, MD

Smaller Cerebellar Growth and Poorer Neurodevelopmental Outcomes in Very Preterm Infants Exposed to Neonatal Morphine

Zwicker JG, Miller SP, Grunau RE, et al (Univ of British Columbia, Vancouver, Canada; et al)

J Pediatr 172:81-87, 2016

Objective.—To examine the relationship between morphine exposure and growth of the cerebellum and cerebrum in very preterm neonates from early in life to term-equivalent age, as well as to examine morphine exposure and brain volumes in relation to neurodevelopmental outcomes at 18 months corrected age (CA).

Study Design.—A prospective cohort of 136 very preterm neonates (24-32 weeks gestational age) was serially scanned with magnetic resonance imaging near birth and at term-equivalent age for volumetric measurements of the cerebellum and cerebrum. Motor outcomes were assessed with the Peabody Developmental Motor Scales, Second Edition and cognitive outcomes with the Bayley Scales of Infant and Toddler Development, Third Edition at 18 months CA. Generalized least squares models and linear regression models were used to assess relationships between morphine exposure, brain volumes, and neurodevelopmental outcomes.

Results.—A 10-fold increase in morphine exposure was associated with a 5.5% decrease in cerebellar volume, after adjustment for multiple clinical confounders and total brain volume ($P = .04$). When infants exposed to glucocorticoids were excluded, the association of morphine was more pronounced, with an 8.1% decrease in cerebellar volume. Morphine exposure was not associated with cerebral volume ($P = .30$). Greater morphine exposure also predicted poorer motor ($P < .001$) and cognitive outcomes ($P = .006$) at 18 months CA, an association mediated, in part, by slower brain growth.

Conclusions.—Morphine exposure in very preterm neonates is independently associated with impaired cerebellar growth in the neonatal period and poorer neurodevelopmental outcomes in early childhood. Alternatives to better manage pain in preterm neonates that optimize brain development and functional outcomes are urgently needed.

▶ Morphine is the most commonly used opiate in the neonatal intensive care unit (NICU), despite concerns for its efficacy and safety. A particular vulnerability of the immature cerebellum and Purkinje cell population has been demonstrated in animal models of morphine exposure. This study reports on a prospective cohort of 136 very preterm neonates (24–32 weeks gestational age) who underwent serial magnetic resonance imaging near birth and at term-equivalent age for volumetric measurements of the cerebellum and cerebrum as well as neurodevelopmental evaluation at 18 months of age. Of these infants, approximately a third received no morphine, a third received morphine at < 2 mg/kg, and a third received > 2 mg/kg throughout their NICU course. The infants in the high morphine exposure were more immature, more than 50% had surgical exposure, received dexamethasone, and had more sepsis. After adjustment for multiple clinical confounders and total brain volume, the authors found that increased morphine exposure was associated with a decrease in cerebellar volume ($P = .04$). Greater morphine exposure also predicted poorer motor ($P < .001$) and cognitive outcomes ($P = .006$) at 18 months corrected age. Morphine exposure was not associated with cerebral volume ($P = .30$). These findings suggest that morphine exposure in very preterm neonates is independently associated with impaired cerebellar growth in the neonatal period and poorer neurodevelopmental outcomes in early childhood. These data support that morphine exposure should be limited to intermittent use during recognized painful procedures and that alternatives to better manage distress and anxiety in preterm infants are urgently needed.

T. E. Inder, MD

A Randomized Clinical Trial of Therapeutic Hypothermia Mode During Transport for Neonatal Encephalopathy

Akula VP, Joe P, Thusu K, et al (Stanford Univ School of Medicine and Lucile Packard Children's Hosp Stanford, Palo Alto, CA; Children's Hosp and Res Ctr, Oakland, CA; Children's Hosp Central California, Madera; et al)

J Pediatr 166:856-861, 2015

Objective.—To determine if temperature regulation is improved during neonatal transport using a servo-regulated cooling device when compared with standard practice.

Study Design.—We performed a multicenter, randomized, nonmasked clinical trial in newborns with neonatal encephalopathy cooled during transport to 9 neonatal intensive care units in California. Newborns who met institutional criteria for therapeutic hypothermia were randomly assigned to receive cooling according to usual center practices vs device servo-regulated cooling. The primary outcome was the percentage of temperatures in target range (33°-34°C) during transport. Secondary outcomes included percentage of newborns reaching target temperature any time during transport, time to target temperature, and percentage of newborns in target range 1 hour after cooling initiation.

Results.—One hundred newborns were enrolled: 49 to control arm and 51 to device arm. Baseline demographics did not differ with the exception of cord pH. For each subject, the percentage of temperatures in the target range was calculated. Infants cooled using the device had a higher percentage of temperatures in target range compared with control infants (median 73% [IQR 17-88] vs 0% [IQR 0-52], $P < .001$). More subjects reached target temperature during transport using the servo-regulated device (80% vs 49%, $P < .001$), and in a shorter time period (44 ± 31 minutes vs 63 ± 37 minutes, $P = .04$). Device-cooled infants reached target temperature by 1 hour with greater frequency than control infants (71% vs 20%, $P < .001$).

Conclusions.—Cooling using a servo-regulated device provides more predictable temperature management during neonatal transport than does usual care for outborn newborns with neonatal encephalopathy.

▶ Hypothermic neuroprotection has become a standard of care for the treatment of acute neonatal encephalopathy following intrapartum asphyxia. Current thought is that the sooner the desired temperature is reached, the better will be the outcome. Unfortunately, many infants who might benefit from cooling are born in settings where cooling is not offered, and transport to a center that provides cooling becomes necessary. Many cooling centers, my own included, will recommend initiation by passive cooling (turning off the radiant warmer) and maintaining this during the duration of transport. Others have tried active cooling, using ice, gel packs, or cold-water gloves in contact with the baby. These are inexact and, as we have seen, can result in overshoot and significant hypothermia. This study evaluated the use of a servo-regulated system applied during transport. Not surprisingly, infants randomized to the device had a much better temperature profile than those treated manually. Whether this ultimately leads to better outcomes remains to be seen, but it does show that the technology is a lot more accurate and targeted than manual management. The authors did not provide information regarding the cost of the device.

S. M. Donn, MD

Injury to the Cerebellum in Term Asphyxiated Newborns Treated with Hypothermia

Kwan S, Boudes E, Gilbert G, et al (McGill Univ, Montreal, Quebec, Canada; Philips Healthcare, Montreal, Quebec, Canada)
AJNR Am J Neuroradiol 36:1542-1549, 2015

Background and Purpose.—Until now, most studies of brain injury related to term neonatal encephalopathy have focused on the cerebrum and ignored the cerebellum. We sought to evaluate whether cerebellar injury occurs in term asphyxiated neonates.

Materials and Methods.—Asphyxiated neonates treated with hypothermia were enrolled prospectively. Severity of brain injury in the cerebrum was scored on each MR imaging obtained during the first month of life; cerebellar injury was recorded when mentioned in the imaging or autopsy report. In addition, for some of the neonates, the ADC and fractional anisotropy were measured in 4 regions of interest in the cerebellum.

Results.—One hundred seventy-two asphyxiated neonates met the criteria for hypothermia. Cerebellar injury was visible only on conventional imaging of 4% of the neonates for whom brain imaging was available, but it was reported in the autopsy report of 72% of the neonates who died. In addition, 41 of the asphyxiated neonates had a total of 84 ADC and fractional anisotropy maps. Neonates with brain injury described only in the cerebrum demonstrated ADC and fractional anisotropy changes similar to those of the neonates with brain injury in the cerebrum and cerebellum—increased ADC around day 10 of life and decreased fractional anisotropy on day 2–3 of life, around day 10 of life, and around 1 month of age.

Conclusions.—The cerebellum may be injured in term neonates after birth asphyxia. These cerebellar injuries are only rarely visible on conventional imaging, but advanced neuroimaging techniques may help to identify them.

▶ The cerebellum is the "black box" of the neonatal brain. Compared with the cerebrum, much less is known regarding mechanisms of hypoxic-ischemic injury, and limitations of standard neuroimaging techniques have continued the mystery. This article describes cerebellar injury in term asphyxiated newborns with hypoxic-ischemic encephalopathy severe enough to warrant hypothermic neuroprotection. The investigators prospectively studied 172 cooled newborns and found that conventional imaging revealed cerebellar injury in only 4% of cases. Postmortem evaluation of nonsurvivors demonstrated a 72% incidence of cerebellar involvement. Apparent diffusion coefficient mapping and fractional anisotropy, where performed, showed similar changes in the cerebrum and cerebellum. It is difficult to discern whether the much higher incidence of cerebellar injury on the postmortem series is representative of the entire population or whether it signifies an agonal event, but the message from this study is that we need to be more cognizant of the potential vulnerability of the cerebellum to hypoxic-ischemic injury, and more sophisticated imaging will be necessary to diagnose it. This should also be taken into account, both in future studies of hypothermic neuroprotection and in designing appropriate follow-up studies to test for cerebellar dysfunction.

S. M. Donn, MD

Moderate hypothermia within 6 h of birth plus inhaled xenon versus moderate hypothermia alone after birth asphyxia (TOBY-Xe): a proof-of-concept, open-label, randomised controlled trial

Azzopardi D, Robertson NJ, Bainbridge A, et al (King's College London, UK; Univ College London, UK; UCL Hosps NHS Foundation Trust, UK; et al)

Lancet Neurol 2015 [Epub ahead of print]

Background.—Moderate cooling after birth asphyxia is associated with substantial reductions in death and disability, but additional therapies might provide further benefit. We assessed whether the addition of xenon gas, a promising novel therapy, after the initiation of hypothermia for birth asphyxia would result in further improvement.

Methods.—Total Body hypothermia plus Xenon (TOBY-Xe) was a proof-of-concept, randomised, open-label, parallel-group trial done at four intensive-care neonatal units in the UK. Eligible infants were 36–43 weeks of gestational age, had signs of moderate to severe encephalopathy and moderately or severely abnormal background activity for at least 30 min or seizures as shown by amplitude-integrated EEG (aEEG), and had one of the following: Apgar score of 5 or less 10 min after birth, continued need for resuscitation 10 min after birth, or acidosis within 1 h of birth. Participants were allocated in a 1:1 ratio by use of a secure web-based computer-generated randomisation sequence within 12 h of birth to cooling to a rectal temperature of 33·5°C for 72 h (standard treatment) or to cooling in combination with 30% inhaled xenon for 24 h started immediately after randomisation. The primary outcomes were reduction in lactate to N-acetyl aspartate ratio in the thalamus and in preserved fractional anisotropy in the posterior limb of the internal capsule, measured with magnetic resonance spectroscopy and MRI, respectively, within 15 days of birth. The investigator assessing these outcomes was masked to allocation. Analysis was by intention to treat. This trial is registered with ClinicalTrials.gov, number NCT00934700, and with ISRCTN, as ISRCTN08886155.

Findings.—The study was done from Jan 31, 2012, to Sept 30, 2014. We enrolled 92 infants, 46 of whom were randomly assigned to cooling only and 46 to xenon plus cooling. 37 infants in the cooling only group and 41 in the cooling plus xenon group underwent magnetic resonance assessments and were included in the analysis of the primary outcomes. We noted no significant differences in lactate to N-acetyl aspartate ratio in the thalamus (geometric mean ratio 1·09, 95% CI 0·90 to 1·32) or fractional anisotropy (mean difference −0·01, 95% CI −0·03 to 0·02) in the posterior limb of the internal capsule between the two groups. Nine infants died in the cooling group and 11 in the xenon group. Two adverse events were reported in the xenon group: subcutaneous fat necrosis and transient desaturation during the MRI. No serious adverse events were recorded.

Interpretation.—Administration of xenon within the delayed timeframe used in this trial is feasible and apparently safe, but is unlikely to enhance the neuroprotective effect of cooling after birth asphyxia.

▶ Although induced hypothermia is the standard of care for neonatal hypoxic-ischemic encephalopathy (HIE), it is only moderately effective. Approximately 25% of infants with moderate to severe HIE who undergo treatment with induced hypothermia die, and 20% of surviving infants have evidence of neurodevelopmental impairment. A number of adjuvant therapies have been proposed; however, the resources needed to test even the most promising of these therapies in large randomized clinical trials far outstrip those available, particularly if neurodevelopmental outcome in early childhood is a component of the primary outcome.

To ascertain the utility of using xenon as an adjuvant therapy, the investigators in this clinical trial used a proof-of-concept design. Magnetic resonance biomarkers of acute brain injury were used to assess whether adding xenon therapy to induced hypothermia could further improve neurological outcomes after moderate to severe neonatal HIE. Because there was no difference in the biomarkers between the 2 groups, the investigators concluded that xenon when given by 12 hours of age and for 24 hours does not have additional neuroprotective effects compared with induced hypothermia alone.

As noted by the authors, perhaps xenon treatment needs to be given before 12 hours of age, at a higher dose or for a longer duration, to be beneficial. A more compelling explanation for the lack of efficacy relates to the severity of the encephalopathy; 85% of the infants in the cooling group and 87% of those in the in the cooling plus xenon group had amplitude electroencephalogram (aEEG) changes classified as severe encephalopathy. Thus, it may be that the study infants were too severely asphyxiated and had little prospect of benefit from any intervention after birth.

L. A. Papile, MD

MRI obtained during versus after hypothermia in asphyxiated newborns

Boudes E, Tan X, Saint-Martin C, et al (McGill Univ, Montreal, Quebec, Canada; McGill Univ Health Centre, Montreal, Quebec, Canada; et al)

Arch Dis Child Fetal Neonatal Ed 100:F238-F242, 2015

Objective.—To assess whether the brain MRI results obtained during hypothermia identify the later brain injury observed in asphyxiated newborns after therapy is completed.

Patients and Methods.—Asphyxiated newborns treated with hypothermia were prospectively enrolled in this study if they had at least one MRI performed during hypothermia treatment and then another MRI performed around day 10 of life.

Results.—A total of 129 MRI scans were obtained from 43 asphyxiated newborns treated with hypothermia. Sixty per cent developed brain injury; all the brain injuries observed on the late scans were already present on day 2–3 of life during hypothermia, and the extent of injury was similar between the early and late scans. The brain MRI on day 2–3 of life had a sensitivity of 100% (95% CI 84% to 100%) and a specificity of 100% (95% CI 77% to 100%) to identify the presence and extent of later brain injury.

Conclusions.—The brain MRIs performed during hypothermia already permit an accurate definition of the presence and extent of brain injury that later develop in asphyxiated newborns despite treatment. These results may have research and clinical implications for the care of these newborns.

▶ In this observational study, the investigators compared the results of brain magnetic resonance imaging (MRI) from day 2 or 3 with that done around day 10 in a population of infants undergoing therapeutic hypothermia for hypoxic-ischemic encephalopathy. It appears that there was good concordance between the 2 studies, with the day 2–3 study predicting the day 10 result. The authors suggest important research and clinical implications by doing the earlier examination. I would argue the opposite: that we do far too many MRIs on this population of infants. If the studies are essentially no different, why subject the infant to the rigors of a transport to the MRI suite? Many of these infants are still on life support, receiving infusions of vasoactive drugs, and will be subjected to less stable thermal environments.

Our own group recently published a study that demonstrated that most cooled infants will have a normal MRI unless their clinical course was compromised by seizure activity or the inability to achieve full oral feeding by 7 days.[1] This begs the question as to whether every "cooled" baby needs an MRI study.

Perhaps less is more.

S. M. Donn, MD

Reference

1. Sarkar S, Donn SM, Bapuraj JR, Bhagat I, Dechert RE, Barks JD. Does clinical evaluation one week after therapeutic hypothermia predict brain MRI abnormalities? *J Perinatol.* 2013;33:538-542.

Treating EEG Seizures in Hypoxic Ischemic Encephalopathy: A Randomized Controlled Trial

Srinivasakumar P, Zempel J, Trivedi S, et al (Washington Univ in St Louis, MO; et al)

Pediatrics 136:e1302-e1309, 2015

Background.—The impact of treating electrographic seizures in hypoxic ischemic encephalopathy (HIE) is unknown.

Methods.—Neonates ≥36 weeks with moderate or severe HIE were randomly assigned to either treatment of electrographic seizures alone (ESG) or treatment of clinical seizures (CSG). Conventional EEG video was monitored in both groups for up to 96 hours. Cumulative electrographic seizure burden (SB) was calculated in seconds and converted to log units for analysis. MRI scans were scored for severity of brain injury. Infants underwent neurodevelopmental evaluation at 18 to 24 months. Statistical analyses were performed by using SAS 9.3 version (SAS Institute, Inc, Cary, NC).

Results.—Thirty-five of 69 neonates (51%) who were randomly assigned and included in the study developed seizures (15 in ESG and 20 in CSG). Excluding infants with status epilepticus, median SB (interquartile range) in seconds in ESG ($n = 10$) was lower than in CSG ($n = 16$) (449 [113–2070] vs 2226 [760–7654]; $P = .02$). ESG had fewer seizures with shorter time to treatment ($P = .04$). Twenty-four of 30 (80%) surviving infants with seizures underwent neurodevelopmental evaluation at 18 to 24 months. Increasing SB in the combined cohort was significantly associated with higher brain injury scores ($P < .03$) and lower performance scores across all 3 domains on BSID III ($P = .03$).

Conclusions.—In neonates with HIE, EEG monitoring and treatment of electrographic seizures results in significant reduction in SB. SB is associated with more severe brain injury and significantly lower performance scores across all domains on BSID III.

▶ The American Clinical Neurophysiology Society recommends electroencephalographic (EEG) monitoring for at least 24 hours in infants with neonatal hypoxic/ischemic encephalopathy (HIE) to detect seizure activity that may not be evident clinically.[1] However, there is no direct evidence available that neonatal EEG monitoring, seizure identification, or treatment of seizures in infants with HIE impacts clinical outcomes.

The objective of this single-center randomized clinical trial was to monitor and treat electrographic seizures in infants with moderate to severe HIE. As part of usual care, all of the infants underwent continuous conventional EEG video monitoring which was not visible to the bedside caregivers. Infants were then randomized to either the electrographic seizure group or the clinical seizure group. The electrographic seizure group received additional seizure monitoring with limited channel bedside amplitude electroencephalography (aEEG) containing automatic seizure detecting software that alerted caregivers with a change in color on the monitor display panel. If an infant in the clinical seizure group had seizures detected by the epileptologist on continuous conventional EEG video monitoring, she or he was unblinded to receive antiepileptic therapy. It is interesting to note that 20 of the 34 infants (59%) randomized to the clinical seizure group fell into this category.

Despite a reduced total accumulative seizure burden and a shorter time to treatment from seizure onset, the aEEG group had cognitive, motor, and composite language scores on the Bayley Scales of Infant development (BSID-III) similar to those of the clinical seizure cohort. In fact, the BSID-III composite scores for both groups did not differ significantly from those of infants without seizures. When an analysis of the whole cohort was performed increasing seizure burden correlated significantly with both worse injury on MRI and lower performance scores on the BSID, suggesting that infants with the most severe HIE have seizures intractable to treatment. Unfortunately the results of the above study do little to answer questions regarding the utility of continuous neonatal EEG monitoring.

L. A. Papile, MD

Cerebral palsy after neonatal encephalopathy: do neonates with suspected asphyxia have worse outcomes?

Garfinkle J, On Behalf of the Canadian Cerebral Palsy Registry (Montreal Children's Hosp-McGill Univ Health Ctr, Quebec, Canada; et al)

Dev Med Child Neurol 58:189-194, 2016

Aim.—We sought to investigate how brain injury and severity, and neurological subtype of cerebral palsy (CP) differed in term-born children with CP after neonatal encephalopathy, between those with suspected birth asphyxia and those without.

Method.—Using the Canadian CP Registry, which included 1001 children, those with CP born at ≥ 36 wks after moderate or severe neonatal encephalopathy, were dichotomized according to the presence or absence of suspected birth asphyxia. Gross Motor Function Classification System (GMFCS) scores, neurological subtypes, comorbidities, and magnetic resonance imaging findings were compared.

Results.—Of the 147 term-born children with CP (82 males, 65 females; median age 37 months, interquartile range [IQR] 26–52.5) who after moderate or severe neonatal encephalopathy had the required outcome data, 61 (41%) met criteria for suspected birth asphyxia. They had a higher frequency of non-ambulatory GMFCS status (odds ratio [OR] 3.4, 95% confidence interval [CI] 1.72–6.8), spastic quadriplegia (OR 2.8, 95% CI 1.4–5.6), nonverbal communication skills impairment (OR 4.2, 95% CI 2.0–8.6), isolated deep grey matter injury (OR 4.1, 95% CI 1.8–9.5), a lower frequency of spastic hemiplegia (OR 0.17, 95% CI 0.07–0.42), focal injury (OR 0.20; 95% CI 0.04–0.93), and more comorbidities ($p = 0.017$) than those who did not meet criteria.

Interpretation.—Term-born children who develop CP after neonatal encephalopathy with suspected birth asphyxia have a greater burden of disability than those without suspected birth asphyxia.

► The selection criteria for therapeutic hypothermia include evidence of fetal and/or neonatal asphyxia and clinical signs of moderate to severe encephalopathy. The elements of both criteria were selected to provide treatment to those infants most likely to benefit from the therapy. In this study the authors suggest that the criteria may be too restrictive.

The study used data extracted from Canadian Cerebral Palsy Registry. The registry captures cases of cerebral palsy (CP) identified through both pediatric rehabilitation centers and university hospitals for the birth years of 1999 through 2011. Once cases are identified, parental consent is obtained and the maternal and child's records are reviewed. To be enrolled in the registry children must be at least 2 years old and meet diagnostic consensus criteria for CP. Only children who met the gestational age and birth weight criteria for therapeutic hypothermia were included. An additional criterion was evidence of moderate to severe neonatal encephalopathy (NE) based on the Sarnat score during the first week after birth. Clinical criteria were derived from the National Institute of Child Health and Human Development randomized controlled trial of hypothermia and the Positions Statement of the Canadian Pediatric Society.

There are several limitations to the authors' estimated 5.1% of CP after NE that may be prevented with therapeutic hypothermia. First, the estimate does not take into consideration that 11 of the 64 infants with NE who met cooling criteria actually were cooled. Additionally, infants who developed NE at any point within the first week of age were included. Seizures were the most common manifestation of NE among infants who did not meet the clinical criteria for cooling (68/91; 75%). It is highly likely that the majority of the seizures would have occurred after 6 hours, and thus beyond the optimal window for effective therapy.

The current criteria for therapeutic hypothermia represent our best estimate of the infants most likely to benefit from this therapy. Despite this, the practice of extending the treatment to infants who do not meet criteria is becoming more widespread. It may be that the criteria for therapeutic hypothermia needs to be broadened. To do so without additional clinical trials assessing the risks and benefits is ill advised.

L. A. Papile, MD

Fetal and Neonatal Effects of N-Acetylcysteine When Used for Neuroprotection in Maternal Chorioamnionitis

Jenkins DD, Wiest DB, Mulvihill DM, et al (Med Univ of South Carolina, Charleston; et al)

J Pediatr 168:67-76, 2016

Objective.—To evaluate the clinical safety of antenatal and postnatal N-acetylcysteine (NAC) as a neuroprotective agent in maternal chorioamnionitis in a randomized, controlled, double-blinded trial.

Study Design.—Twenty-two mothers >24 weeks gestation presenting within 4 hours of diagnosis of clinical chorioamnionitis were randomized with their 24 infants to NAC or saline treatment. Antenatal NAC (100 mg/kg/dose) or saline was given intravenously every 6 hours until delivery. Postnatally, NAC (12.5-25 mg/kg/dose, n = 12) or saline (n = 12) was given every 12 hours for 5 doses. Doppler studies of fetal umbilical and fetal and infant cerebral blood flow, cranial ultrasounds, echocardiograms, cerebral oxygenation, electroencephalograms, and serum cytokines were evaluated before and after treatment, and 12, 24, and 48 hours after birth. Magnetic resonance spectroscopy and diffusion imaging were performed at term age equivalent. Development was followed for cerebral palsy or autism to 4 years of age.

Results.—Cardiovascular measures, cerebral blood flow velocity and vascular resistance, and cerebral oxygenation did not differ between treatment groups. Cerebrovascular coupling was disrupted in infants with chorioamnionitis treated with saline but preserved in infants treated with NAC, suggesting improved vascular regulation in the presence of neuroinflammation. Infants treated with NAC had higher serum anti-inflammatory interleukin-1 receptor antagonist and lower proinflammatory vascular endothelial growth factor over time vs controls. No adverse events related to NAC administration were noted.

Conclusions.—In this cohort of newborns exposed to chorioamnionitis, antenatal and postnatal NAC was safe, preserved cerebrovascular regulation, and increased an anti-inflammatory neuroprotective protein.

Trial Registration.—ClinicalTrials.gov: NCT00724594.

▶ This study illustrates the obstacles encountered by investigators who wish to conduct interventional clinical trials in the setting of labor and delivery suites. The investigators were given a waiver by their Institutional Review Board to obtain prequalifying consent from women in preterm labor or with ruptured membranes. Enrollment/randomization was initiated only if inclusion criteria were met. Of the 78 women who were eligible for the study, 72% were not included because of inadequate time between qualifying and infant delivery to initiate the protocol. Thus, a total of 22 pregnant women were enrolled over a 16-month period with 12 allocated to the treatment group.

A total of 24 infants, including 2 sets of twins, were born to enrolled women. Of these, 1 infant in the control group died, and 9 and 12, respectively, of the control and the study infants were available for follow-up to 3 to 4 years of age. Two children in each group had a developmental delay. Although the sample size is limited, it appears that N-acetylcysteine does not afford neuroprotection to preterm and term infants exposed to chorioamnionitis. A previous study evaluating the usefulness of N-acetylcysteine to prevent bronchoplumonary dysplasia demonstrated similar findings.[1]

L. A. Papile, MD

Reference

1. Ahola T, Lapatto R, Raaivo KO, et al. N-acetylcysteine does not prevent bronchopulmonary dysplasia in immature infants; a randomized controlled trial. *J Pediatr.* 2003;203:713-719.

Prenatal Factors in Singletons with Cerebral Palsy Born at or near Term

Nelson KB, Blair E (Natl Insts of Health, Bethesda, MD; Children's Natl Med Ctr, Washington, DC)

N Engl J Med 373:946-953, 2015

Background.—Cerebral palsy is a disorder of movement caused by nonprogressive cerebral defects acquired early in life. It is often accompanied by disorders of intellectual function, epilepsy, and sensory disturbances. No cure is available so efforts have been focused on prevention, which necessitates an understanding of the causal pathways. Two thirds of those with cerebral palsy are born at or after 35 weeks of gestation, although extremely preterm survivors are at much higher risk for the disorder. However, few of these neonates born before 28 weeks of gestation survive. Preventive efforts have included continuous electronic fetal monitoring during labor to identify fetal asphyxia, but even with the extensive use of fetal monitoring the numbers of live births with cerebral palsy has not declined in 3 decades. Investigation into prenatal antecedents related to cerebral palsy has identified several determinants of the risk of cerebral palsy for children in developed countries who are born at or near term.

Birth Defects.—Birth defects are more common in persons with cerebral palsy than in those without this disorder. Major malformations, including cerebral defects, may be the primary factor linked to cerebral palsy. Although early detection of these defects has improved, some do not manifest until after the newborn period, so infants at risk should be observed for an extended period. Preterm infants are more likely to have birth defects than term infants, but among infants with cerebral palsy, major malformations are more common in infants born at term or at normal birth weight. The risk of a birth defect associated with cerebral palsy is increased by a factor of 9 among term or near term infants compared with preterm infants.

The types of defects most often associated with cerebral palsy involve the brain, with cardiac lesions the next most common. Brain defects include structural abnormalities, aberrant growth, and prenatal destructive lesions. Congenital microcephaly is the most common birth defect in those with cerebral palsy.

Fetal Growth Restriction.—Marked fetal growth restriction is associated with an increased risk for cerebral palsy. Neonates with poor growth are also more likely to have birth defects and infants with birth defects are more likely to have growth restrictions. Having major birth defects and fetal growth restriction increases cerebral palsy risk.

Thrombotic States.—Low blood flow in the placenta, brain, or other organs predisposes to clotting. Thromboembolism, vascular disruption, and major hemodynamic shifts can contribute to malformations, possibly causing brain lesions in early fetal life or cerebral infarction in later fetal life. Perinatal stroke is linked to hemiplegic cerebral palsy, which is the most common type found in term birth or near-term birth infants.

Placental Conditions.—Pathologic processes of the placenta are linked to cerebral palsy, growth restriction, and some birth defects. Embolization from the placenta near delivery can cause perinatal stroke. Fetal thrombotic vasculopathy is linked to term stillbirth, fetal growth restriction, birth defects, neonatal encephalopathy, and cerebral palsy.

Genetic Factors.—Some infants with cerebral palsy are suspected to have a genetic component to the disorder. One population-based study showed the risk of cerebral palsy was increased by a factor of 11 in single births at term who had an affected older sibling and a factor of 15 in twin births who had an affected co-twin. Studies are needed in this area because of the complexity of conditions related to the same genetic mutation.

Conclusions.—The evidence indicates that prenatal factors can play a major factor in increasing the risk of cerebral palsy. Special management of infants with fetal growth restriction may permit the identification of birth defects and warn of a higher risk of cerebral palsy. Intrauterine infections, teratogens, and genetic syndromes should be evaluated to determine the joint occurrence of such problems with cerebral palsy. Placental investigations and microanalyses of biochemical and genetic markers may someday be able to identify neonates at increased risk and provide treatment options.

▶ Significant abnormalities in neurodevelopment, such as cerebral palsy (CP), likely represent the adverse outcomes parents most fear and physicians dread. For decades, CP was attributed largely to perinatal complications, such as hypoxic-ischemic encephalopathy and traumatic brain injury. Because the diagnosis of CP often is not made until age 18 months or beyond, the possible late identification of the disorder and the threat of associated medical-legal action has been a long-standing burden to our obstetrical colleagues and other perinatal caregivers. In recent years, however, the medical and scientific communities have come to appreciate that other important exposures, including preterm birth, are contributing factors for the majority of infants who later develop CP. In this scholarly review that should be on the must-read list for all neonatologists and neonatal-perinatal medicine trainees, Drs Nelson and Blair review the trends in CP from 1980 through 2009 among infants of all birth weights, showing a relatively stable CP rate, despite climbing rates of elective and emergency cesarean deliveries. The authors provide an in-depth view of antenatal factors that are associated with CP, including anomalies (even those outside of the central nervous system), genetic factors, low gestational age, growth restriction, and evidence of intrauterine inflammation. Their co-occurrence almost certainly further increases CP risk. The knowledge that the onset of CP might begin with certain pregnancy complications, such as fetal growth restriction, should fuel obstetrical efforts toward early identification, prevention, and innovation in management of these disorders, as well as in engagement and communication with neonatology colleagues when these challenging cases arise. It should, likewise, provide pediatricians and neonatologists with strong motivation to increase vigilance for anomalies when performing physical exams on both normal and growth-restricted term and late preterm infants, enhance attention to placental pathology, and encourage engagement in rigorous identification of fetal or neonatal growth restriction and its underlying cause(s), as well as ensure appropriate neurodevelopmental follow-up when 1 or more CP risk factor is identified,.

L. J. Van Marter, MD, MPH

Impaired cognitive performance in premature newborns with two or more surgeries prior to term-equivalent age

Gano D, Andersen SK, Glass HC, et al (Univ of California–San Francisco; Queens Univ, Kingston, Ontario, Canada)

Pediatr Res 78:323-329, 2015

Background.—Anesthesia in early childhood is associated with adverse neurodevelopmental outcome; however, it is not known if age at exposure affects the risk of adverse outcome. Our objective was to evaluate the association of the number and timing of anesthetic exposures for surgery with cognitive outcome in a cohort of premature newborns.

Methods.—A cohort study of exposure to anesthesia for surgery in premature newborns (<33 wk gestation) prospectively evaluated with neonatal magnetic resonance imaging (MRI) and neurodevelopmental testing at 3-6 y was employed. Exposure to anesthesia for surgery was classified as before term-equivalent age (TEA, <42 wk postmenstrual age) or after (≥42 wk). Multivariate regression was performed to analyze the association of composite IQ scores with the number of surgeries before and after TEA.

Results.—Among 137 newborns, 25 (18.2%) had one surgery before TEA and 18 (13.1%) had ≥2 surgeries. Two or more surgeries before TEA were associated with significantly reduced composite IQ scores at 4.6 ± 0.6 y after adjusting for gestational age and illness severity. Neither the number of surgeries after TEA nor sedation for MRI was associated with cognitive outcome.

Conclusions.—More than one surgery prior to TEA is independently associated with impaired cognitive performance in premature newborns (Fig 1).

▶ "Brain injury in premature infants is of enormous public health importance because of the large number of such infants who survive with serious neurodevelopmental disability, including major cognitive deficits and motor disability. This type of brain injury is generally thought to consist primarily of periventricular leukomalacia (PVL), a distinctive form of cerebral white matter injury.

PVL is frequently accompanied by neuronal/axonal disease, affecting the cerebral white matter, thalamus, basal ganglia, cerebral cortex, brain stem, and cerebellum. This constellation of PVL and neuronal/axonal disease is sufficiently distinctive to be termed 'encephalopathy of prematurity.' The encephalopathy of prematurity is a complex amalgam of primary destructive disease and secondary maturational and trophic disturbances."[1] Surgery and anesthesia may trigger both delays in maturation as well as destruction.

Gano et al add convincing data to the story that neonates undergoing surgery, and particularly those exposed to multiple surgeries and anesthetic agents, are at risk for poorer neurodevelopmental outcomes. Fig 1 illustrates the global effects very well.

Children who required neonatal surgery have previously been reported to have an increased risk of neurosensory impairment[2]; worse academic

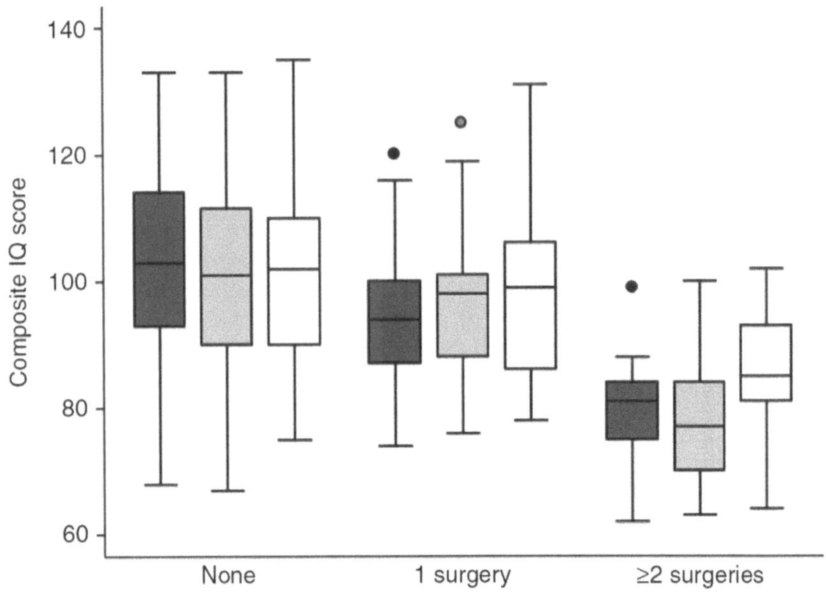

FIGURE 1.—Composite IQ scores by number of surgeries prior to term-equivalent age. Box plot demonstrating composite full-scale (dark gray), performance (light gray), and verbal (white) IQ scores in children by the number of surgeries prior to term-equivalent age (TEA). Circles represent outliers. (Reprinted from Gano D, Andersen SK, Glass HC, et al. Impaired cognitive performance in premature newborns with two or more surgeries prior to term-equivalent age. *Pediatr Res.* 2015;78:323-329, with permission from International Pediatric Research Foundation, Inc.)

performance in adolescence compared with controls[3]; and impaired neurodevelopment in infancy.[4] None of these studies accounted for surgeries required after the neonatal period. A large multicenter cohort study,[4] involving 2186 infants, has recently shown that major surgery in very-low-birth-weight infants was independently associated with a 52% increased risk of death or neurodevelopmental impairment at 18 to 22 months' corrected age. Patients classified as having minor surgery had no increased adjusted risk. However, the number and timing of exposures to anesthesia for surgery was not evaluated, the study population excluded newborns who required patent ductus arteriosus ligation, and only severe cystic white matter injury detected by ultrasound was adjusted for in the analysis. They did, however, note that "the role of general anesthesia is implicated but remains unproven." That is indeed a good summation of the state of the art. There is an indisputable association between surgery and poorer neurodevelopmental outcome for infants operated on before term. It remains an association until causality is determined.

A. A. Fanaroff, MD

References

1. Volpe JJ. Brain injury in premature infants: a complex amalgam of destructive and developmental disturbances. *Lancet Neurol.* 2009;8:110-124.

2. Kabra NS, Schmidt B, Roberts RS, Doyle LW, Papile L, Fanaroff A. Trial of Indomethacin Prophylaxis in Preterms Investigators. Neurosensory impairment after surgical closure of patent ductus arteriosus in extremely low birth weight infants: results from the Trial of Indomethacin Prophylaxis in Preterms. *J Pediatr.* 2007; 150:229-234. 234.e1.
3. Ludman L, Spitz L, Wade A. Educational attainments in early adolescence of infants who required major neonatal surgery. *J Pediatr Surg.* 2001;36:858-862.
4. Morriss FH Jr, Saha S, Bell EF, et al. Eunice Kennedy Shriver National Institute of Child Health and Human Development Neonatal Research Network. Surgery and neurodevelopmental outcome of very low-birthweight infants. *JAMA Pediatr.* 2014;168:746-754.

Neonatal Morphine Exposure in Very Preterm Infants—Cerebral Development and Outcomes

Steinhorn R, McPherson C, Anderson PJ, et al (Washington Univ in St Louis, MO; Brigham and Women's Hosp, Boston, MA; The Univ of Melbourne, Carlton, Australia; et al)
J Pediatr 166:1200-1207, 2015

Objective.—To investigate the association of morphine exposure in very preterm infants with cerebral volumes and neurodevelopmental outcome from birth through middle childhood.

Study Design.—Observational study of very preterm infants in the Victorian Infant Brain Study cohort. A total of 230 infants born <30 weeks' gestational age or <1250 g were recruited from all admissions to the neonatal intensive care unit of the Royal Women's Hospital. Fifty-seven (25%) infants received morphine analgesia during their neonatal intensive care unit stay at the attending physician's discretion. Primary outcomes were regional brain volumes at term and 7 years; neurobehavioral performance at term; and cognitive, motor, emotional, behavioral, communication, and executive function scores at age 2 and 7 years. Linear regressions were used to compare outcomes between participants who did and did not receive morphine.

Results.—At term, preterm infants who received morphine had similar rates of gray matter injury to no-morphine infants, but a trend toward smaller cortical volumes in the orbitofrontal (*P*left = .002, *P*right = .01) and subgenual (*P*left = .01) regions. At 7 years, cortical volumes did not differ between groups. At 2 years, morphine-exposed children were more likely to show behavioral dysregulation (*P* = .007) than no-morphine children, but at 7 years no detrimental impacts of morphine on neurobehavioral outcome were observed.

Conclusions.—Low-dose morphine analgesia received during neonatal intensive care was associated with early alterations in cerebral structure and short-term neurobehavioral problems that did not persist into childhood.

▶ Chronic exposure to morphine in animal studies produces neuronal degeneration, reduced cortical neuron number and density, and reduced basilar dendritic growth. In human studies, reports on the neurologic consequences of morphine exposure have been inconsistent. Neonatal exposure to continuous morphine infusions to reduce pain did not result in neurodevelopmental benefit. This observational study of 230 very preterm infants born < 30 weeks' gestational age or < 1250 g describes 57 of these infants (25%) receiving morphine analgesia during their neonatal intensive care unit (NICU) stay at the attending physician's discretion. The infants received a median cumulative dose 0.79 mg/kg (interquartile range 0.12–0.95 mg/kg, range 0.1–5.3 mg/kg). Thirty-two participants received only boluses, 21 received a mixture of boluses and infusion, and 4 received an infusion only; no clinical factors differed between these 3 subgroups. One hundred sixty-six infants received no sedative or analgesic medication while in the NICU. The infants who received morphine were only slightly more immature (1 week gestation), with higher illness severity and length of ventilation. At term, the preterm infants who received morphine had similar rates of gray matter injury to no-morphine infants, but a trend toward smaller cortical volumes in the orbitofrontal (Pleft = .002, Pright = .01) and subgenual (Pleft = .01) regions. At 7 years, cortical volumes did not differ between groups. At 2 years, morphine-exposed children were more likely to show behavioral dysregulation ($P = .007$) than no-morphine children, but at 7 years, no detrimental impacts of morphine on neurobehavioral outcome were observed. This study would support that the use of low-dose morphine analgesia during neonatal intensive care was not associated with long-term alterations in cerebral structure or adverse neurobehavioral outcomes. Low-dose targeted morphine use as an analgesic may not carry long-term adverse consequences for the very preterm infant.

T. E. Inder, MD

The whole spectrum of cystic periventricular leukomalacia of the preterm infant: results from a large consecutive case series

Resch B, Resch E, Maurer-Fellbaum U, et al (Med Univ of Graz, Austria)
Child's Nerv Syst 31:1527-1532, 2015

Purpose.—The purpose of this study is to describe features of cystic periventricular leukomalacia (PVL) in a large consecutive cohort study including long-term neurodevelopmental follow-up.

Methods.—We performed a retrospective single-centre cohort study including all preterm infants ≤35 weeks of gestational age with PVL diagnosed by ultrasound scans (US) from a tertiary care university hospital between 1988 and 2012.

Results.—The majority of 160 consecutively diagnosed cases had a gestational age between 28 and 32 weeks (60.6 %), and male sex was predominant (60.6 %). The most common associated clinical findings included respiratory distress syndrome, preterm premature rupture of the membranes, and chorioamnionitis (57.5, 49.4, and 39.4 %, respectively). Infants presented with apnoeas in 66.3 and neonatal seizures in

23.1 %. Any kind of respiratory support was present in 75.0 %. Associated low-grade intraventricular haemorrhage was evident in 33.1, high-grade haemorrhage in 9.4 %. Cysts were located on both hemispheres in 75 % and PVL grades 3 and 4 were predominant (75.6 %). Neurodevelopmental follow-up of 146 cases at a median age of 72 months revealed normal development in 11.0, mental retardation in 50.0, and cerebral palsy in 83.6 %. Visual impairment was diagnosed in 21.9% and hearing impairment in one case. A quarter of cases (27.4 %) developed seizure disorders. Outcome data were significantly better in unilateral compared to bilateral PVL.

Conclusions.—Long-term neurodevelopmental outcome of bilateral PVL always was adverse and different from unilateral PVL. The latter might be negatively influenced by associated intra- and periventricular haemorrhages.

► Cystic periventricular leukomalacia (PVL) refers to the spectrum of white matter damage by inflammation, excitotoxicity, hypoxia-ischemia, or exposure to free radicals. This article from Graz, Austria, encompasses a 25-year time span during which 160 cases of PVL were encountered. Of note, a third of these patients also had low-grade intraventricular hemorrhage (IVH), and almost 10% had severe IVH. There was nothing remarkable about the cohort with regard to risk factors, gestational age, and clinical courses. Not surprisingly, outcomes at age 6 years were worse in the patients with bilateral PVL.

To gain perspective on the changes in germinal matrix hemorrhage with IVH (GMH-IVH) over a period of hundred years, we turn to this remarkable paper from Hefti and associates.[1] They noted, "The care of premature infants in the 20th century is remarkable for technical advances that have dramatically improved survival, but little is known about temporal changes in the neuropathology of the premature infant over this time frame." They hypothesized that the autopsy rate of GMH-IVH would reflect changes in clinical interventions that would be both beneficial and harmful.

From 345 autopsies on premature infants, they observed that the incidence of GMH-IVH increased from 4.7% before 1960 to 50.0% from 1975 to 1980, and then decreased to 12.5% after 2005 ($P < .001$).

The incidence of GMH-IVH increased more than 3-fold around the time of the introduction of positive pressure ventilation into premature intensive care in the mid-1960s.

They speculated that the increased incidence of GMH-IVH in the 1970s and 1980s likely reflects respiratory and hemodynamic imbalances complicating mechanical ventilation, and the subsequent decreased incidence of GMH-IVH likely reflects stabilization of respiratory function with improvements in ventilators and in ventilator management beginning in the 1970s and the use of surfactant and antenatal steroids in the 1980s.

The most effective strategy for prevention of IVH is prevention of preterm birth, a goal that has not yet been met. Clinical care designed to minimize rates of GMH-IVH include prompt resuscitation; avoidance of fluctuations in oxygen and carbon dioxide that affect cerebral blood flow; stabilization of blood pressure, including optimal timing of cord clamping; maintaining normal blood sugar levels; and avoidance of packed red blood cell transfusions early in life. Numerous therapies including antenatal vitamin K and phenobarbital; postnatal vitamin E, indomethacin, heparin, and recombinant clotting have failed to effectively prevent IVH. However the combination of antenatal corticosteroids and attention to the factors mentioned above has effectively reduced the rates of severe IVH. Although the incidence of IVH in very low birth weight infants (birth weight [BW] <1500 g) has declined from rates as high as 40% to 50% in the late 1970s to 20% to 25% in 2010, the absolute numbers of infants with IVH remain significant. This is because of the increased survival rate of premature infants, especially in the extremely low birth weight category (BW <1000 g) who continue to be at risk for IVH.

A. A. Fanaroff, MD

Reference

1. Hefti MM, Trachtenberg FL, Haynes RL, Hassett C, Volpe JJ, Kinney HC. A century of germinal matrix intraventricular hemorrhage in autopsied premature infants: a historical account. *Pediatr Dev Pathol.* 2016;19:108-114.

Voice problems in school-aged children following very preterm birth

Reynolds V, Meldrum S, Simmer K, et al (Univ of Western Australia, Perth, Australia)

Arch Dis Child 101:556-560, 2016

Background and Objective.—Very preterm children may be at risk of voice abnormalities (dysphonia). Risk factors previously identified in extremely preterm children include female gender, multiple intubations, complicated intubation and very low birth weight. This study sought to identify the prevalence of dysphonia in very preterm children, at school age.

Methods.—Children born between 23 and 32 weeks' gestation were included in this prospective observational study. Participants were randomly selected from a sample stratified by gestational age and number of intubations, and were aged between 5 and 12 years at the time of assessment. Clinical voice assessments were conducted by a speech pathologist, and a diagnosis of dysphonia was made based on the presence and severity of disturbance to the voice. Retrospective chart review identified medical and demographic characteristics.

Results.—178 participants were assessed. The prevalence of dysphonia in this cohort was 61%. 31% presenting with significant dysphonia, that is, voice disturbance of greater than mild in severity. Female gender ($p = 0.009$), gestational age ($p = 0.031$) and duration of intubation ($p = 0.021$) were significantly associated with dysphonia although some preterm children with dysphonia were never intubated.

Conclusions.—Significant voice abnormalities were observed in children born at up to 32 weeks' gestation, with intubation a major contributing factor.

Trial Registration Number.—ACTRN12613001015730.

▶ As illustrated by this observational study, the consequences of being born very preterm are wide ranging. The study investigated the influence of demographic variables and intubation characteristics on functional voice outcomes in very preterm children. Clinical assessment consisted of the administration of a perceptual rating scale, the Consensus-Auditory Perceptual Evaluation of Voice and an objective acoustic assessment, the Acoustic Voice Quality Index. Visualization of laryngeal structures was not performed as part of the clinical assessment.

Of particular interest is the association between factors unrelated to intubation and voice quality. In children who were never intubated, females were more susceptible to severe dysphonia than males. There were no significant differences between males and females on any demographic characteristic, suggesting that sex-related factors may underlie this increased risk. The authors suggest that a possible explanatory variable is sex or thyroid hormones, both of which are associated with voice changes. In the intubation cohort, chronic conditions such as bronchopulmonary dysplasia and the use of medications such as inhaled corticosteroids, both of which are associated with dysphonia, were not included in the analysis. In addition, for both groups, other medical interventions that may be associated with pharyngoesophageal injury, and subsequent voice difficulties were not included. Nevertheless, the study points out that very preterm infants may be at risk of significant dysphonia at school age and that routine screening for voice difficulties needs to be considered.

L. A. Papile, MD

Association Between Intermittent Hypoxemia or Bradycardia and Late Death or Disability in Extremely Preterm Infants

Poets CF, for the Canadian Oxygen Trial Investigators (Tuebingen Univ Hosp, Germany; et al)

JAMA 314:595-603, 2015

Importance.—Extremely preterm infants may experience intermittent hypoxemia or bradycardia for many weeks after birth. The prognosis of these events is uncertain.

Objective.—To determine the association between intermittent hypoxemia or bradycardia and late death or disability.

Design, Setting, and Participants.—Post hoc analysis of data from the inception cohort assembled for the Canadian Oxygen Trial in 25 hospitals in Canada, the United States, Argentina, Finland, Germany, and Israel, including 1019 infants with gestational ages of 23 weeks 0 days through 27 weeks 6 days who were born between December 2006 and August

2010 and survived to a postmenstrual age of 36 weeks. Follow-up assessments occurred between October 2008 and August 2012.

Exposures.—Episodes of hypoxemia (pulse oximeter oxygen saturation <80%) or bradycardia (pulse rate <80/min) for 10 seconds or longer. Values were sampled every 10 seconds within 24 hours after birth until at least 36 weeks' postmenstrual age.

Main Outcomes and Measures.—The primary outcome was a composite of death after 36 weeks' postmenstrual age, motor impairment, cognitive or language delay, severe hearing loss, or bilateral blindness at 18 months' corrected age. Secondary outcomes were motor impairment, cognitive or language delay, and severe retinopathy of prematurity.

Results.—Downloaded saturation and pulse rate data were available for a median of 68.3 days (interquartile range, 56.8-86.0 days). Mean percentages of recorded time with hypoxemia for the least and most affected 10% of infants were 0.4%and 13.5%, respectively. Corresponding values for bradycardia were 0.1% and 0.3%. The primary outcome was ascertained for 972 infants and present in 414 (42.6%). Hypoxemic episodes were associated with an estimated increased risk of late death or disability at 18 months of 56.5% in the highest decile of hypoxemic exposure vs 36.9% in the lowest decile (modeled relative risk, 1.53; 95% CI, 1.21-1.94). This association was significant only for prolonged hypoxemic episodes lasting at least 1 minute (relative risk, 1.66; 95% CI, 1.35-2.05 vs for shorter episodes, relative risk, 1.01; 95% CI, 0.77-1.32). Relative risks for all secondary outcomes were similarly increased after prolonged hypoxemia. Bradycardia did not alter the prognostic value of hypoxemia.

Conclusions and Relevance.—Among extremely preterm infants who survived to 36 weeks' postmenstrual age, prolonged hypoxemic episodes during the first 2 to 3 months after birth were associated with adverse 18-month outcomes. If confirmed in future studies, further research on the prevention of such episodes is needed.

▶ Desaturation and bradycardia episodes, with or without associated apnea, are very common among the very low birth weight infants in our neonatal intensive care units. Because they are difficult or impossible to eradicate, we tolerate them in our patients to some extent, despite a lingering anxiety that episodes that are too frequent, prolonged, or severe may have lasting adverse neurodevelopmental consequences. Evidence to better frame or assuage that concern has been surprisingly difficult to acquire, and analyses to date have been limited by the necessity of reliance on nursing documentation of these occurrences. Despite that limitation, at least 1 report has described a strong association between adverse outcomes (death or severe handicap) and severity of apnea and bradycardia of prematurity as measured using a scoring system in which deeper desaturation (<80%) and more prolonged (>45 seconds) episodes were heavily weighted.[1] The advent of automated capture of monitoring data, initially for clinical trials of oxygen saturation targeting and now increasingly into the electronic medical record, has permitted analyses based on more complete data, such as that acquired in the Canadian Oxygen Trial as reported here.

This analysis confirms that more severe hypoxemic episodes (SpO_2 < 80%) are associated with significantly greater risk of death or disability at 18 months of age, as previously suspected, but episodes of bradycardia were not. These data do not demonstrate that the relationship is causal, however, as it may simply reflect an increased risk of poor long-term outcomes along with more frequent or severe desaturation episodes in the sickest babies or a predilection for hypoxemic spells in babies with evolving CNS injuries. The very important observation that compromised outcomes are significantly associated only with episodes that were 1 minute or longer in duration provides a target for intervention trials to determine whether efforts to prevent such episodes might lead to better long-term outcomes, and such trials should be supported. Until those results are in, efforts to optimize outcomes for very low birth weight infants should be based on interventions with known efficacy, such as antenatal steroids and magnesium sulfate, early postnatal caffeine, and postdischarge developmental interventions. In addition, we can more confidently reassure anxious parents that the brief desaturation and bradycardia episodes that we are often obliged to tolerate are not associated with worse developmental outcomes.

W. E. Benitz, MD

Reference

1. Pillekamp F, Hermann C, Keller T, et al. Factors influencing apnea and bradycardia of prematurity - implications for neurodevelopment. *Neonatology.* 2007;91: 155-161.

Antenatal factors modulate hearing screen failure risk in preterm infants

Leung JC, Cifra CL, Agthe AG, et al (Univ of Maryland School of Medicine, Baltimore; Univ of Iowa Carver College of Medicine)

Arch Dis Child Fetal Neonatal Ed 101:F56-F61, 2016

Objective.—The objective of this study was to characterise the effects of antenatal inflammatory factors and maternal therapies on neonatal hearing screen outcomes in very low birthweight infants.

Methods.—We conducted a retrospective study of a cohort of infants <33 weeks' gestational age and <1501 g birth weight prospectively enrolled between 1999 and 2003 for whom placental pathology, cord blood interleukin (IL) 6, IL-1β, tumour necrosis factor-α and neonatal hearing screen results were available.

Results.—Of 289 infants with documented hearing screen results, 244 (84%) passed and 45 (16%) failed the hearing screen (unilateral, N = 25 (56%); bilateral, N = 20 (44%)). In the final logistic model, the fetal inflammatory response syndrome defined as the presence of fetal vasculitis and/or cord serum IL-6>18.2 pg/mL was the factor with greatest risk for hearing screen failure (OR 3.62, 95% CI 1.38 to 9.5). A patent ductus arteriosus treated with indomethacin significantly increased the risk (OR 3.3, 95% CI 1.3 to 8.26), while combined maternal steroid and magnesium sulfate exposure (0.37, 95% CI 0.11 to 0.81) reduced the risk for hearing screen failure.

Conclusions.—Intrauterine infection with a fetal inflammatory response is a risk factor for neonatal hearing loss while maternal therapies significantly reduced the risk of neonatal hearing loss in very low birthweight infants.

▶ This study examined the effects of antenatal inflammatory factors including placental pathology, cord blood interleukin (IL)-6, IL-1ß, tumor necrosis factor-α, and maternal therapies on neonatal hearing screen outcomes. In logistic modeling, fetal inflammatory response syndrome (FIRS) defined as the presence of fetal vasculitis and/or cord serum IL-6 >18.2 pg/mL provided the greatest risk for hearing screen failure (odds ratio: 3.62, 95% confidence interval: 1.38–9.5). The authors conclude that intrauterine infection with a fetal inflammatory response is a risk factor for neonatal hearing loss, whereas receipt of betamethasone and magnesium sulfate significantly reduce the risk of neonatal hearing loss in very low birth weight infants. The findings are of interest as a possible marker of specific early perinatal findings of inflammation to predict risk of a hearing screen fail. Before we jump to conclusions regarding the efficacy of this finding to predict permanent hearing loss, one should note a number of limitations of the study. First, 70% of the 463 eligible were enrolled, and 62% of those eligible survived and had the 2-stage hearing screen. The significance of the failed screen remains unclear, because an automated auditory brainstem response (AABR) fail can represent a transient conductive hearing loss, permanent conductive hearing loss, permanent sensorineural hearing loss, or auditory neuropathy. In addition, a diagnostic follow-up assessment was not obtained. Although the authors state that the likelihood of a failed diagnostic assessment increases after 2 failed AABR screens, the screen fail rate in this study was high at 16%. Others have reported rates of hearing loss confirmed by a diagnostic assessment in extremely preterm infants of 3.1%,[1] 2%,[2] and 1% to 3%[3] in cohorts followed for 3 years, 5 years, and 18 to 22 months. Schmidt et al[2] have shown a strong relationship among neonatal morbidities associated with inflammation including BPD, severe brain injury, and severe retinopathy of prematurity with permanent hearing loss. In addition, a strong stepwise relationship was reported between decreasing gestational age and increasing rates of permanent hearing loss diagnosis ranging from 1.2% at 31 weeks to 7.5% at 24 weeks using 2 stage AABR.[4] It can be assumed that a significant percent of the failed screens in this study reflect middle ear effusion. This does have relevance. Doyle et al[5] have shown that neonatal middle ear fluid predicts later chronic otitis media in preterm infants. The Leung data suggest that mechanisms involved with clinical and placental infection remain unclear because rates of maternal histologic chorioamnionitis and other infections were similar in the pass and fail groups. The FIRS association with a failed hearing screen suggests that assessment of fetal vasculitis and cord blood IL-6 may has greater sensitivity than a clinical report of maternal infection. Of interest to both obstetricians and neonatologists was that administration of both betamethasone and magnesium sulfate significantly reduced the risk of a failed hearing screen by 63%. These maternal interventions are known to be associated with improved clinical and neurologic outcomes in preterm infants. One fact that was reaffirmed was that preterm infants with greater degree of immaturity and greater illness severity reflected by multiple neonatal morbidities and markers of inflammation are at increased risk of failing the newborn hearing screen. The ability of FIRS to predict permanent hearing loss remains to be determined.

B. Vohr, MD

References

1. Robertson CM, Howarth TM, Bork DL, Dinu IA. Permanent bilateral sensory and neural hearing loss of children after neonatal intensive care because of extreme prematurity: a thirty-year study. *Pediatrics.* 2009;123:e797-e807.
2. Schmidt B, Roberts RS, Davis PG, et al. Prediction of late death or disability at age 5 years using a count of 3 neonatal morbidities in very low birth weight infants. *J Pediatr.* 2015;167:982-986. e982.
3. Morris BH, Oh W, Tyson JE, et al. Aggressive vs. conservative phototherapy for infants with extremely low birth weight. *N Engl J Med.* 2008;359:1885-1896.
4. van Dommelen P, Verkerk PH, van Straaten HL, Dutch Neonatal Intensive Care Unit Neonatal Hearing Screening Working Group. Hearing loss by week of gestation and birth weight in very preterm neonates. *J Pediatr.* 2015;166:840-843. e841.
5. Doyle KJ, Kong YY, Strobel K, Dallaire P, Ray RM. Neonatal middle ear effusion predicts chronic otitis media with effusion. *Otol Neurotol.* 2004;25:318-322.

Effect of Early Prophylactic High-Dose Recombinant Human Erythropoietin in Very Preterm Infants on Neurodevelopmental Outcome at 2 Years: A Randomized Clinical Trial

Natalucci G, the Swiss EPO Neuroprotection Trial Group (Univ of Zurich, Switzerland; et al)
JAMA 315:2079-2085, 2016

Importance.—Very preterm infants are at risk of developing encephalopathy of prematurity and long-term neurodevelopmental delay. Erythropoietin treatment is neuroprotective in animal experimental and human clinical studies.

Objective.—To determine whether prophylactic early high-dose recombinant human erythropoietin (rhEPO) in preterm infants improves neurodevelopmental outcome at 2 years' corrected age.

Design, Setting, and Participants.—Preterm infants born between 26weeks 0 days' and 31 weeks 6 days' gestation were enrolled in a randomized, double-blind, placebo-controlled, multicenter trial in Switzerland between 2005 and 2012. Neurodevelopmental assessments at age 2 years were completed in 2014.

Interventions.—Participants were randomly assigned to receive either rhEPO (3000 IU/kg) or placebo (isotonic saline, 0.9%) intravenously within 3 hours, at 12 to 18 hours, and at 36 to 42 hours after birth.

Main Outcomes and Measures.—Primary outcome was cognitive development assessed with the Mental Development Index (MDI; norm, 100 [SD, 15]; higher values indicate better function) of the Bayley Scales of Infant Development, second edition (BSID-II) at 2 years corrected age. The minimal clinically important difference between groups was 5 points (0.3 SD). Secondary outcomes were motor development (assessed with the Psychomotor Development Index), cerebral palsy, hearing or visual impairment, and anthropometric growth parameters.

Results.—Among 448 preterm infants randomized (mean gestational age, 29.0 [range, 26.0-30.9] weeks; 264 [59%] female; mean birth weight, 1210 [range, 490-2290] g), 228 were randomized to rhEPO and 220 to placebo. Neurodevelopmental outcome data were available for 365 (81%) at a mean age of 23.6 months. In an intention-to-treat analysis, mean MDI was not statistically significantly different between the rhEPO group (93.5 [SD, 16.0] [95%CI, 91.2 to 95.8]) and the placebo group (94.5 [SD, 17.8] [95%CI, 90.8 to 98.5]) (difference, −1.0 [95% CI, −4.5 to 2.5]; $P = .56$). No differences were found between groups in the secondary outcomes.

Conclusions and Relevance.—Among very preterm infants who received prophylactic early high-dose rhEPO for neuroprotection, compared with infants who received placebo, there were no statistically significant differences in neurodevelopmental outcomes at 2 years. Follow-up for cognitive and physical problems that may not become evident until later in life is required.

Trial Registration.—clinicaltrials.gov Identifier: NCT00413946.

▶ There has been a resurgence of interest in recombinant human erythropoietin (rhEPO) therapy for preterm infants focused on its potential neuroprotective properties. This study is the first published, large randomized clinical trial assessing the efficacy of rhEPO therapy in mitigating brain injury in very preterm infants, and the results are not auspicious, at least for the population studied. The mean Mental Development Index in the placebo group was 94.5, and survival without severe neurodevelopmental impairment occurred in 87%. Given the remarkably intact neurodevelopmental outcome of the placebo group, it is not surprising that no beneficial effect of EPO therapy was found.

Exclusion criteria for the study included a gestational age less that 26 weeks or greater than 31 weeks, severe intraventricular hemorrhage (IVH) before randomization, and a priori palliative care. The exclusion of infants with moderate to severe IVH before the third dose was added after the study was temporarily suspended for safety concerns. Although not stated explicitly in the article, the data in the study flow chart indicate that 46% of potentially eligible infants were excluded because the parents were not approached; this group included parents who elected before delivery to provide primary nonintervention and palliative care after delivery. Overall, the study population was relatively free of medical issues; the median days on mechanical ventilation for both groups was 0 and the rates of severe IVH and bronchopulmonary dysplasia were 5%

to 6% and 34% to 37%, respectively. Moreover, approximately 10% of study infants received additional rhEPO to treat anemia.

In the discussion, the authors suggest that the results of the study may be due to the timing and duration of rhEPO administration. However, a more likely explanation is that the population studied had a low risk for neurodevelopmental problems. A large ongoing large clinical trial (PENUT; NCT01378273) has been designed to analyze the neuroprotective role of rhEPO in extremely low gestational age infants, a group that is at high risk for neurodevelopmental morbidity. However, data relating to the primary outcome of death of severe neurodevelopmental impairment at 24 to 26 months corrected age will not be forthcoming for several years.

L. A. Papile, MD

Safety of Early High-Dose Recombinant Erythropoietin for Neuroprotection in Very Preterm Infants

Fauchère JC, on behalf of the Swiss Erythropoietin Neuroprotection Trial Group (Univ Hosp Zurich, Switzerland; et al)

J Pediatr 167:52-57, 2015

Objective.—To investigate the safety and short term outcome of high dose recombinant human erythropoietin (rhEpo) given shortly after birth and subsequently over the first 2 days for neuroprotection to very preterm infants.

Study Design.—Randomized, double masked phase II trial. Preterm infants (gestational age 26 0/7-31 6/7 weeks) were given rhEpo ($n_t = 229$; 3000 U/kg body weight) or NaCl 0.9% ($n_c = 214$) intravenously at 3, 12-18, and 36- 42 hours after birth.

Results.—There were no relevant differences between the groups for short-term outcomes such as mortality, retinopathy of prematurity, intraventricular hemorrhage, sepsis, necrotizing enterocolitis, and bronchopulmonary dysplasia. At day 7-10, we found significantly higher hematocrit values, reticulocyte, and white blood cell counts, and a lower platelet count in the rhEpo group.

Conclusions.—Early high-dose rhEpo administration to very premature infants is safe and causes no excess in mortality or major adverse events.

Trial Registration.—ClinicalTrials.gov: NCT00413946.

▶ Erythropoietin administration to stimulate red cell production in preterm and term infants was first evaluated 1989. In the mid-1990s researchers began exploring potential nonhematopoietic effects of erythropoiesis stimulating agents (ESAs) such as erythropoietin (Epo) and Darbepoetin alfa (Darbe), a long-acting ESA. A number of animal models provided evidence that higher ESA dosing might be the ideal neuroprotective treatment to improve neurodevelopmental outcomes in preterm infants.[1] In January 2006, Fauchere and colleagues[2] began enrolling preterm infants in a high-dose Epo study (3000 U/kg given at 3-4 hours, 12-18 hours, and 36-42 hours of age), designed to evaluate neurodevelopmental outcomes at 2 years' corrected age. The eligibility criteria were based on the Swiss Study Group's previous pilot study,[2] with 2 exceptions: infants 24 0/7 to 25 6/7 weeks of gestational age and any infants with grade III/IV intracranial hemorrhage were excluded. The resulting 443 preterm infants randomly selected to Epo or placebo had an average weight greater than 1200 g and a gestational age greater than 29 weeks, somewhat larger than the extremely preterm infants who are the focus of many outcomes studies in the United States.

Clinical outcomes in this study were similar between treatment groups, including the incidence of greater than stage 2 retinopathy of prematurity (ROP). ROP became a specific focus of Epo investigators after publication of a Cochrane review in 2006[3] which linked early Epo administration with an increased incidence of greater than stage 2 ROP. A revised review was published in 2014,[4] which reversed the original conclusion but still cautioned use of Epo in preterm infants. With the addition of Fauchere's study and a recent Epo study performed by Zhu and colleagues in China,[5] the incidence of ROP in Epo-treated and placebo-treated infants is approximately equal: 119 of 988 (12.0%) of Epo-treated infants versus 128 of 959 (13.3%) of placebo-treated infants have been reported with greater than stage 2 ROP ($P = .414$).

The switch in focus from blood/transfusion effects to potential brain/neuroprotection effects has rejuvenated interest in the use of Epo in the neonatal intensive care unit. Studies based on cranial magnetic resonance imaging of a subset of infants in Fauchere's study suggest that Epo may mitigate brain injury. Leuchter and colleagues[6] reported decreased white matter and gray matter injury in Epo-treated infants compared with their placebo-treated counterparts, while O'Gorman and colleagues[7] reported improved fractional anisotropy and white matter development in Epo-treated compared with placebo-treated infants. These studies support ESAs as potential neuroprotective agents in preterm infants.

R. K. Ohls, MD

References

1. Messier AM, Ohls RK. Neuroprotective effects of erythropoiesis-stimulating agents in term and preterm neonates. *Curr Opin Pediatr.* 2014;26:139-145.
2. Fauchere JC, Dame C, Vonthein R, et al. An approach to using recombinant erythropoietin for neuroprotection in very preterm infants. *Pediatrics.* 2008;122:375-382.
3. Ohlsson A, Aher SM. Early erythropoietin for preventing red blood cell transfusion in preterm and/or low birth weight infants. *Cochrane Database Syst Rev.* 2006;(3):CD004863.
4. Ohlsson A, Aher SM. Early erythropoietin for preventing red blood cell transfusion in preterm and/or low birth weight infants. *Cochrane Database Syst Rev.* 2014;(4):CD004863.
5. Zhu C, Song J, Sun H, et al. Recombinant human erythropoietin improves neurological outcomes in very preterm infants. *E-PAS.* 2016;3130:3.
6. Leuchter RH, Gui L, Poncet A, et al. Association between early administration of high-dose erythropoietin in preterm infants and brain MRI abnormality at term equivalent age. *JAMA.* 2014;312:817-824.

7. O'Gorman RL, Bucher HU, Held U, et al. Tract-based spatial statistics to assess the neuroprotective effect of early erythropoietin on white matter development in preterm infants. *Brain.* 2015;138:388-397.

Retinal and Optic Nerve Hemorrhages in the Newborn Infant: One-Year Results of the Newborn Eye Screen Test Study

Callaway NF, Ludwig CA, Blumenkranz MS, et al (Stanford Univ School of Medicine, Palo Alto, CA)

Ophthalmology 123:1043-1052, 2016

Purpose.—To report the birth prevalence, risk factors, characteristics, and location of fundus hemorrhages (FHs) of the retina and optic nerve present in newborns at birth.

Design.—Prospective cohort study at Stanford University School of Medicine.

Participants.—All infants who were 37 weeks postmenstrual age or older and stable were eligible for screening. Infants with known or suspected infectious conjunctivitis were excluded.

Methods.—Infants born at Lucile Packard Children's Hospital (LPCH) from July 25, 2013, through July 25, 2014, were offered universal newborn screening via wide-angle digital retinal photography in the Newborn Eye Screen Test study. Maternal, obstetric, and neonatal factors were obtained from hospital records. The location, retinal layer, and laterality of FH were recorded by 1 pediatric vitreoretinal specialist.

Main Outcome Measures.—Birth prevalence of FH. Secondary outcomes included rate of adverse events, risk factors for FH, hemorrhage characteristics, and adverse events.

Results.—The birth prevalence of FH in this study was 20.3% (41/202 infants). Ninety-five percent of FHs involved the periphery, 83% involved the macula, and 71% involved multiple layers of the retina. The fovea was involved in 15% of FH cases (birth prevalence, 3.0%). No cases of bilateral foveal hemorrhage were found. Fundus hemorrhages were more common in the left eye than the right. Fundus hemorrhages were most commonly optic nerve flame hemorrhages (48%) and white-centered retinal hemorrhages (30%). Retinal hemorrhages were found most frequently in all 4 quadrants (35%) and more often were multiple than solitary. Macular hemorrhages most often were intraretinal (40%). Among the risk factors examined in this study, vaginal delivery compared with cesarean section (odds ratio [OR], 9.34; 95% confidence interval [CI], 2.57–33.97) showed the greatest level of association with FH. Self-identified ethnicity as Hispanic or Latino showed a protective effect (OR, 0.43; 95% CI, 0.20–0.94). Other study factors were not significant.

Conclusions.—Fundus hemorrhages are common among newborns. They often involve multiple areas and layers of the retina. Vaginal delivery was associated with a significantly increased risk of FH, whereas self-identified Hispanic or Latino ethnicity was protective against FH in this study. The long-term consequences of FH on visual development remain unknown.

▶ The Retcam and other such models have facilitated examination of the retina in newborns. In addition to screening for retinopathy of prematurity, it is useful for diagnosing other ocular conditions, including retinal hemorrhage. A number of investigators have revisited this condition with similar findings and observations to those presented by Li et al in the 2013 YearBook.[1] Remember that in addition to birth-related retinal hemorrhage, they are common in asphyxiated infants, those with hemorrhagic disease of the newborn, other coagulopathies, and sepsis in addition to retinopathy of prematurity. Be aware that scleral depression to examine premature infants with retinopathy has been associated with hemorrhage.

Callaway presents the 1-year results of the first universal retinal image screening performed in healthy term infants in the United States. Overall approximately 20% to 30% of newborns exhibit retinal hemorrhages, and they are present in both eyes in almost 75% of the subjects. The hemorrhages are of various shapes and distribution. To no one's surprise, more infants delivered with vacuum assist and per vaginam have hemorrhages than those delivered by cesarean delivery. Those delivered by emergency cesarean delivery have a higher incidence of hemorrhage than elective section. If an infant has a cephalohematoma, accompanying retinal hemorrhage is almost certain.[2] It is of interest that Callaway noted self-identified Hispanic or Latino ethnicity had a protective effect (56%) against retinal hemorrhage. Reasons for this remain to be determined, but pelvic size, head circumference, and vessel elasticity were some factors to be considered.

Two-thirds of hemorrhages have cleared by 1 week after birth in term infants, but some resolve at a slower pace. All should resolve within a month. The main significance of this report perhaps lies in the next phase of the study, in which these children will be followed to determine whether hemorrhage in vital areas may interfere with the visual pathways lead to visual deprivation and amblyopia. These lesions could then be identified at birth rather than at the school examination. Although there is no therapy for the hemorrhage, early identification of those at risk for visual impairment could receive early intervention including patching, cycloplegics, and correcting refractive errors, which would optimize the child's vision potential.

A. A. Fanaroff, MD

References

1. Li LH, Li N, Zhao JY, et al. Findings of perinatal ocular examination performed on 3573, healthy full-term newborns. *Br J Ophthalmol.* 2013;97:588-591.
2. Zhao Q, Zhang Y, Yang Y, et al. Birth-related retinal hemorrhages in healthy full-term newborns and their relationship to maternal, obstetric, and neonatal risk factors. *Graefes Arch Clin Exp Ophthalmol.* 2015;253:1021-1025.

Population Outcomes of Three Approaches to Detection of Congenital Hearing Loss

Wake M, Ching TYC, Wirth K, et al (Childrens Res Inst, Parkville, Australia; Natl Acoustic Laboratories, North Ryde, Australia; et al)
Pediatrics 137:e20151722, 2016

Background.—Universal newborn hearing screening was implemented worldwide largely on modeled, not measured, long-term benefits. Comparative quantification of population benefits would justify its high cost.

Methods.—Natural experiment comparing 3 population approaches to detecting bilateral congenital hearing loss (>25 dB, better ear) in Australian states with similar demographics and services: (1) universal newborn hearing screening, New South Wales 2003–2005, $n = 69$; (2) risk factor screening (neonatal intensive care screening + universal risk factor referral), Victoria 2003–2005, $n = 65$; and (3) largely opportunistic detection, Victoria 1991–1993, $n = 86$. Children in (1) and (2) were followed at age 5 to 6 years and in (3) at 7 to 8 years. Outcomes were compared between states using adjusted linear regression.

Results.—Children were diagnosed younger with universal than risk factor screening (adjusted mean difference −8.0 months, 95% confidence interval −12.3 to −3.7). For children without intellectual disability, moving from opportunistic to risk factor to universal screening incrementally improved age of diagnosis (22.5 vs 16.2 vs 8.1 months, $P < .001$), receptive (81.8 vs 83.0 vs 88.9, $P = .05$) and expressive (74.9 vs 80.7 vs 89.3, $P < .001$) language and receptive vocabulary (79.4 vs 83.8 vs 91.5, $P < .001$); these nonetheless remained well short of cognition (mean 103.4, SD 15.2). Behavior and health-related quality of life were unaffected.

Conclusions.—With new randomized trials unlikely, this may represent the most definitive population-based evidence supporting universal newborn hearing screening. Although outperforming risk factor screening, school entry language still lagged cognitive abilities by nearly a SD. Prompt intervention and efficacy research are needed for children to reach their potential.

▶ This report provides population-based evidence of the benefits of earlier age of screening, diagnosis, and intervention on school-age outcomes of children with bilateral permanent hearing loss. Strengths of this work are that it is a population-based study of 3 protocols; children in the 3 study cohorts had similar degrees of hearing loss and nonverbal IQ; there was a high consent rate; families received a full range of amplification and intervention services; annual assessment of hearing aid gain with adjustments was made as needed; examiners were blinded to degree of hearing loss; and school-age follow-up occurred at 5 to 8 years. The findings are consistent with studies demonstrating benefits of early intervention[1,2] on early childhood outcomes of children with permanent hearing loss. In the Wake et al study, age of diagnosis for children without intellectual disability was the youngest for the universal newborn hearing screening (UNHS) group, intermediate for the risk factor group and oldest for the opportunistic group (8.1 vs 16.2 vs 22.5 months, $P < .001$), respectively. In addition, the relationship between language outcomes and intervention protocols was similar. Earlier age of diagnosis was consistently associated with higher receptive language (88.9 vs 83.0 vs 81.8, $P = .05$), expressive language (89.3 vs 80.7 vs 74.9, $P < .001$) and receptive vocabulary scores (91.5 vs 83.8 vs 79.4 $P < .001$) for the UNHS, risk factor, and opportunistic groups, respectively. The authors point out, however, that scores were consistently lower than their cognitive scores (mean 103.4, SD 15.2). The bottom line is that earlier age of diagnosis of a permanent hearing loss and access to communication result in more optimal language development. Why is earlier better? Language is processed in the brain. During the first 3 years of life, the brain grows and matures in complexity at an incredible rate, in part mediated by the language sensory environment to which the infant is exposed. The central auditory pathway, which delivers auditory information to the brain, matures and develops during this time. Sharma et al[3] have shown that earlier implantation of a cochlear implant is associated with optimal development of the auditory pathway to the cortex. Children who are deaf and born to deaf parents have early exposure to visual language (ASL). The majority of children born deaf/hard of hearing, however, are born to hearing parents and do not have immediate access to visual language or auditory language. Therefore, early access to language and early intervention that meets the communication needs of the family is the key. Hart and Risley[4] have shown that the amount and quality of language that children are exposed to in the home varies significantly, and the greater the input of child directed quality language, the better the child's language and cognitive outcomes. The Wake et al study confirms that universal newborn hearing screening programs are succeeding in earlier screening, which results in significantly improved language outcomes at school age. Language skills in the UNHS children, however, were not commensurate with their cognitive ability. There is more to be done. The next challenge is to shorten the time line of early hearing detection and quality intervention from screening at 1 month, diagnosis at 3 months and intervention at 6 months to a goal of 1, 2 and 3 months so that every infant with a permanent hearing loss has the same opportunity to achieve language and academic success as his or her hearing peers.

B. Vohr, MD

References

1. Yoshinaga-Itano C, Coulter D, Thomson V. Developmental outcomes of children with hearing loss born in Colorado hospitals with and without universal newborn hearing screening programs. *Semin Neonatol.* 2001;6:521-529.
2. Moeller MP. Early intervention and language development in children who are deaf and hard of hearing. *Pediatrics.* 2000;106:E43.
3. Sharma A, Dorman MF, Kral A. The influence of a sensitive period on central auditory development in children with unilateral and bilateral cochlear implants. *Hear Res.* 2005;203:134-143.
4. Hart B, Risley TR. *Meaningful Differences in the Everyday Experience of Young American Children.* Baltimore, MD: P.H. Brookes; 1995.

Follow-up of infants with congenital cytomegalovirus and normal fetal imaging

Amir J, Atias J, Linder N, et al (Schneider Children's Med Ctr of Israel, Petach Tikva; Tel Aviv Univ, Israel)

Arch Dis Child Fetal Neonatal Ed F1-F5, 2016

Objective.—To evaluate the outcome of infants with congenital cytomegalovirus (CMV) infection and normal fetal imaging.

Design.—Retrospective cohort study.

Setting.—Tertiary paediatric medical centre.

Patients.—98 infants born to mothers with primary CMV infection in the first and second trimesters (diagnosed by positive amniotic fluid findings) and normal fetal imaging.

Methods.—Initial evaluation included confirmatory urine culture, complete blood count, liver and kidney function tests, funduscopy, brain ultrasound and hearing test. Follow-up included periodic neurological and developmental evaluation, hearing tests until age 5 and Bayley-III Developmental Scale (in some patients).

Main Outcome Measures.—The presence and rate of sequelae of congenital CMV.

Results.—52 (53.1%) infants received early antiviral treatment for central nervous system symptoms or signs, mainly lenticulostriatal vasculopathy on postnatal ultrasonography (88.5%). Sensorineural hearing loss was found on first examination in 16 infants (25 ears), of whom 10 also had cranial ultrasound findings; another five with late-onset hearing loss were also treated. The median follow-up time was 32 (12–83) months. Most infants with moderate and severe hearing loss were infected in the first trimester (10 vs 2, $p = 0.053$). At the last assessment, eight children (10 ears) still had hearing loss, including two with bilateral loss who underwent a cochlear implant. The mean Bayley-III score was 102.6 ± 10.3 (range 85–127). All 98 children attended regular educational institutions.

Conclusions.—Congenital CMV infection acquired from primary maternal infection with normal fetal imaging is associated with a high rate of subtle signs and symptoms after birth. Overall, intermediate-term outcome is good with a low rate of sequelae.

▶ In Israel it is common for women who are pregnant to be screened for cytomegalovirus infection (CMV) during the first trimester. Women who have a positive result undergo additional testing, and, if they are determined to have a primary CMV infection, amniocentesis is performed to detect fetal CMV infection after 21 completed weeks of gestation and at least 7 weeks after the assumed date of infection. Fetal CMV infection is diagnosed when the virus is detected in the amniotic fluid by both polymerase chain reaction amplification and rapid shell-vial culture. If a woman opts to continue her pregnancy, follow-up fetal imaging including repeated detailed transabdominal and transvaginal ultrasound scan and fetal brain MRI at 33 to 34 weeks of gestation is done. All infants undergo a confirmatory urine culture (shell-vial), brainstem-evoked response audiometry, cranial ultrasonography (HUS) and fundoscopy.

In the above retrospective study, the investigators describe the outcome of a cohort of infants who were born to women whose amniotic fluid was positive for CMV and had normal findings on fetal imaging by both ultrasonography and MRI. Infants who had a hearing loss or an abnormal HUS after birth were treated with ganciclovir/valganciclovir. There were 101 infants with a primary CMV infection, of whom, 3 were lost to follow-up. Sixty of the 98 infants (61.2%) exhibited early postnatal signs possibly related to congenital CMV, and 46 (46.9%) had abnormal HUS findings, most of which was lenticulostriate vasculopathy (95.7%). Sensorineural hearing loss on initial screening was noted in 16 infants, 10 of whom also had abnormal HUS findings. An additional 5 infants who were noted to have sensorineural hearing loss after the newborn period were treated and subsequently recovered. Overall, 58.2% of the infants received antiviral therapy.

The authors' conclusion that the intermediate-term outcome of these infants is good with a low rate of sequelae needs to be viewed within the context of their data. Only 27% of the affected infants underwent formal neurodevelopmental assessment with the Bayley Scales of Infant Development III. In addition, the statement that all of the infants attended regular educational institutions needs to be qualified; most were in day care centers (54%) or attended kindergarten (41%).

L. A. Papile, MD

Posterior fossa tumors in infants and neonates

Spennato P, Nicosia G, Quaglietta L, et al (Santobono-Pausilipon Children's Hosp, Naples, Italy; et al)

Childs Nerv Syst 31:1751-1772, 2015

Introduction.—Management of posterior fossa tumors in infants and neonates is challenging. The characteristics of the young babies make surgery very difficult, sometimes precluding a safe complete removal.

Methods.—A review of the literature was undertaken to examine the incidence, histology, surgical aspects, and prognosis of posterior fossa tumors in the first year of life. Therapeutical strategies of the most frequent tumor types are also discussed in detail.

Results.—Histology is dominated by tumors with aggressive behavior, such as medulloblastomas, atypical teratoid/rhabdoid tumors, and anaplastic ependymomas. The most important surgical considerations in small children are the small circulating blood volume; the poor thermoregulation; and incomplete maturation of the brain, of the skull, and of the soft tissue. Treatment toxicity is inversely related to the age of the patients. Radiation therapy is usually considered as contraindicated in young children, with few exceptions. Proton therapy is a promising tool, but access to this kind of treatment is still limited. The therapeutic limitations of irradiation render resection of this tumor and adjuvant chemotherapy often the only therapeutic strategy in many cases.

Conclusions.—The overall prognosis remains dismal because of the prevalent aggressive histologies, the surgical challenges, and the limitations of adjuvant treatment. Nevertheless, the impressive improvements in anesthesiology and surgical techniques allow, in the vast majority of the cases, complete removal of the lesions with minor sequelae in high-volume referral pediatric centers.

▶ This article is a literature review of the infratentorial (posterior fossa) brain tumors of neonates and young infants, as well as the personal perspective of the authors who have extensive experience in their treatment at a single large Italian institution. The review includes discussion of the protean clinical manifestations with which these infants present and of their predominantly more malignant spectrum of tumor pathology, both of which differ from that of older children. It also discusses the age-specific approach to treatment, addressing the unique difficulties encountered in the surgical and medical management of posterior fossa tumors in young infants and the limitations of such treatment in terms of survival and of late-effects of therapy.

The general discussion of current optimal therapy for these tumors in young infants is fairly comprehensive, well written, and useful. There is particularly in-depth analysis of the issues confronting the neurosurgeon attempting to manage and operate on posterior fossa tumors in very young children. The viewpoint of the experienced pediatric neurosurgeon-authors is probably most useful to other neurosurgeons. However, it is also informative and of practical value to neonatologists in that it emphasizes the indications for urgent neurosurgical intervention and the importance of referring such infants to high-volume pediatric centers for definitive surgical therapy.

As well, the article reviews specific therapies for individual types of tumor and updates current knowledge of the molecular mechanisms of tumorigenesis. Going forward, this will drive more targeted therapy that could mitigate neurotoxicity to the developing brain. Although the details of this information do not pertain to the usual daily practice of neonatology/perinatology, nevertheless, overview of the general approach to treatment of these tumors, both current and future, is valuable information.

P. L. Robertson, MD

Bladder Function After Fetal Surgery for Myelomeningocele

Brock JW III, for the MOMS Investigators (Vanderbilt Univ Med Ctr, Nashville, TN; et al)

Pediatrics 136:e906-e913, 2015

Background.—A substudy of the Management of Myelomeningocele Study evaluating urological outcomes was conducted.

Methods.—Pregnant women diagnosed with fetal myelomeningocele were randomly assigned to either prenatal or standard postnatal surgical repair. The substudy included patients randomly assigned after April 18, 2005. The primary outcome was defined in their children as death or the need for clean intermittent catheterization (CIC) by 30 months of age characterized by prespecified criteria. Secondary outcomes included bladder and kidney abnormalities observed by urodynamics and renal/bladder ultrasound at 12 and 30 months, which were analyzed as repeated measures.

Results.—Of the 115 women enrolled in the substudy, the primary outcome occurred in 52% of children in the prenatal surgery group and 66% in the postnatal surgery group (relative risk [RR]: 0.78; 95% confidence interval [CI]: 0.57–1.07). Actual rates of CIC use were 38% and 51% in the prenatal and postnatal surgery groups, respectively (RR: 0.74; 95% CI: 0.48–1.12). Prenatal surgery resulted in less trabeculation (RR: 0.39; 95% CI: 0.19–0.79) and fewer cases of open bladder neck on urodynamics (RR: 0.61; 95% CI: 0.40–0.92) after adjustment by child's gender and lesion level. The difference in trabeculation was confirmed by ultrasound.

Conclusions.—Prenatal surgery did not significantly reduce the need for CIC by 30 months of age but was associated with less bladder trabeculation and open bladder neck. The implications of these findings are unclear now, but support the need for long-term urologic follow-up of patients with myelomeningocele regardless of type of surgical repair.

▶ The results of the landmark Management of Myelomeningocele Study (MOMS) continue to come in. In the initial report of this study, Adzick et al described significant reductions in hindbrain herniation (64% in the prenatal group vs 96% in the postnatal surgery group) and need for ventriculoperitoneal shunt placement in the first 12 months after birth (40% vs 82%), as well as improved mental development and rates of independent ambulation (42% vs 21%) at 30 months of age for infants managed with fetal surgery compared with those in the postnatal surgery group.[1] These benefits were offset by maternal and fetal complications including rupture of amniotic membranes (46% in the prenatal group vs 8% in the postnatal surgery group), oligohydramnios (21% vs 4%), preterm birth (79% vs 15%), and respiratory distress syndrome (21% vs 6%). More than a third of mothers in the prenatal surgery group showed dehiscence or a very thin uterine wall at the hysterotomy site. These results required assembly of highly skilled and trained multidisciplinary teams at a small number of dedicated centers. Some commentators immediately questioned whether the number-needed-to-treat of 5 maternal-fetal surgeries to achieve 1 additional ambulatory child was low enough to justify the expense and associated maternal and neonatal morbidities.[2] This concern remains cogent because the extent to which early benefits will be sustained into adulthood is still uncertain.

In this important follow-up study, the MOMS investigators report on the urological outcomes at age 12 and 30 months in their trial cohort. Although there were statistically significant differences in ultrasonography and urodynamics, with fewer abnormal findings in the fetal surgery group, those did not translate to a significant reduction in the need for clean intermittent catheterization for management of neurogenic bladder function. The authors speculate that functional differences may become apparent at a later age but emphasize the necessity of ongoing urological monitoring of bladder function following fetal surgery.

It is notable that this report, as well as the broader literature on this topic, is replete with descriptions of "fetal repair of meningomyelocele." This report, and the less-than-perfect results achieved with respect to other outcomes, should make it readily evident that fetal surgery does not result in a "repair," any more than postnatal surgical closure of the defect does. For women carrying an affected fetus, who should have the opportunity to consider prenatal intervention at a well-qualified center, decisions about how to proceed will not be well served by continued use of this misnomer.

W. E. Benitz, MD

References

1. Adzick NS, Thom EA, Spong CY, et al. A randomized trial of prenatal versus postnatal repair of myelomeningocele. *N Engl J Med.* 2011;364:993-1004.
2. Simpson JL, Greene MF. Fetal surgery for myelomeningocele? *N Engl J Med.* 2011;364:1076-1077.

9 Gastrointestinal Health and Nutrition

Bifidobacterium breve BBG-001 in very preterm infants: a randomised controlled phase 3 trial

Costeloe K, on behalf of The Probiotics in Preterm Infants Study Collaborative Group (Barts and the London School of Medicine and Dentistry, UK; et al)

Lancet 387:649-660, 2016

Background.—Probiotics may reduce necrotising enterocolitis and late-onset sepsis after preterm birth. However, there has been concern about the rigour and generalisability of some trials and there is no agreement about whether or not they should be used routinely. We aimed to test the effectiveness of the probiotic *Bifidobacterium breve* BBG-001 to reduce necrotising enterocolitis, late-onset sepsis, and death in preterm infants.

Methods.—In this multicentre, randomised controlled phase 3 study (the PiPS trial), we recruited infants born between 23 and 30 weeks' gestational age within 48 h of birth from 24 hospitals in southeast England. Infants were randomly assigned (1:1) to probiotic or placebo via a minimisation algorithm randomisation programme. The probiotic intervention was *B breve* BBG-001 suspended in dilute elemental infant formula given enterally in a daily dose of 8·2 to 9·2 $\log_{10}$ CFU; the placebo was dilute infant formula alone. Clinicians and families were masked to allocation. The primary outcomes were necrotising enterocolitis (Bell stage 2 or 3), blood culture positive sepsis more than 72 h after birth; and death before discharge from hospital. All primary analyses were by intention to treat. This trial is registered with ISRCTN, number 05511098 and EudraCT, number 2006-003445-17.

Findings.—Between July 1, 2010, and July 31, 2013, 1315 infants were recruited; of whom 654 were allocated to probiotic and 661 to placebo. Five infants had consent withdrawn after randomisation, thus 650 were analysed in the probiotic group and 660 in the placebo group. Rates of the primary outcomes did not differ significantly between the probiotic and placebo groups. 61 infants (9%) in the probiotic group had necrotising enterocolitis compared with 66 (10%) in the placebo group (adjusted risk ratio 0·93 (95% CI 0·68–1·27); 73 (11%) infants in the probiotics group had sepsis compared with 77 (12%) in the placebo group (0·97 (0·73–1·29); and 54 (8%) deaths occurred before discharge home in the probiotic group compared with 56 (9%) in the placebo group (0·93 [0·67–1·30]). No probiotic-associated adverse events were reported.

Interpretation.—There is no evidence of benefit for this intervention in this population; this result does not support the routine use of *B breve* BBG-001 for prevention of necrotising enterocolitis and late-onset sepis in very preterm infants.

▶ Whether to use probiotics routinely in preterm neonates to prevent necrotizing enterocolitis (NEC) or sepsis has been a major controversy in neonatology for the past several years. Numerous underpowered studies have been done with different probiotic agents, and meta-analyses of these studies have suggested a benefit, including a recent Cochrane review, which uncharacteristically recommended a change in practice suggesting routine use of these agents.[1] Others have suggested caution[2,3] because of the heterogeneity of studies comprising the meta-analyses, the lack of a pharmaceutical grade agent, and lack of efficacy in babies less than 1000 grams (the population at highest risk for NEC) in the existing studies. Safety concerns have been underlined by the death of a neonate associated with a contaminated batch of probiotic (http://www.philly.com/philly/blogs/healthy_kids/CDC-advisory-infant-death-caused-by-probiotic-powder.html).

The study by Costeloe and colleagues is a randomized, controlled, very well-designed multicentered study powered to evaluate the effect of a single probiotic on the development of NEC. The results of this study show there are clearly no differences in NEC as a primary outcome or other secondary outcomes that were evaluated.

Although probiotics are already being routinely used in many parts of the world including the United States, this study raises the possibility that the Cochrane review (as well as several of the other meta-analyses) is being incorrectly interpreted. It is still not clear which probiotic should be used and what dose is really effective. Should probiotics be limited to babies greater than 1000 grams? It also appears that many neonatologists in the United States are using probiotic preparations for preterms that have not yet been studied in this population. More large trials are currently being done.

J. Neu, MD

References

1. Robinson J. Cochrane in context: probiotics for prevention of necrotizing enterocolitis in preterm infants. *Evid Based Child Health.* 2014;9:672-674.
2. Neu J. Routine probiotics for premature infants: let's be careful! *J Pediatr.* 2011;158:672-674.
3. Abrahamsson TR, Rautava S, Moore AM, Neu J, Sherman PM. The time for a confirmative necrotizing enterocolitis probiotics prevention trial in the extremely low birth weight infant in North America is now! *J Pediatr.* 2014;165:389-394.

Bifidobacterium breve BBG-001 in very preterm infants: a randomised controlled phase 3 trial

Costeloe K, on behalf of The Probiotics in Preterm Infants Study Collaborative Group (Barts and the London School of Medicine and Dentistry, UK; et al)

Lancet 387:649-660, 2016

Background.—Probiotics may reduce necrotising enterocolitis and late-onset sepsis after preterm birth. However, there has been concern about the rigour and generalisability of some trials and there is no agreement about whether or not they should be used routinely. We aimed to test the effectiveness of the probiotic *Bifidobacterium breve* BBG-001 to reduce necrotising enterocolitis, late-onset sepsis, and death in preterm infants.

Methods.—In this multicentre, randomised controlled phase 3 study (the PiPS trial), we recruited infants born between 23 and 30 weeks' gestational age within 48 h of birth from 24 hospitals in southeast England. Infants were randomly assigned (1:1) to probiotic or placebo via a minimisation algorithm randomisation programme. The probiotic intervention was *B breve* BBG-001 suspended in dilute elemental infant formula given enterally in a daily dose of 8·2 to 9·2 $\log_{10}$ CFU; the placebo was dilute infant formula alone. Clinicians and families were masked to allocation. The primary outcomes were necrotising enterocolitis (Bell stage 2 or 3), blood culture positive sepsis more than 72 h after birth; and death before discharge from hospital. All primary analyses were by intention to treat. This trial is registered with ISRCTN, number 05511098 and EudraCT, number 2006-003445-17.

Findings.—Between July 1, 2010, and July 31, 2013, 1315 infants were recruited; of whom 654 were allocated to probiotic and 661 to placebo. Five infants had consent withdrawn after randomisation, thus 650 were analysed in the probiotic group and 660 in the placebo group. Rates of the primary outcomes did not differ significantly between the probiotic and placebo groups. 61 infants (9%) in the probiotic group had necrotising enterocolitis compared with 66 (10%) in the placebo group (adjusted risk ratio 0·93 (95% CI 0·68–1·27); 73 (11%) infants in the probiotics group had sepsis compared with 77 (12%) in the placebo group (0·97 (0·73–1·29); and 54 (8%) deaths occurred before discharge home in the probiotic group compared with 56 (9%) in the placebo group (0·93 [0·67–1·30]). No probiotic-associated adverse events were reported.

Interpretation.—There is no evidence of benefit for this intervention in this population; this result does not support the routine use of *B breve* BBG-001 for prevention of necrotising enterocolitis and late-onset sepis in very preterm infants.

▶ Meta-analysis of probiotic delivery in preterm infants for the prevention of necrotizing enterocolitis favored treatment, and, as a result, there was a call to incorporate probiotics into the standard of care despite the heterogeneity of the included studies. This was even accompanied by some to view the decision not to provide probiotics to preterm infants as unethical. Such claims were made even though the meta-analysis answered none of the questions needed to develop safe and justified medical practices such as, what probiotic(s), what dosage, when to start, for how long, and so on. The use of probiotics has also been tempered by reports of bacteremia and death in a few preterm infants receiving probiotics, a consequence of administering live organisms to an uncompromised host and the lack of a pharmaceutical grade probiotic available for use.

Costeloe et al conducted a large, high-quality, multicenter, double-blind randomized clinical trial to evaluate the effectiveness of *Bifidobacterium breve* BBG-001 in the prevention of necrotizing enterocolitis, late-onset sepsis, and mortality. This study used a pharmaceutical grade product and enrolled more than 1300 infants between 23 and 30 weeks of gestation. The infants who received *B breve* showed no difference in clinical outcomes compared with infants who did not receive the probiotic. The study was a critical undertaking, and the investigators should be commended for completing this thoughtful, high-quality study. The results reinforce several principles: (1) large randomized clinical trials remain the gold standard and should not be replaced by meta-analyses; (2) for a multitude of reasons, it is not uncommon for results of large, adequately powered phase III trials to refute positive findings observed in smaller studies; and (3) large, high-quality clinical trials of pharmaceutical grade probiotics still are needed to investigate other strains or combination of strains to conclusively determine the role of probiotic treatment of preterm infants. All probiotics are not the same.

Probiotics may find a role in the neonatal intensive care unit. However, we should demand for the quality of evidence needed to ensure safe and effective therapies in this vulnerable population. Giving a drug that may be potentially harmful and one with unknown long-term side effects is a high price to pay without evidence of its overall health benefits despite these risks.

C. Martin, MD

***Bifidobacterium breve* BBG-001 in very preterm infants: a randomised controlled phase 3 trial**

Costeloe K, on behalf of The Probiotics in Preterm Infants Study Collaborative Group (Barts and the London School of Medicine and Dentistry, UK; et al)

Lancet 387:649-660, 2016

Background.—Probiotics may reduce necrotising enterocolitis and late-onset sepsis after preterm birth. However, there has been concern about the rigour and generalisability of some trials and there is no agreement about whether or not they should be used routinely. We aimed to test the effectiveness of the probiotic *Bifidobacterium breve* BBG-001 to reduce necrotising enterocolitis, late-onset sepsis, and death in preterm infants.

Methods.—In this multicentre, randomised controlled phase 3 study (the PiPS trial), we recruited infants born between 23 and 30 weeks' gestational age within 48 h of birth from 24 hospitals in southeast England. Infants were randomly assigned (1:1) to probiotic or placebo via a minimisation algorithm randomisation programme. The probiotic intervention was *B breve* BBG-001 suspended in dilute elemental infant formula given enterally in a daily dose of 8·2 to 9·2 $\log_{10}$ CFU; the placebo was dilute infant formula alone. Clinicians and families were masked to allocation. The primary outcomes were necrotising enterocolitis (Bell stage 2 or 3), blood culture positive sepsis more than 72 h after birth; and death before discharge from hospital. All primary analyses were by intention to treat. This trial is registered with ISRCTN, number 05511098 and EudraCT, number 2006-003445-17.

Findings.—Between July 1, 2010, and July 31, 2013, 1315 infants were recruited; of whom 654 were allocated to probiotic and 661 to placebo. Five infants had consent withdrawn after randomisation, thus 650 were analysed in the probiotic group and 660 in the placebo group. Rates of the primary outcomes did not differ significantly between the probiotic and placebo groups. 61 infants (9%) in the probiotic group had necrotising enterocolitis compared with 66 (10%) in the placebo group (adjusted risk ratio 0·93 (95% CI 0·68–1·27); 73 (11%) infants in the probiotics group had sepsis compared with 77 (12%) in the placebo group (0·97 (0·73–1·29); and 54 (8%) deaths occurred before discharge home in the probiotic group compared with 56 (9%) in the placebo group (0·93 [0·67–1·30]). No probiotic-associated adverse events were reported.

Interpretation.—There is no evidence of benefit for this intervention in this population; this result does not support the routine use of *B breve* BBG-001 for prevention of necrotising enterocolitis and late-onset sepis in very preterm infants (Table 4).

▶ From my point of view, too many research articles commence with the statement that necrotizing enterocolitis (NEC) remains the major gastrointestinal disorder in preterm infants. More disturbingly, NEC still accounts for extensive mortality and long-term morbidity. I want to read that we have eliminated NEC as a problem in the neonatal intensive care unit. The focus of attention has tended to shift from feeding volumes to the composition of the intestinal microbiota and how to modify it. Promising NEC prevention strategies that alter the intestinal microbiota include probiotics, prebiotics, lactoferrin, and human milk The movement to exclusive use of human milk and human milk products appears to have reduced the incidence of NEC in those units that do this, but the data remain anecdotal at this point.

The literature on the benefits of probiotics is confusing. If you are a strong believer in meta-analyses, you will be convinced that they are effective.

Hence the Cochrane review from Alfaleh[1] including 27 quasi-randomized trials reported that enteral supplementation of probiotics prevents severe NEC and all cause mortality in preterm infants. "Our updated review of available evidence strongly supports a change in practice. Head to head comparative studies are required to assess the most effective preparations, timing, and length of therapy to be utilized."

TABLE 4.—Analysis of Stool Culture and PCR Results on Stools Collected at 2 Weeks' Postnatal and 36 Weeks' Postmenstrual Age

	Bifidobacterium breve BBG-001 Probiotic (n = 650)	Placebo (n = 660)	Adjusted* Risk Ratio
Stool culture at 2 weeks' postnatal age†			
B breve	436 (74%)	122 (21%)	3·51 (2·83–4·34)
MRSA	1 (<1%)	2 (<1%)	Too few data
VRE	0	1 (<1%)	Too few data
ESβL	18 (3%)	20 (3%)	0·76 (0·36–1·61)
Stool PCR at 2 weeks' postnatal age			
PCR positive§	416 (84%)	177 (35%)	2·42 (2·06–2·85)
B breve positive by culture or PCR	505 (85%)	219 (37%)	2·30 (1·99–2·66)
Stool culture at 36 weeks' postmenstrual age‡			
B breve	438 (84%)	253 (49%)	1·69 (1·50–1·91)
MRSA	1 (<1%)	0	Too few data
VRE	3 (1%)	1 (<1%)	2·97 (0·15–57·67)
ESβL	19 (4%)	18 (4%)	0·98 (0·44–2·18)

Data are n (% of received). MRSA=meticillin-resistant *Staphlococcus aureus*. VRE=vancomycin-resistant enterococcus. ESβL=extended spectrum β lactamase- producing Gram-negative bacteria.

*Adjusted for sex, gestational age at birth, and randomisation within 24 h of birth. Adjustment by centre was excluded because the model did not converge. Allowances for correlations between multiple births are accounted for.

†Includes 1266 infants alive, 1186 (94%) stools received.

‡Includes 1245 infants alive, 1043 (84%) stools received.

§Of 1186 stools received at 2 weeks' postnatal age, there was sufficient material available to do PCR to detect *B breve* BBG-001 in addition to culture on 1007.

Reprinted from Costeloe K, on behalf of The Probiotics in Preterm Infants Study Collaborative Group. *Bifidobacterium breve* BBG-001 in very preterm infants: a randomised controlled phase 3 trial. *Lancet*. 2016;387:649-660.

Ohlsen[2] included only 12 studies with 10 800 premature neonates (5144 receiving prophylactic probiotics and 5656 controls). The meta-analysis showed a significant 45% decline in the incidence of NEC and 28% reduction in mortality. Sepsis did not differ significantly between the 2 groups. They quite naturally concluded that "Probiotic supplementation reduces the risk of NEC and mortality in preterm infants. The effect sizes are similar to findings in meta-analyses of RCTs. However, the optimal strain, dose and timing need further investigation."

Jacobs et al[3] in a randomized trial enrolled 1099 preterm infants in Australia and New Zealand and tested the combined probiotics B infantis, *Streptococcus thermophilus*, and *Bifidobacterium lactis*. They reported a significantly reduced NEC of Bell stage ≥2 in very preterm infants, but not definite late-onset sepsis or mortality.

The Italian group[4] included 26 trials and reported a 52% reduction in the incidence of NEC most notably with *Bifidobacteria* and probiotic mixtures. They did point out that there was insufficient data for extremely low birth weight infants in addition to the specific probiotic strain to be used, issues that need to be resolved before widespread use of these products could be recommended.

In an excellent trial with sufficient power, Costeloe and colleagues have unequivocally answered the question with regard to *Brevibacillus brevi*, and the answer is there were no benefits detected with regard to the primary or secondary outcomes (Table 4). Of concern was their finding that 49% of the placebo group became colonized with the same *B brevi* strain as the intervention group. This occurred at all participating sites. This may have diluted the benefits; on the other hand, if these live organisms have the potential to do harm, then many infants who would not be targeted for the probiotics will become colonized with them. Because of the size of the trial, they are of the opinion that their results are generalizable.

So we have the accumulated evidence of the many small trials using multiple probiotics suggesting that probiotics are effective, safe, and reduce necrotizing enterocolitis. The 2 large trials from Jacobs and Costeloe show no short-term harm but also no benefit with regard to NEC, sepsis, or mortality. We remain at a point in time where much more testing is needed. Costeloe suggested that different strains and combinations should be investigated separately. She concluded, "The importance of the microbiome in the complex pathogenesis of necrotizing enterocolitis is widely accepted. As understanding progresses so the rationale for the choice of probiotics that might have a therapeutic role either alone or in combination, and of which infants might benefit, strengthen. In the meantime, the evidence from this trial does not support the routine administration of probiotics to the preterm infant and the validity of combining trials of different probiotics to perform meta-analyses must be questioned." Strong words and right on point.

A. A. Fanaroff, MD

References

1. Alfaleh K, Anabrees J, Bassler D, Al-Kharfi T. Probiotics for prevention of necrotizing enterocolitis in preterm infants. *Cochrane Database Syst Rev.* 2014;(3): CD005496.

2. Olsen R, Greisen G, Schrøder M, Brok J. Prophylactic probiotics for preterm infants: a systematic review and meta-analysis of observational studies. *Neonatology.* 2016;109:105-112.
3. Jacobs SE, Tobin JM, Opie GF, et al. Probiotic effects on late-onset sepsis in very preterm infants: a randomized controlled trial. *Pediatrics.* 2013;132:1055-1062.
4. Aceti A, Gori D, Barone G, et al. Italian Society of Neonatology. Probiotics for prevention of necrotizing enterocolitis in preterm infants: systematic review and meta-analysis. *Ital J Pediatr.* 2015;41:89.

Probiotic Supplementation and Late-Onset Sepsis in Preterm Infants: A Meta-Analysis

Rao SC, Athalye-Jape GK, Deshpande GC, et al (King Edward Memorial Hosp for Women, Perth, Western Australia; Nepean Hosp, Kingswood, New South Wales, Australia)

Pediatrics 137:e20153684, 2016

Context.—Late-onset sepsis (LOS) is a major cause of mortality and morbidity in preterm infants. Despite various preventive measures, its incidence continues to remain high, hence the urgent need for additional approaches. One such potential strategy is supplementation with probiotics. The updated Cochrane Review (2014) did not find benefits of probiotics in reducing the risk of LOS in preterm infants (19 studies, $N = 5338$). Currently there are >30 randomized controlled trials (RCTs) of probiotics in preterm infants that have reported on LOS.

Objectives.—To conduct a systematic review including all relevant RCTs.

Data Sources.—PubMed, Embase, Cochrane Central Register of Controlled Trials, Cumulative Index of Nursing and Allied Health Literature, and E-abstracts from the Pediatric Academic Society meetings and other pediatric and neonatal conference proceedings were searched in June and August 2015.

Study Selection.—RCTs comparing probiotics versus placebo/no probiotic were included.

Data Extraction.—Relevant data were extracted independently by 3 reviewers.

Results.—Pooled results from 37 RCTs ($N = 9416$) using fixed effects model meta analysis showed that probiotics significantly decreased the risk of LOS (675/4852 [13.9%] vs 744/4564 [16.3%]; relative risk, 0.86; 95% confidence interval, 0.78–0.94; $P = .0007$; $I^2 = 35\%$; number needed to treat, 44). The results were significant even after excluding studies with high risk of bias.

Conclusions.—Probiotic supplementation reduces the risk of LOS in preterm infants.

▶ More than 20 published studies have focused on the impact of probiotic treatment of preterm infants. A meta-analysis[1] of these studies supports a significant reduction in both mortality and severe necrotizing enterocolitis

(NEC), attributable to probiotic treatment of this population. In many newborn intensive care units (NICUs), most prominently those outside of the United States, probiotics are used commonly to enhance the intestinal microbiome of the preterm infant with the goal of optimizing survival and preventing gastrointestinal complications of prematurity. The current meta-analysis may be the first to show a reduction also in late-onset sepsis among preterm infants—clearly a scourge we endeavor to eliminate. Two factors stand in the way of broad adoption of probiotic prophylaxis across NICUs in the United States: the rare report of neonatal infection with an organism found in a probiotic preparation and the frequent discrepancy between reported and actual bacterial species or subspecies in probiotic products—a factor important in both metabolic and colonization capacity. This heterogeneity was well demonstrated in another recent study of commercially available probiotic products,[2] which showed that in only 1 of 16 preparations was there a perfect match between the bifidobacterial species on the product label and samples tested; furthermore, both pill-to-pill and lot-to-lot variations were observed. I'm just one of many eagerly awaiting a pharmaceutical-grade probiotic preparation available in the United States that can be used to assist microbiome and overall health among our most vulnerable patients. Can't at least 1 pharmaceutical company step up and lead this effort?

L. J. Van Marter, MD, MPH

References

1. AlFaleh K, Anabrees J. Probiotics for prevention of necrotizing enterocolitis in preterm infants. *Cochrane Database Syst Rev.* 2014;(4):CD005496.
2. Lewis Z, Shani G, Masarweh, et al. Validating bifidobacterial species and subspecies identity in commercial probiotic products. *Pediatr Res.* 2016;79:445-452.

Buccal administration of human colostrum: Impact on the oral microbiota of premature infants

Sohn K, Kalanetra KM, Mills DA, et al (Univ of California Davis, Sacramento)
J Perinatol 36:106-111, 2016

Objective.—To determine whether the administration of mother's colostrum into the buccal pouch in the first days of life alters the oral microbiota compared with control infants.

Study Design.—In this pilot study, 12 very low birth weight (VLBW) infants were randomly assigned to receive either colostrum from their mothers directly into the buccal pouch every 2 h for 46 h or standard care. We analyzed the oral microbiota at initiation and 48 and 96 h later using next-generation sequencing.

Result.—The oral microbiota changed markedly over the 96 h period in all babies. Patterns of colonization differed between groups with Planococcaceae, the dominant family at 48 and 96 h in the colostrum group, and Moraxellaceae and Staphylococcaceae, the dominant families at 48 and 96 h, respectively, in the control group.

Conclusion.—Buccal administration of mother's colostrum to VLBW infants influenced the colonization of the oral cavity with differences persisting 48 h after completion of the intervention.

▶ It has not been my preference to select articles that have randomized so few infants. However, I am intrigued by the properties of colostrum and the many downstream effects of even minute doses when placed in the cheek pouch of preterm infants. Additionally, this is the first randomized controlled clinical trial to evaluate changes that occur in the oral microbiota of very low birth weight infants after the administration of mother's colostrum into the buccal pouch.

Not surprisingly, there were no significant differences between groups in clinical outcomes in this study, which was not powered to determine differences in these outcomes. The results of this pilot study support the hypothesis that the oral microbiota of preterm infants is altered by colostrum administration, although the differences between groups were not as significant as the changes in the entire group over time. Inclusion of analysis of the oral microbiota and changes in markers of the innate and adaptive immune systems in future studies may help shed light on possible mechanisms of protection. Colostrum is rich in cytokines and other immune agents that provide bacteriostatic bactericidal, antiviral, antiinflammatory and immunomodulatory protection against infection.

In 2015, we reported on the randomized controlled trial involving 48 preterm infants with gestational age <28 weeks, reported by Lee.[1] Subjects received 0.2 mL of their mother's colostrum or sterile water via oropharyngeal route every 3 hours for 3 days beginning at 48 to 96 hours of life. Urinary levels of secretory immunoglobulin A at 1 and 2 weeks and lactoferrin at 1 week were significantly higher in colostrum group. Urine interleukin-1β level was significantly lower in colostrum group at 2 weeks. Salivary transforming growth factor-β1 and interleukin-8 were significantly lower at 2 weeks in the colostrum group. A significant reduction in the incidence of clinical sepsis was noted in colostrum group (50% vs 92%), but these rates are exceptionally high in both groups. Overall, there is evidence of stepped up immune function with quieting of proinflammatory cytokines and reduced sepsis.

Larger studies, powered to determine differences in sepsis, chronic lung disease, and pneumonia are indicated and required before widespread adoption of this intervention. However, it is a simple enough intervention that should be offered more often.

A. A. Fanaroff, MD

Reference

1. Lee J, Kim HS, Jung YH, et al. Oropharyngeal colostrum administration in extremely premature infants: an RCT. *Pediatrics*. 2015;135:e357-e366.

Association of Cesarean Delivery and Formula Supplementation With the Intestinal Microbiome of 6-Week-Old Infants

Madan JC, Hoen AG, Lundgren SN, et al (Children's Hosp at Dartmouth, Lebanon, NH; The Geisel School of Medicine at Dartmouth, Hanover, NH; et al)

JAMA Pediatr 170:212-219, 2016

Importance.—The intestinal microbiome plays a critical role in infant development, and delivery mode and feeding method (breast milk vs formula) are determinants of its composition. However, the importance of delivery mode beyond the first days of life is unknown, and studies of associations between infant feeding and microbiome composition have been generally limited to comparisons between exclusively breastfed and formula-fed infants, with little consideration given to combination feeding of both breast milk and formula.

Objective.—To examine the associations of delivery mode and feeding method with infant intestinal microbiome composition at approximately 6 weeks of life.

Design, Setting, and Participants.—Prospective observational study of 102 infants followed up as part of a US pregnancy cohort study.

Exposures.—Delivery mode was abstracted from delivery medical records, and feeding method prior to the time of stool collection was ascertained through detailed questionnaires.

Main Outcomes and Measures.—Stool microbiome composition was characterized using next-generation sequencing of the 16S rRNA gene.

Results.—There were 102 infants (mean gestational age, 39.7 weeks; range, 37.1-41.9 weeks) included in this study, of whom 70 were delivered vaginally and 32 by cesarean delivery. In the first 6 weeks of life, 70 were exclusively breastfed, 26 received combination feeding, and 6 were exclusively formula fed. We identified independent associations between microbial community composition and both delivery mode ($P < .001$; $Q < .001$) and feeding method ($P = .01$; $Q < .001$). Differences in microbial community composition between vaginally delivered infants and infants delivered by cesarean birth were equivalent to or significantly larger than those between feeding groups ($P = .003$). Bacterial communities associated with combination feeding were more similar to those associated with exclusive formula feeding than exclusive breastfeeding ($P = .002$). We identified 6 individual bacterial genera that were differentially abundant between delivery mode and feeding groups.

Conclusions and Relevance.—The infant intestinal microbiome at approximately 6 weeks of age is significantly associated with both delivery mode and feeding method, and the supplementation of breast milk feeding with formula is associated with a microbiome composition that resembles that of infants who are exclusively formula fed. These results may inform feeding choices and shed light on the mechanisms behind the lifelong health consequences of delivery and infant feeding modalities.

▶ Research over the last few years suggests major differences in the intestinal microbiota of infants who were delivered by cesarean section (C-section) versus vaginal delivery. This finding may be of critical importance for several reasons, which include the fact that early intestinal microbial colonization is a crucial factor for development of the immune system. Epidemiologic studies suggest that the odds of the development of type 1 diabetes, allergies, asthma, celiac disease, and even obesity is higher in individuals who were previously delivered by C-section. The C-section rates in certain parts of the world are also very high and may not be based on medical reasons. The subsequent effects on the individual may thus outweigh benefits of the C-section.

This study evaluates the effects of mode of delivery on the fecal microbiome of term infants and simultaneously evaluates the effects of breast feeding, formula feeding, and mixed feeding in infants born by C-section versus vaginal delivery. The findings associated mode of delivery with differences in the fecal microbiome as well as dietary effects.

Before publication of this study, previous studies found that the fecal microbiota differ at various periods after C-section versus vaginal delivery. Despite showing clear differences, it is important that these studies be critiqued in depth. First, many women undergoing C-sections (routine or emergency) receive antibiotics either shortly before or immediately after cutting the umbilical cord. This regimen is not done routinely with vaginal deliveries. Such antibiotic treatment could have a significant effect on the infant either through transplacental passage or via the breast milk and could confound the results of a comparative study. Mothers of C-section–born infants often are note able to breast feed their infants as shortly after birth as are mothers who delivery their infants vaginally. Such a lag in the introduction of milk could also be a confounding factor. These confounding factors as well as several others were not rigorously controlled in the studies we have thus far and, despite these intriguing results, leave a nagging question of whether the differences between vaginal and C-section delivery are actually owing to whether the infant passed through the birth canal or these confounding factors.

The effect of diet in this study is also interesting. At least one previous study suggests modulation of the effects of C-section delivery on the microbiome with breast feeding.[1] Four months after birth, breast-fed babies fecal microbes' taxa looked similar whether the babies were delivered by C-section or vaginal delivery, whereas those infants receiving formula still differed. However, the numbers in that study were very small.

In the Madan study,[1] formula was introduced at a mean age of 3.1 weeks in the mixed group. Taxonomic identification showed that exclusively formula-fed infants differed markedly from breast-fed infants, but taxa from those on a mixed diet appeared more like those in the formula-fed group. It is known that changes in diet can markedly affect the microbiota. From the information provided, it was not clear whether the infants who were on the mixed diet were actually receiving mainly formula at the time of evaluation or were actually receiving some feedings of mother's milk and some feedings of formula. Thus, the authors' interpretation of their results supporting the World Health Organization Baby Friendly Initiative is entirely correct. This initiative promotes exclusive breast milk feeding beginning at birth—and avoidance of formulas. The authors state that their findings provide new evidence for pediatricians who may be considering incorporating formula into their infant's diet. This study did not compare formula versus breast milk feeding in which formula was started first, then breast milk was introduced later. Hence, from a strictly experimental viewpoint, an extrapolation to clinical practice based on microbiome data is not warranted.

The microbiome field is moving forward rapidly. This study evaluated taxonomy of microbes using 16S sequencing technology. This method tells us the relative abundance of microbes present in a given sample, but not what they are doing (function). Future studies should be designed to provide this information using metagenomics and metabolomics.

J. Neu, MD

Reference

1. Azad MB, Konya T, Maughan H, et al. Gut microbiota of healthy Canadian infants: profiles by mode of delivery and infant diet at 4 months. *CMAJ*. 2013; 185:385-394.

Decreased cost and improved feeding tolerance in VLBW infants fed an exclusive human milk diet

Assad M, Elliott MJ, Abraham JH (Herman and Walter Samuelson Children's Hosp at Sinai, Baltimore, MD)

J Perinatol 36:216-220, 2016

Objective.—Human milk is the best form of nutrition for preterm infants and has been associated with a lower incidence of necrotizing enterocolitis (NEC). Infants that develop NEC have a higher incidence of feeding intolerance and longer hospitalizations. The combination of a donor milk bank and donor milk-derived fortifier has changed feeding practices in neonatal intensive care units (NICU). The purpose of this study is to assess the benefits and cost of an exclusive human milk (EHM) diet in very low birth weight (VLBW) infants in a community level III NICU.

Study Design.—This is a retrospective study including preterm infants ≤28 weeks and/or VLBW (≤1500 g) who were enrolled from March 2009 until March 2014. Infants were grouped as follows: group H (entirely human milk based, born March 2012 to 2014), group B (bovine-based fortifier and maternal milk, born March 2009 to 2012), group M (mixed combination of maternal milk, bovine-based fortifier and formula, born March 2009 to 2012) and group F (formula fed infants, born March 2009 to 2012). Baseline characteristics among the four groups were similar.

Result.—The study included 293 infants between gestational ages 23 to 34 weeks and birth weights between 490 and 1700 g. Feeding intolerance occurred less often ($P < 0.0001$), number of days to full feeds was lower ($P < 0.001$), incidence of NEC was lower ($P < 0.011$), and total hospitalization costs were lower by up to $106,968 per infant ($P < 0.004$) in those fed an EHM diet compared with the other groups. Average weight gain per day was similar among the four groups (18.5 to 20.6 g per day).

Conclusions.—Implementing an EHM diet in our VLBW infants has led to a significant decrease in the incidence of NEC. Other benefits of this diet include: decreased feeding intolerance, shorter time to full feeds, shorter length of stay, and lower hospital and physician charges for extremely premature and VLBW infants (Fig 4).

▶ It is a virtual article of faith that maternal breast milk is the optimal source of nutrition for babies, particularly for very preterm infants, but bovine milk–based products continue to have a place in the marketplace, even for the latter group of very high-risk infants. Reasons for this finding appear to be largely historical and include arguments that the benefits of donor milk and human milk–derived supplements have not been adequately shown in randomized trials or that the high cost has not been justified by definitive cost-benefit analyses. Although retrospective and nonrandomized, this report of experience at a single center helps address both of these concerns. For this analysis, the authors appropriately set aside infants fed exclusively bovine formula who were significantly more mature than those fed a diet that consisted at least partially of human milk. Perhaps the most remarkable finding is the much lower rate of necrotizing enterocolitis among infants fed an exclusively human milk diet compared with those whose diet was supplemented with either bovine milk–based formula or bovine-derived milk fortifier (1% vs 10%; Fig 4). This difference undoubtedly accounts for the differences in length of stay (22.9 more hospital days for human milk–fed infants exposed to bovine fortifier or formula) and charges ($27 388 and $106 968 more per infant in human milk–fed infants who were also exposed to bovine fortifier or formula, respectively). These results, along with similar reports from other institutions, leave one to wonder how these data would be interpreted if the historical context was one in which bovine fortifiers were introduced as less expensive and more readily produced alternatives to previously established exclusive use of human milk–based products. Under those circumstances, we surely would not tolerate a 10-fold increase in the rate of necrotizing enterocolitis and 5- to 6-digit increases in charges for care to decrease costs for this single item. Nonetheless, there will continue to be significant impetus to make exactly that choice as long as the health care payment system is structured so that higher costs of human milk–based supplements accrue to the provider (hospital), while savings from shorter, less-complicated hospitalizations accrue to third-party payors. As this misalignment of incentives is reduced or eliminated by transition to case-based or capitated compensation schemes, we should expect a parallel transition to exclusive use of human milk products in very low birth weight (and certainly in extremely low birth weight) infants. Use of bovine milk–derived

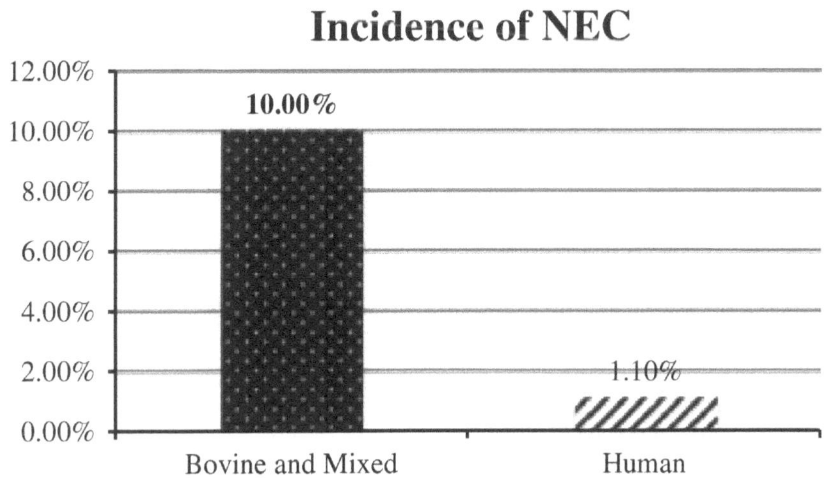

FIGURE 4.—Using Fisher's exact test ($P < 0.011$), $N = 263$. Formula group excluded from analysis (statistically older group), medical NEC represents 1% of bovine and mixed group, all others were surgical. (Reprinted from Assad M, Elliott MJ, Abraham JH. Decreased cost and improved feeding tolerance in VLBW infants fed an exclusive human milk diet. *J Perinatol*. 2016;36:216-220, with permission from Nature America, Inc.)

products should be reserved for those in whom adequately powered trials show safety profiles equivalent to the gold standard.

W. E. Benitz, MD

Early versus Delayed Human Milk Fortification in Very Low Birth Weight Infants—A Randomized Controlled Trial

Shah SD, Dereddy N, Jones TL, et al (Univ of Florida, Jacksonville; Univ of Tennessee Health Science Ctr, Memphis; et al)

J Pediatr 174:126-131.e1, 2016

Objective.—To compare the effect of initiating human milk fortification at 2 different feeding volumes on feeding intolerance and the time to reach full feeding volume.

Study Design.—Very low birth weight infants (n = 100) were prospectively randomized to early fortification (EF) (beginning at a feeding volume of 20 mL/kg/d) or delayed fortification (at a feeding volume of 100 mL/kg/d). We employed a standardized feeding protocol and parenteral nutrition guidelines for the nutritional management of all study infants.

Results.—The median days to reach full feeding volumes were equivalent in the 2 groups (20 vs 20, $P = .45$). No significant difference was observed in the total number of episodes of feeding intolerance (58 vs 57). Two cases of necrotizing enterocolitis (Bell stage ≥2) and deaths occurred in each group. Median daily protein intake (g/kg/d) was higher in EF group in week 1 (3.3 [3.2, 3.5] vs 3.1 [2.9, 3.3], $P < .001$), week 2 (3.6 [3.5, 3.8] vs 3.2 [2.9, 3.4], $P < .001$), and week 3 (3.7 [3.4, 3.9] vs 3.5 [2.8, 3.8], $P = .006$). Cumulative protein intake (g/kg) in the first 4 weeks of life was higher in EF group (98.6 [93.8, 104] vs 89.6 [84.2, 96.4], $P < .001$).

Conclusions.—Very early human milk fortification may improve early protein intake in very low birth weight infants without increasing frequencies of adverse events.

Trial Registration.—ClinicalTrials.gov: NCT01988792.

▶ Providing adequate nutrition to very low birth weight (VLBW) infants, particularly during the first month after birth, is a daunting task. Despite efforts to improve early nutrition, many VLBW infants exhibit extrauterine growth restriction at 36 to 40 weeks of corrected gestational age. In this single-center, randomized, clinical study, the investigators compared the clinical outcomes and growth of VLBW infants who received fortified human milk at 2 different feeding volumes (20 mL/kg/d vs 100 mL/kg/d).

Oral nutrition was started on the third postnatal day in both groups, and full feeding volumes were achieved in the same interval. The rate of feeding intolerance, defined as enteral feedings held for at least 24 hours secondary to emesis/aspirates or abdominal distension, was similar, as was the rate of metabolic acidosis. In addition, the rate and severity necrotizing enterocolitis did not differ, with one infant in each group requiring surgical intervention, and there was no difference in growth velocity between the 2 groups at 1 month of age and 36 weeks of corrected age. Approximately 70% of the infants in both groups were small for gestational age (<10th percentile) at the time of discharge to home. Although the cohort that received fortified breast milk early had a significantly higher cumulative protein intake over the first month after birth, the actual difference was only 9 g, apparently an insufficient amount to have a beneficial effect on growth.

L. A. Papile, MD

Effect of Donor Milk on Severe Infections and Mortality in Very Low-Birth-Weight Infants: The Early Nutrition Study Randomized Clinical Trial

Corpeleijn WE, de Waard M, Christmann V, et al (Emma Children's Hosp-Academic Med Ctr, Amsterdam, the Netherlands; VU Univ Med Ctr, Amsterdam, the Netherlands; Radboud Univ Med Ctr, Nijmegen, the Netherlands; et al)

JAMA Pediatr 170:654-661, 2016

Importance.—Infections and necrotizing enterocolitis, major causes of mortality and morbidity in preterm infants, are reduced in infants fed their own mother's milk when compared with formula. When own mother's milk is not available, human donor milk is considered a good alternative, albeit an expensive one. However, most infants at modern neonatal intensive care units are predominantly fed with own mother's milk. The benefits of add-on donor milk over formula are not clear.

Objective.—To determine whether providing donor milk instead of formula as supplemental feeding whenever own mother's milk is insufficiently available during the first 10 days of life reduces the incidence of serious infection, necrotizing enterocolitis, and mortality.

Design, Settings, and Participants.—The Early Nutrition Study was a multicenter, double-blind randomized clinical trial in very low-birth-weight infants (birth weight <1500 g) admitted to 1 of 6 neonatal intensive care units in the Netherlands from March 30, 2012, through August 17, 2014. Intent-to-treat analysis was performed.

Interventions.—Infants received pasteurized donor milk or preterm formula during the first 10 days of life if own mother's milk was not (sufficiently) available.

Main Outcomes and Measures.—The primary end point was cumulative occurrence of serious infection (sepsis or meningitis), necrotizing enterocolitis, or mortality during the first 60 days of life.

Results.—A total of 930 infants were screened for inclusion; 557 were excluded, resulting in 373 infants (183 receiving donor milk and 190 receiving formula) who were evaluated by intent-to-treat analysis (median birth weight, 1066 g; mean gestational age, 28.4 weeks). Own mother's milk comprised 89.1%and 84.5%of total mean intake during the intervention period for the donor milk and formula groups, respectively. The incidence of the combined outcome was not different (85 [44.7%] [formula] vs 77 [42.1%] [donor milk]; mean difference, 2.6%; 95% CI, −12.7% to 7.4%). The adjusted hazard ratio was 0.87 (95% CI, 0.63-1.19; *P* =.37).

Conclusions and Relevance.—In the current study, pasteurized donor milk and preterm formula as supplemental feeding during the first 10 days of life yielded similar short-term outcomes in very low-birth-weight infants regarding safety and efficacy when own mother's milk availability was insufficient. Future studies investigating longer duration of use of human donor milk on short-term and long-term outcomes are necessary

Trial Registration.—trialregister.nl Identifier: NTR3225.

▶ In 2012, the American Academy of Pediatrics guidelines stated that "the potent benefits of human milk are such that all preterm infants should receive human milk. Mother's own milk, fresh or frozen, should be the primary diet, and should be fortified appropriately for the infant born weighing less than 1.5 kg. If mother's own milk is unavailable despite significant lactation support, pasteurized donor milk should be used. Quality control of pasteurized donor milk is important and should be monitored."[1] This statement led to the widespread use of the donor milk in many neonatal intensive care units in the United States. Donor milk is relatively expensive, and even though its benefits have been touted, many questions remain. Donor milk in the United States undergoes pasteurization, a process that decreases some and actually eliminates several bioactive components including lipase activity, alkaline phosphatase activity, and other enzymes. It eliminates microbial components that may have beneficial bioactive roles, but these have not yet been determined. Furthermore, when pooled, donor milk has been found to be relatively low in protein, and thus babies receiving nonfortified donor milk grow at a lower rate than those infants provided formula.

This study evaluates the effect of donor milk versus formula in a randomized clinical trial with the major outcomes being severe infections such as sepsis or meningitis, necrotizing enterocolitis, or mortality during the first 60 days after birth. This is a multicenter, double-blind, randomized clinical trial performed on very low birth weight infants weighing less than 1500 g at birth 373 infants were randomized to receive only donor milk versus formula during the first 10 days after birth. The results showed similar short-term outcomes regarding safety and efficacy when own mother's milk availability was insufficient.

Does this mean that it's time to close the donor milk banks in the United States and ignore the AAP guidelines for the use of donor milk for very low birth weight infants? The current answer to this should be no! However, we need to be aware that donor human milk has many deficiencies. Available studies show that to obtain proper growth and neurodevelopment for the most susceptible preterm infants, unfortified donor milk is not optimal. The available meta-analyses that evaluate necrotizing enterocolitis include studies that were done more than 20 years ago, and the quality of the individual studies on which these are based (eg, diagnostic criteria used to identify NEC) need to be questioned.

This study by Corpeleijn et al raises important questions about the efficacy of donor milk in the prevention of severe infections and mortality when used short term. Obviously, more extensive studies are needed as suggested by the authors. In the meantime, we should note that pooled donor milk is not a good substitute for baby's own mother's milk when the latter is available. An emphasis needs to be placed on helping the mother provide her milk for her own infant.

J. Neu, MD

Reference

1. Section on Breastfeeding. Breastfeeding and the use of human milk. *Pediatrics.* 2012;129:e827-e841.

Human Milk Analyser shows that the lactation period affects protein levels in preterm breastmilk

Kreissl A, Zwiauer V, Repa A, et al (Med Univ of Vienna, Austria)

Acta Paediatr 105:635-640, 2016

Aim.—This study measured the composition of preterm human breastmilk, particularly the protein content, with the MIRIS Human Milk Analyser, compared our results with published values and determined the relationship between protein content and lactation period.

Methods.—We analysed 83 samples of 24-hour pooled human milk from 76 mothers who delivered preterm infants weighing under 1500 g at less than 32 weeks of gestational age. The milk's protein, fat and energy were measured by the MIRIS Human Milk Analyser and compared to reference values. The relationship between protein content and lactation period was quantified.

Results.—On average, the samples contained 1.1 ± 0.37 g (0.2–2.2 g) of protein, 3.2 ± 0.85 g (range 1.1–6.1 g) of fat, 6.6 ± 0.34 g of lactose (5.5–8.0 g) and 60 ± 11 kcal (39–94 kcal) of energy per 100 mL. The wide variations in macronutrient content were not influenced by the gestational age of the infant and the lactation day results from 70 of the mothers correlated inversely with the protein content ($p < 0.0001$; $r = -0.42$). The MIRIS proved useful, but some adjustments are needed.

Conclusion.—Variations in macronutrients were high in the breastmilk of women who delivered preterm babies and the protein content decreased with lactation. With adjustments, the MIRIS might provide a helpful tool for individualised fortification.

▶ It is well known that the protein requirements for very low birth weight infants are relatively high compared with those for full-term infants. When using pooled term banked donor milk for these infants, the quantity of the protein present per 100 mL is low; therefore, a large volume of milk would be required to provide the protein needed for these babies. Such volumes range between 300 and 400 mL/kg/d; therefore, most preterm babies would be unable to tolerate such heart high intake volumes. Furthermore, there are other nutrients that to are found to be lacking such as calcium and phosphorus when human milk, especially donor human milk, is provided. Thus, fortification of human milk has become an adjunct to the nutritional support of these preterm infants. To provide optimal personalization for providing such nutrients, it is thought that having a technique that will accurately and rapidly measure the amount of the protein present in samples would provide an enhanced ability to provide sufficient macronutrients that will optimally support these infants' nutritional needs.

This study used a commercial milk analyzer to quantify the amount of the macronutrients in samples of milk from the different stages of lactation. As is already well known, during the early stages of lactation in preterm infants, the milk contains higher levels of protein, which subsequently decreases over time. When these quantities were evaluated and compared with values found in the literature, the method used in this study showed slightly lower levels of the macronutrients, especially protein. The ranges of the protein in the donor human milk were very high, 0.2 to 2.2 g/100 mL. Such a range does suggest that measurement of the protein and other macronutrient composition of human milk may be helpful to personalize the amount of protein for feeding these infants.

However, this study does not answer the question of whether simple supplementation of all donor milk samples with fortifiers without measurement of the macronutrient composition would actually be inferior to the more personalized approach one might achieve with measuring the composition and, more specifically, adding the fortifiers to a certain predefined level. A head-to-head comparison of the nonmeasured human milk versus measured human milk and a determination of how this would result in the patient outcome characteristics such as growth and biochemical outcomes are needed.

J. Neu, MD

Human milk oligosaccharides in premature infants: absorption, excretion, and influence on the intestinal microbiota

Underwood MA, Gaerlan S, De Leoz ML, et al (Univ of California Davis, Sacramento; Univ of California Davis)
Pediatr Res 78:670-677, 2015

Background.—Human milk oligosaccharides (HMOs) shape the intestinal microbiota in term infants. In premature infants, alterations in the intestinal microbiota (dysbiosis) are associated with risk of necrotizing enterocolitis (NEC) and sepsis, and the influence of HMOs on the microbiota is unclear.

Methods.—Milk, urine, and stool specimens from 14 mother–premature infant dyads were investigated by mass spectrometry for HMO composition. The stools were analyzed by next-generation sequencing to complement a previous analysis.

Results.—Percentages of fucosylated and sialylated HMOs were highly variable between individuals but similar in urine, feces, and milk within dyads. Differences in urine and fecal HMO composition suggest variability in absorption. Secretor status of the mother correlated with the urine and fecal content of specific HMO structures. Trends toward higher levels of *Proteobacteria* and lower levels of *Firmicutes* were noted in premature infants of nonsecretor mothers. Specific HMO structures in the milk, urine, and feces were associated with alterations in fecal *Proteobacteria* and *Firmicutes*.

Conclusion.—HMOs may influence the intestinal microbiota in premature infants. Specific HMOs, for example those associated with secretor mothers, may have a protective effect by decreasing pathogens associated with sepsis and NEC, while other HMOs may increase dysbiosis in this population.

▶ Studies of the intestinal microbiome and various disease states are a hot topic in contemporary medical and scientific circles. In neonatology, specific patterns in the intestinal microbiome have been linked to risk of sepsis and necrotizing enterocolitis (NEC). A healthy microbiome is fostered by certain human milk oligosaccharides (HMOs), potentially offering one explanation as to why human milk–fed infants are at lower risk of NEC than those receiving cow's milk–based formula. The current study explored the relationship of HMOs to microbiome in biological samples from mother–premature infant dyads. What this study adds to our knowledge is the recognition that both infants' absorption of HMOs and mothers' secretory status differs among individuals and that specific HMOs produced by "secretor" mothers foster a healthier neonatal microbiome. Perhaps one day, we'll be able to screen mother's milk for and/or supplement infants with these healthy HMOs and thereby enhance the preterm infant's gastrointestinal and immunological competence—just another step in our NEC eradication campaign! For a terrific review of the relationship between intestinal microbiota and NEC, see Ravi Patel and Patricia Denning's recent publication.[1]

L. J. Van Marter, MD, MPH

Reference

1. Patel RM, Denning PW. Intestinal microbiota and its relationship with necrotizing enterocolitis. *Pediatr Res.* 2015;78:232-238.

Independent Predictors of Human Milk Receipt at Neonatal Intensive Care Unit Discharge

Brownell EA, Lussier MM, Hagadorn JI, et al (Connecticut Children's Med Ctr, Hartford)

Am J Perinatol 31:891-898, 2014

Objective.—The aim of this study is to construct a predictive model for very low birth weight (VLBW) infants' receipt of mother's own milk within 24 hours before neonatal intensive care unit (NICU) discharge.

Study Design.—Vermont Oxford Network (VON) clinical data were analyzed retrospectively for VLBW infants admitted between 2002 and 2012 at an inner city, level IV NICU with a well-established lactation program. Bivariate analyses compared infant characteristics between recipients and nonrecipients of human milk before 24 hours of NICU discharge. Independent predictors identified in the bivariate analyses ($p \leq 0.05$), were eligible for inclusion into a multivariable logistic regression model.

Results.—We observed a 60.4% human milk feeding rate at NICU discharge. Multiple independent maternal (black race and Hispanic ethnicity) and clinical factors (need for mechanical ventilation, patent ductus arteriosus, late-onset sepsis, or discharge to home on a cardiorespiratory monitor) positively predicted the outcome.

Conclusions.—Our results were inconsistent with previous studies and suggest that a strong NICU lactation program in combination with a community-based peer counselor program may increase rates of human milk receipt among VLBW infants born to black/ Hispanic mothers and those with more complicated neonatal courses.

▶ Friendship is born at that moment when one person says to another:

"What! You too? I thought I was the only one."—C.S. Lewis

Scientific evidence regarding the multiple benefits of human milk feedings for premature infants continues to expand. However, despite improved initiation rates, many very low birth weight (VLBW) infants do not receive human milk at the time of neonatal intensive unit (NICU) discharge.[1] This study aimed to develop a model that predicts which factors independently affect the VLBW infants' receipt of mother's own milk within 24 hours of NICU discharge. In contrast to other studies, the model in this study predicted that black race, Hispanic ethnicity, and infants with more severe illnesses were more likely to receive maternal human milk within 24 hours of discharge. These characteristics have been shown previously to be negative predictive factors.[2,3] The authors concluded that their individual NICU's strong lactation assistance, breastfeeding peer counseling program, and community support were contributors to the study's unique findings. This conclusion is important because it associates the power of peer support and a unified team culture in promoting the benefits of maternal human milk.

Throughout time, breastfeeding support for new mothers has been provided by other mothers. The La Leche League was developed in 1957 by a group of 7 young mothers with breastfeeding infants.[4] Today, it has grown into an international mother-mother support group and educational community that consistently promotes the importance of breastfeeding among all maternal-infant dyads.[4] Breastfeeding peer counselor programs that have been instituted in multiple NICUs across the country are an extension of the La Leche League for the premature patient. NICU breastfeeding peer counselors are not only mothers who are trained in lactation support; they are also mothers of premature infants who have experienced firsthand the unique nuances of an NICU. Through shared experiences, evidence indicates that new mothers of premature infants value the education, assistance, and support that only a "peer" can provide.[5] New mothers report a sense of empowerment, hope, and connection that goes beyond demographics, socioeconomic status or ethnicity.[5,6] In addition, a breastfeeding peer counselor is able to send a consistent message regarding the importance of human milk for the premature infant via one-on-one time with the mother and family.[6] Thus, a breastfeeding peer counselor serves as both a cheerleader and an educator who promotes a positive human milk culture for the entire NICU team.

Although this study is based on retrospective data from a single center and the conclusions are speculative, I believe it demonstrates how the uniqueness of unit culture can affect individual NICU outcomes that may not always follow traditional predictive models. As individual NICUs implement new programs to enhance human milk use, I encourage units to evaluate their own data and culture. Barriers to the use of human milk that in the past may have been viewed as fixed patient characteristics such as race, ethnicity, and illness may be overcome by something as simple as having a friend and finding common ground.

K. P. Stanley, MD

Variability of Criteria for Pasteurized Donor Human Milk Use: A Survey of U.S. Neonatal Intensive Care Unit Medical Directors

Hagadorn JI, Brownell EA, Lussier MM, et al (Connecticut Children's Med Ctr, Hartford; et al)

JPEN J Parenter Enteral Nutr 40:326-333, 2016

Background.—Use of donor human milk (DHM) is increasing, but criteria for its use are not well defined.

Materials and Methods.—We conducted a 34-question Internet-based survey of medical directors of U.S. level 3 and level 4 neonatal intensive care units (NICUs), with the goal of describing specifics of policies developed to guide DHM use in U.S. NICUs. Respondents reported NICU characteristics and details of policies concerning DHM use. Policy-specified criteria for DHM use, if any, were described. Bivariate and multivariate analyses were used to identify NICU characteristics associated with DHM use.

Results.—Respondents returned 153 (33%) surveys, with use of DHM reported by 91 (59%). Donor human milk use was more likely with more than 100 annual admissions <1500 g at birth (odds ratio [OR], 2.2; 95% confidence interval [CI], 1.1–4.7) and with Vermont-Oxford Network participants (OR, 4.6; 95% CI, 1.8–11.6). Among 72 NICUs reporting a written policy, criteria for providing DHM required birth weights varying from <1000 to <1800 g and/or gestational ages from <28 to <34 completed weeks, but criteria were reportedly waived in many circumstances. Policies regarding duration of DHM therapy were similarly varied.

Conclusions.—Criteria for initiating and continuing DHM vary widely among U.S. level 3 and level 4 NICUs. Donor human milk use is more frequent in NICUs with many very low-birth-weight admissions and among Vermont-Oxford Network participants. Further research is needed to define short- and long-term outcomes and cost benefits of DHM use in subgroups of NICU patients, particularly for uses other than necrotizing enterocolitis prevention (Fig 1).

▶ This article is of interest in that using an Internet-based survey of medical directors of US level 3 and 4 neonatal intensive care units (NICUs), it documents widely varying criteria for donor human milk use. The busiest units caring for the most preterm infants appeared to have the greatest usage of donor milk. There was a high variability in gestational age as well as birth weight criteria and when to stop donor milk usage was also variable. Of interest is that the most common reasons for providing donor milk was to reduce necrotizing enterocolitis and, secondarily, to improve feeding tolerance. Reduction of allergies, family request, reduction of nosocomial infections were relatively uncommon reasons (Fig 1A). Reasons provided to not use donor milk were primarily based on the high expense (Fig 1B).

High usage of donor milk has partially also been the result of recommendations from the American Academy of Pediatrics, the World Health Organization, and the US Surgeon General, again based largely on the reduction of necrotizing

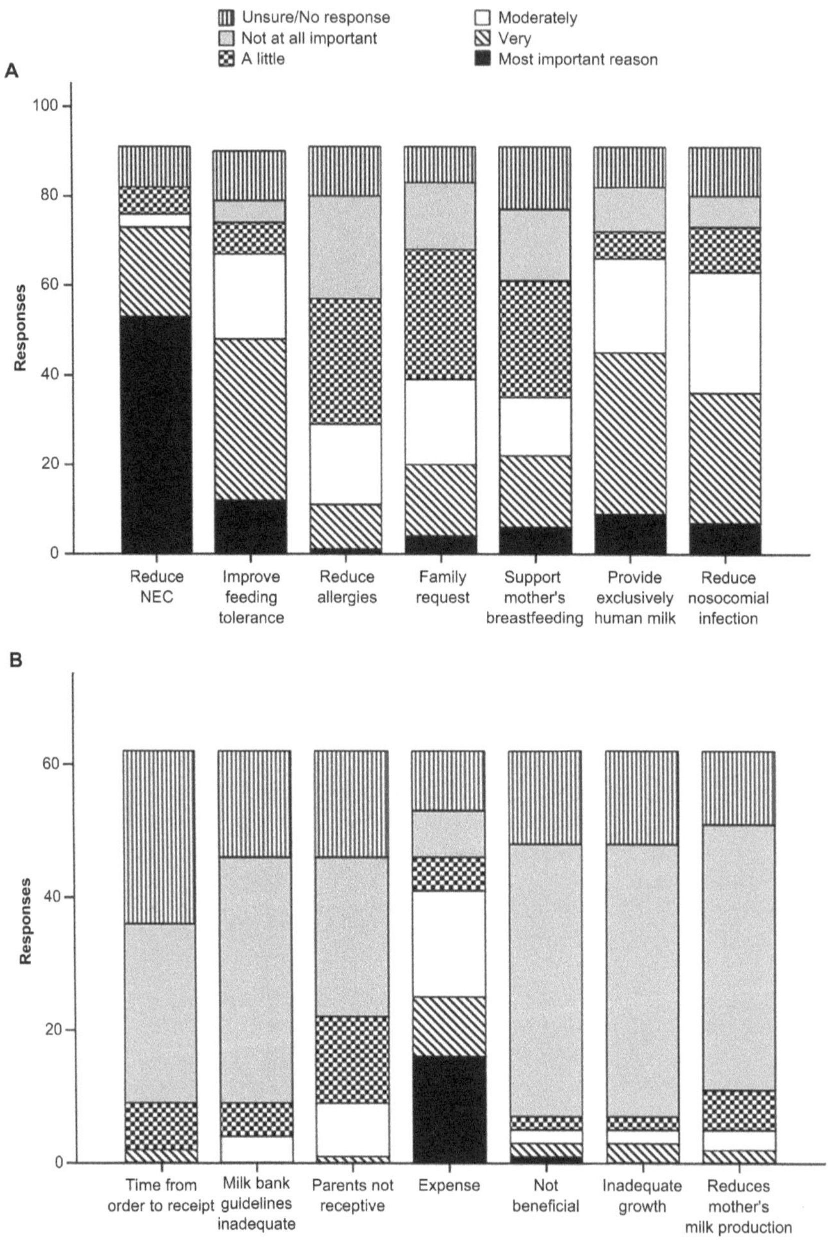

FIGURE 1.—Reasons for (A) providing (n = 91) and (B) not providing (n = 62) pasteurized banked donor human milk, as reported by sampled U.S. level 3 or level 4 neonatal intensive care unit medical directors. NEC, necrotizing enterocolitis. (Reprinted from Hagadorn JI, Brownell EA, Lussier MM, et al. Variability of criteria for pasteurized donor human milk use: a survey of U.S. neonatal intensive care unit medical directors. *JPEN J Parenter Enteral Nutr.* 2016;40:326-333, with permission from American Society for Parenteral and Enteral Nutrition.)

enterocolitis (NEC) based primarily from 3 studies.[1-3] Of interest is that in the Cochrane review,[3] some of the studies were done more than 20 years ago, and none of the individual studies showed clinically significant decreases in NEC with the use of donor milk. The other 2 studies[1,2] were not powered to evaluate NEC and found differences in post hoc analyses with baseline levels that were considerably higher than seen in most NICUs. The variability in use as described in this study as well as the quality of the studies on which the recommendations are based, that is, prevention of NEC raises the need for reevaluation of the current studies, better controlled prospective trials, and perhaps more extensive cost-benefit analyses that also take into account the need to fortify donor milk and the consequences that the patients incur if not adequately fortified.

J. Neu, MD

References

1. Sullivan S, Schanler RJ, Kim JH, et al. An exclusively human milk-based diet is associated with a lower rate of necrotizing enterocolitis than a diet of human milk and bovine milk-based products. *J Pediatr.* 2010;156:562-567.e1.
2. Cristofalo EA, Schanler RJ, Blanco CL, et al. Randomized trial of exclusive human milk versus preterm formula diets in extremely premature infants. *J Pediatr.* 2013; 163:1592-1595.e1.
3. Quigley M, McGuire W. Formula versus donor breast milk for feeding preterm or low birth weight infants. *Cochrane Database Syst Rev.* 2014;(4):CD002971.

Breastmilk from obese mothers has pro-inflammatory properties and decreased neuroprotective factors

Panagos PG, Vishwanathan R, Penfield-Cyr A, et al (Tufts Med Ctr, Boston, MA; Tufts Univ, Boston, MA; Brigham and Women's Hosp, Boston, MA; et al)
J Perinatol 36:284-290, 2016

Objective.—To determine the impact of maternal obesity on breastmilk composition.

Study Design.—Breastmilk and food records from 21 lean and 21 obese women who delivered full-term infants were analyzed at 2 months postpartum. Infant growth and adiposity were measured at birth and 2 months of age.

Result.—Breastmilk from obese mothers had higher omega-6 to omega-3 fatty acid ratio and lower concentrations of docosahexaenoic acid, eicosapentaenoic acid, docasapentaenoic acid and lutein compared with lean mothers ($P < 0.05$), which were strongly associated with maternal body mass index. Breastmilk saturated fatty acid and monounsaturated fatty acid concentrations were positively associated with maternal dietary inflammation, as measured by dietary inflammatory index. There were no differences in infant growth measurements.

Conclusion.—Breastmilk from obese mothers has a pro-inflammatory fatty acid profile and decreased concentrations of fatty acids and carotenoids that have been shown to have a critical role in early visual and neurodevelopment. Studies are needed to determine the link between these early-life influences and subsequent cardiometabolic and neurodevelopmental outcomes.

▶ The advantages of breast feeding are well documented throughout the literature. It is also known that obesity is a pro-inflammatory state that is associated with differences in dietary intake, which can influence inflammation. This study was designed to determine whether maternal obesity has an impact on breast milk composition, especially in terms of the anti- and pro-inflammatory mediators. The design of this study was to evaluate food records and breast milk from 21 lean and 21 obese women who delivered full-term infants. The milk samples were analyzed for 2 months postpartum.

Although no short-term differences in growth or adiposity of the infants were seen, the most salient feature from this study was that there was a correlation between maternal body mass index and the omega-6 to omega-3 long-chain fatty acid ratio. This ratio is one that reflects pro-inflammatory mediators compared with anti-inflammatory potential of these lipids. A different statistical analysis also found that the obese mothers had a higher omega-6 to omega-3 ratio, which differed at a *P* value of .0034. Several other mediators such as carotenoid compositions differed; specifically, milk lutein was significantly lower in obese mothers compared with lean mothers at a *P* value of .006. Lutein is a carotenoid that is known to protect the eyes via oxidative stress mechanisms.

This article is, to my knowledge, the first showing that the composition of breast milk from obese women differs from that of the lean women in terms of the inflammatory fatty acid ratios as well as carotenoids and various fatty acid concentrations. The maternal diet composition that reflects a dietary inflammatory index also relates to maternal obesity and some of the components that comprise breast milk that may be highly active in terms of inflammatory potential, as shown in this study. Additional research is needed on interventions in the maternal diet, which may, in turn, affect obesity and breast milk fatty acid pro-inflammatory anti-inflammatory ratios as well as other potentially neuroprotective substances and their effects on subsequent development of the newborn.

J. Neu, MD

Early Detection Tool of Intestinal Dysfunction: Impact on Necrotizing Enterocolitis Severity

Fox JR, Thacker LR, Hendricks-Muñoz KD (Virginia Commonwealth Univ, Richmond)

Am J Perinatol 32:927-932, 2015

Objective.—The aim of this study is to determine the use of an early clinical signs and symptoms warning tool in early identification of intestinal dysfunction as a clinical strategy to decrease necrotizing enterocolitis (NEC) severity.

Design.—Using signs and symptoms of 297 infants, of which 33 infants were diagnosed with stage II and III EC intestinal dysfunction, a five clinical category scoring tool (Neonatal Necrotizing Enterocolitis Early Detection Score [NeoNEEDS]) and strategy with abdominal X-ray alert was developed. The categories included behavior, cardiac, respiratory, gastrointestinal, and feeding tolerance. The strategy was tested in a prospective cohort of 72 infants < 1,500 g, utilizing 532 observations between 10/2012 and 9/1/2013. The statistical analysis utilized the Statistical Analysis Software (SAS).

Results.—The earliest signs and symptoms of intestinal dysfunction (Stage I NEC) were cardiorespiratory baseline changes, $p < 0.001$. Abdominal distension and/or feeding intolerance were late findings associated with stage II or III NEC. Tool scores ≥ 5 predicted intestinal dysfunction ($p < 0.00$). Sensitivity was high (95%) with specificity of 82% and positive and negative predictive values of 76% and 95%, respectively. Use of the tool during the study period was associated with decreased NEC severity rates (Bell NEC stage II and III).

Conclusion.—Cardiorespiratory symptoms precede gastrointestinal symptoms of intestinal dysfunction. Targeting signs and symptoms in an early warning tool to identify intestinal dysfunction can impact NEC severity progression.

▶ This study evaluated early and late clinical symptoms associated with necrotizing enterocolitis (NEC). A retrospective review was used to formulate a scoring system that was used as an "abdominal X-ray alert" (score > 5) for prospective use to indicate when the baby should have further x-ray evaluation. Prospectively evaluating this technique, they found high sensitivity, specificity, moderate positive predictive value, and high negative predictive value. Receiver operating characteristics are not provided in this study. There are some significant caveats that need to be considered here. First, Stage 1 NEC was included as a determinant for score development in the retrospective study as well as in the prospective study. "Stage 1 NEC" is highly nonspecific and may simply correspond to instabilities in the patient. So if one correlates an instability (using the scoring system) to another instability, it is not surprising that associations are found. Furthermore, abdominal radiographs provide challenges in the diagnosis of NEC. What sometimes appears as granular pneumatosis may reflect artifacts such as stool in the bowel. When one is led to doing more abdominal x-rays using this tool, artifacts suggesting NEC are more likely to be found, thus leading to unnecessary interventions such as holding feedings and starting antibiotics. In addition, showing a decrease in NEC over a period of a few years is not highly likely to be due to only 1 intervention. Feeding practices, use of guidelines, and other modalities including what we are actually calling NEC (as opposed to spontaneous intestinal perforations and other confounding intestinal problems such as septic ileus), are also changing over time. Whether this tool would be useful in other neonatal intensive care units should also be questioned.

J. Neu, MD

Early Detection of Necrotizing Enterocolitis by Fecal Volatile Organic Compounds Analysis

de Meij TGJ, van der Schee MPC, Berkhout DJC, et al (Vrije Universiteit University Medical Center, Amsterdam, The Netherlands; Academic Med Ctr, Amsterdam, The Netherlands; et al)
J Pediatr 167:562-567, 2015

Objectives.—To test the hypothesis that fecal volatile organic compounds (VOCs) analysis by electronic nose (eNose) allows for early detection of necrotizing enterocolitis (NEC).

Study Design.—In 3 neonatal intensive care units, fecal samples of infants born at gestational age ≤30 weeks were collected daily, up to the 28th day of life. Included infants were allocated in 3 subgroups: NEC, sepsis, and matched controls. Three time windows were defined: (1) $T_{-5,-4}$ (5 and 4 days before diagnosis); (2) $T_{-3,-2}$ (3 and 2 days before diagnosis); and (3) $T_{-1,0}$ (day before and day of diagnosis). Three subgroups were analyzed by eNose.

Results.—Fecal VOC profiles of infants with NEC (n = 13) could significantly be discriminated from matched controls (n = 14) at $T_{-3,-2}$ (area under the curve ± 95% CI, *P* value, sensitivity, specificity: 0.77 ± 0.21, *P* =.02, 83%, 75%); the accuracy increased at $T_{-1,0}$ (0.99 ± 0.04, *P* ≤.001, 89%, 89%). VOC profiles of infants with NEC were also significantly different from those with sepsis (n = 31) at $T_{-3,-2}$ (0.80 ± 0.17, *P* =.004, 83%, 75%), but not at $T_{-1,0}$ (0.64 ± 0.18, *P* =.216, 89%, 57%).

Conclusions.—In this proof of principle study, we observed that fecal VOC profiles of infants with NEC could be discriminated from controls, from 2-3 days predating onset of clinical symptoms. Our observations suggest that VOC-profiling by eNose has potential as a noninvasive tool for the early prediction of NEC.

▶ One of the major problems with necrotizing enterocolitis is its fulminant nature with minimal warning signs. The ability to recognize necrotizing enterocolitis early using noninvasive techniques before development of full-blown disease and the ability to differentiate it from late-onset sepsis has been a significant goal in neonatal intensive care. Noninvasive techniques could include evaluation of the cardiovascular instability, breath analysis, stool sampling for microbes and inflammatory markers and urine sampling for markers of intestinal epithelial breakdown and or markers of the inflammation.[1-3] However, the studies using these techniques have thus far not led to clinical applicability.

This study evaluates a novel technique that involves collection of fecal samples on a longitudinal basis and inducing a known quantity of fecal sample to release volatile fatty acids upon warming. The sensor output of the "E-nose" apparatus is based on electronic detection of groups of volatile fatty acids that produce individual signatures on principal component plots. The volatile fatty acids are evaluated using a technique that has commonly been used for volatile fatty acids produced during degradation of foods, petrochemicals, and other substances.

This study demonstrated that analysis of fecal volatile fatty acids in a small number of patients who developed necrotizing enterocolitis showed differences from controls, especially within 1 day of the development of the disease. The area under the curve (AUC) evaluation between 2 to 5 days before the development of the disease was in the fair range of accuracy for this measurement. The discrimination of necrotizing enterocolitis versus late-onset sepsis also appeared to be in the fair range 2 to 3 days before the diagnosis, but not in a very good range within a day of diagnosis or 4 to 5 days before the diagnosis.

This test is somewhat reminiscent of research that was done a few decades ago evaluating breath hydrogen as a fermentation product of intestinal microbes as a potential biomarker for necrotizing enterocolitis.[4,5] Although intriguing, because of its noninvasive nature, breath hydrogen was found to be highly dependent on the amount of carbohydrate ingested, intestinal motility, and various other factors that confounded this as a highly usable diagnostic tool. Nevertheless, the "E-nose" technique described in this article certainly deserves further scrutiny in larger multicenter studies.

J. Neu, MD

References

1. Nantais-Smith L, Kadrofske M. Noninvasive biomarkers of necrotizing enterocolitis. *J Perinat Neonatal Nurs.* 2015;29:69-80.
2. Young C, Sharma R, Handfield M, Mai V, Neu J. Biomarkers for infants at risk for necrotizing enterocolitis: clues to prevention? *Pediatr Res.* 2009;65:91R-97R.
3. Ng EW, Poon TC, Lam HS, et al. Gut-associated biomarkers L-FABP, I-FABP, and TFF3 and LIT score for diagnosis of surgical necrotizing enterocolitis in preterm infants. *Ann Surg.* 2013;258:1111-1118.
4. Garstin WI, Boston VE. Sequential assay of expired breath hydrogen as a means of predicting necrotizing enterocolitis in susceptible infants. *J Pediatr Surg.* 1987;22:208-210.
5. Cheu HW, Brown DR, Rowe MI. Breath hydrogen excretion as a screening test for the early diagnosis of necrotizing enterocolitis. *Am J Dis Child.* 1989;143:156-159.

Impact of Donor Milk Availability on Breast Milk Use and Necrotizing Enterocolitis Rates

Kantorowska A, Wei JC, Cohen RS, et al (Univ of Rochester School of Medicine and Dentistry, Rochester, NY; Univ of California, Berkeley; Stanford Univ School of Medicine, CA; et al)
Pediatrics 137:e20153123, 2016

Objectives.—To examine the availability of donor human milk (DHM) in a population-based cohort and assess whether the availability of DHM was associated with rates of breast milk feeding at NICU discharge and rates of necrotizing enterocolitis (NEC).

Methods.—Individual patient clinical data for very low birth weight infants from the California Perinatal Quality Care Collaborative were linked to hospital-level data on DHM availability from the Mothers' Milk Bank of

San José for 2007 to 2013. Trends of DHM availability were examined by level of NICU care. Hospitals that transitioned from not having DHM to having DHM availability during the study period were examined to assess changes in rates of breast milk feeding at NICU discharge and NEC.

Results.—The availability of DHM increased from 27 to 55 hospitals during the study period. The availability increased for all levels of care including regional, community, and intermediate NICUs, with the highest increase occurring in regional NICUs. By 2013, 81.3% of premature infants cared for in regional NICUs had access to DHM. Of the 22 hospitals that had a clear transition to having availability of DHM, there was a 10% increase in breast milk feeding at NICU discharge and a concomitant 2.6% decrease in NEC rates.

Conclusions.—The availability of DHM has increased over time and has been associated with positive changes including increased breast milk feeding at NICU discharge and decrease in NEC rates.

▶ This article raises some interesting questions. Although it is near dogma that breast milk is beneficial in decreasing necrotizing enterocolitis (NEC), the effects of donor human milk (compared with babies' own mothers' milk [MOM]) are not as clear. As noted in the article, many of the studies included in meta-analyses of donor milk versus formula in prevention of NEC were done approximately 30 years ago, and questions arise as to the stringency of diagnostic criteria used in some of these studies.

This study, done using data generated from the California Perinatal Quality Care Collaborative, evaluated trends in donor human milk (DHM) use from 2007 through 2013. Of 22 hospitals that showed a clear transition to having availability of DHM, there was a 10% increase in breast feeding (from the mother) at neonatal intensive care unit discharge and a concomitant 2.6% decrease in NEC. The concurrence of these findings raises an important question. Did the donor milk itself have anything to do with the decrease in NEC? Donor milk is widely thought to be a substitute for MOM, but the pasteurization process eliminates or significantly reduces potentially beneficial live microbes, cells, enzymes, immune factors, and growth factors, all potentially beneficial and protective against NEC.

The fact that the use of donor milk in this study was concomitantly associated with an increase in breast feeding and a decrease in NEC is fascinating and begs the question of how this could occur. The authors suggest that DHM availability could foster a breast feeding–friendly environment, as previously suggested by authors of a multicenter study done in Italy.[1] Such a breast feeding–friendly environment appeared to be the basis of the increase in breast feeding at discharge among the California neonatal intensive care units in which DHM became available. Although causality is difficult to prove in such a study, this finding is very intriguing and begs further study pertaining to the efficacy of DHM itself in prevention of NEC. It would be interesting to see if other large cohorts experience similar trends in decreased NEC and if they are related to increased feeding with MOM. If MOM is the major factor, then providing MOM should be emphasized rather than DHM.

J. Neu, MD

Reference

1. Arslanoglu S, Moro GE, Bellu R, et al. Presence of human milk bank is associated with elevated rate of exclusive breastfeeding in VLBW infants. *J Perinat Med.* 2013;41:129-131.

Nil-Per-Os Days and Necrotizing Enterocolitis in Extremely Preterm Infants

Kirtsman M, Yoon EW, Ojah C, et al (Univ of Toronto, Ontario, Canada; Saint John Regional Hosp, New Brunswick, Canada; et al)

Am J Perinatol 32:785-794, 2015

Objective.—This study aims to evaluate the association between nil-per-os (NPO) days and development of necrotizing enterocolitis (NEC) in extremely preterm neonates (<29 weeks gestational age).

Study Design.—A case–control study of 234 extremely preterm neonates who developed stage II or III NEC and 467 matched control infants admitted to participating sites in the Canadian Neonatal Network between 2010 and 2011 was conducted. The number and percentage of NPO days before the development of NEC was compared with the equivalent period in control infants using logistic regression.

Results.—Infants with NEC were NPO on average 5.6 days (28% of days before NEC) versus 3.7 days (19% of equivalent days; $p < 0.01$) among controls. NEC cases required more days of inotropic support, antibiotic use, and had higher rates of patent ductus arteriosus (PDA). After adjusting for inotrope use, PDA, antibiotics, and severity of illness, for each additional NPO day the adjusted odds for NEC increased by 1.08 (95% confidence interval: 1.04–1.12).

Conclusion.—Among extremely preterm neonates, those who developed NEC were NPO for a longer period of time than control infants who were NEC-free. We speculate that delayed initiation or interruption of feeding may be a potent risk factor for NEC.

► It is common practice in neonatal intensive care to withhold feedings for preterm infants for several days after birth. This practice has been based largely on tradition rather than evidence. Reasons to withhold feedings include respiratory distress requiring mechanical ventilation, umbilical catheters, use of vasoactive drugs, and signs of instability. None of these reasons ("excuses") are based on systematic evidence that would contraindicate enteral feedings for these preterm infants. Numerous studies in animals have shown that in the absence of enteral feeding, the intestine grows poorly and physiologic responses such as motility are also delayed. In addition, Cochrane reviews have shown that there is no advantage to withholding feedings for prolonged periods of time shortly after birth in preterm infants.[1] In fact, the most recent Cochrane review evaluating the effects of feeding volumes on necrotizing enterocolitis "suggest that advancing enteral feed volumes at daily increments of 30 to 40 mL/kg (compared to 15 to 24 mL/kg) does not increase the risk of NEC or death in

VLBW infants. Advancing the volume of enteral feeds at slow rates results in several days of delay in establishing full enteral feeds and increases the risk of invasive infection."[2] Recent studies have also shown that withholding feedings for more than 4 days after birth, compared with fewer than 4 days, is associated with increased levels of inflammatory markers at 2 weeks of postnatal age as well as several adverse effects, including increased chronic lung disease and a trend toward increased necrotizing enterocolitis.[3]

The study is a case-control study of the large number of babies who developed Stage II or III necrotizing enterocolitis and matched control infants in the Canadian neonatal network between 2010 and 2011. The results showed that infants with necrotizing enterocolitis were nil per os (NPO) an average of almost 2 days more than the control infants. The authors speculated that the delayed initiation or interruption of feeding may be a potent risk factor for necrotizing enterocolitis.

Although this is not a randomized controlled prospective study, it does add additional information that withholding enteral feedings from preterm infants is likely not to decrease the incidence of necrotizing enterocolitis. Studies in animals have shown that enteral feedings decrease intestinal inflammatory responses,[4] and this has been further supported by recent studies in human preterm infants.[3] One note of caution is that the reasons for placing these infants NPO might have an important role to play in the development of necrotizing enterocolitis, and this would need to be addressed with the additional prospective studies. Nevertheless, the evidence for enteral feeding for these infants seems to be tilting strongly away from previous strategies that involved NPO for prolonged periods shortly after birth and stopping enteral feedings for poorly substantiated reasons.

J. Neu, MD

References

1. Morgan J, Bombell S, McGuire W. Early trophic feeding versus enteral fasting for very preterm or very low birth weight infants. *Cochrane Database Syst Rev.* 2013;(3):CD000504.
2. Morgan J, Young L, McGuire W. Slow advancement of enteral feed volumes to prevent necrotising enterocolitis in very low birth weight infants. *Cochrane Database Syst Rev.* 2015;(10):CD001241.
3. Konnikova Y, Zaman MM, Makda M, D'Onofrio D, Freedman SD, Martin CR. Late enteral feedings are associated with intestinal inflammation and adverse neonatal outcomes. *PLoS One.* 2015;(10):e0132924.
4. Kudsk KA. Current aspects of mucosal immunology and its influence by nutrition. *Am J Surg.* 2002;183:390-398.

Metabolomic and proteomic analysis of serum from preterm infants with necrotising entercolitis and late-onset sepsis

Stewart CJ, Nelson A, Treumann A, et al (Northumbria Univ, Newcastle Upon Tyne, UK; Newcastle Univ, UK; et al)

Pediatr Res 79:425-431, 2016

Background.—Necrotising enterocolitis (NEC) and late-onset sepsis (LOS) are the leading causes of death among preterm infants in the developed world. This study aimed to explore the serum proteome and metabolome longitudinally in preterm infants with NEC or LOS, matched to controls.

Methods.—Nineteen patients (10 cases, 9 controls) were included. A sample 14 d prior to and following, as well as at disease diagnosis, was included for cases. Controls had serum matched at diagnosis for corresponding case. All samples ($n = 39$) underwent shotgun proteomic analysis, and 37 samples also underwent metabolomics analysis using ultra performance liquid chromatography—tandem mass spectrometry.

Results.—The proteomic and metabolomic profiles of serum were comparable between all infants. Eight proteins were associated with NEC and four proteins were associated with LOS. C-reactive protein was increased in all NEC patients at diagnosis.

Conclusion.—No single protein or metabolite was detected in all NEC or LOS cases which was absent from controls; however, several proteins were identified which were associated with disease status. The differing expression of these proteins between diseased infants potentially relates to differing pathophysiology of disease. Thus, it is unlikely a single biomarker exists for NEC and/or LOS.

▶ I applaud the authors of this article in their attempt to longitudinally explore the serum proteome and metabolome in preterm infants who developed necrotizing enterocolitis (NEC) or late-onset sepsis (LOS) when matched to controls. Current biomarkers that are used in common clinical practice are not sensitive or predictive enough to predict NEC or LOS or even to detect these diseases early enough to make a difference in outcome. Most previous attempts to have used targeted approaches to evaluate specific biomarkers such as claudin (a tight junction protein), intestinal fatty acid binding protein (an abundant intestinal epithelial cell cytosolic protein), with mixed but somewhat promising results. Nevertheless, these have not been broadly applied to clinical practice. These investigators, using more of a "shotgun" approach that evaluated a large variety of metabolites and proteins, did find some unique proteins associated with NEC and LOS, but no single protein or metabolite was found that could distinguish these from one another or from controls.

This study underlines several conundrums we have in the diagnosis and/or early detection of NEC and LOS. First, do we have a definition for these diseases? NEC, for example, can represent several different pathways that lead to intestinal necrosis. A baby who develops "NEC" secondary to cardiac left ventricular dysfunction has a different disease that an extremely low birth weight baby who is apparently doing well but suddenly develops "NEC" 6 weeks after birth. Thus, to evaluate biomarkers, as attempted in this study, it is important to first differentiate which form of NEC that is to be evaluated. Second, shotgun "omic"-based studies are excellent ways to evaluate pathways, and the use of systems-based analyses can offer insights into pathogenesis of a disease process as well as provide potential targets for analysis. This study did not provide much in the line of systems analysis. Furthermore, even though a few potential targets (metabolites and proteins that differed between disease and controls) were found, the numbers are very small and thus, as mentioned by the authors, provide little power to be of diagnostic value. A third conundrum is that even if "omic" shotgun techniques provide candidates for diagnostics, these need to be validated using less expensive approaches. For example, a protein found in shotgun proteomics to differ between NEC and control cannot be analyzed by mass spectrometry in a clinically useful and inexpensive manner. Less expensive, perhaps even bedside techniques, such as enzyme-linked immunoassay need to be adapted. But this can only be done after a much larger study that is adequately powered to provide information about sensitivity, specificity, and diagnostic accuracy of a particular test.

Studies such as this using increasingly sophisticated technologies are important first steps, but unfortunately for the clinician caring for these infants, they do not yet provide any additions to our current armamentarium for the diagnosis of NEC and/or LOS.

J. Neu, MD

Association of Red Blood Cell Transfusion, Anemia, and Necrotizing Enterocolitis in Very Low-Birth-Weight Infants

Patel RM, Knezevic A, Shenvi N, et al (Emory Univ School of Medicine & Children's Healthcare of Atlanta, GA; Rollins School of Public Health, Atlanta, GA; et al)

JAMA 315:889-897, 2016

Importance.—Data regarding the contribution of red blood cell (RBC) transfusion and anemia to necrotizing enterocolitis (NEC) are conflicting. These associations have not been prospectively evaluated, accounting for repeated, time-varying exposures.

Objective.—To determine the relationship between RBC transfusion, severe anemia, and NEC.

Design, Setting, and Participants.—In a secondary, prospective, multicenter observational cohort study from January 2010 to February 2014, very low-birth-weight (VLBW, ≤1500 g) infants, within 5 days of birth, were enrolled at 3 level III neonatal intensive care units in Atlanta, Georgia. Two hospitals were academically affiliated and 1 was a community hospital. Infants received follow-up until 90 days, hospital discharge, transfer to a non–study-affiliated hospital, or death (whichever came first). Multivariable competing-risks Cox regression was used, including adjustment for birth weight, center, breastfeeding, illness severity, and duration of initial antibiotic treatment, to evaluate the association between RBC transfusion, severe anemia, and NEC.

Exposures.—The primary exposure was RBC transfusion. The secondary exposure was severe anemia, defined a priori as a hemoglobin level of 8 g/dL or less. Both exposures were evaluated as time-varying covariates at weekly intervals.

Main Outcomes and Measures.—Necrotizing enterocolitis, defined as Bell stage 2 or greater by preplanned adjudication. Mortality was evaluated as a competing risk.

Results.—Of 600 VLBW infants enrolled, 598 were evaluated. Forty-four (7.4%) infants developed NEC. Thirty-two (5.4%) infants died (all cause). Fifty-three percent of infants (319) received a total of 1430 RBC transfusion exposures. The unadjusted cumulative incidence of NEC at week 8 among RBC transfusion-exposed infants was 9.9% (95%CI, 6.9%-14.2%) vs 4.6% (95%CI, 2.6%-8.0%) among those who were unexposed. In multivariable analysis, RBC transfusion in a given week was not significantly related to the rate of NEC (adjusted cause-specific hazard ratio, 0.44 [95%CI, 0.17-1.12]; P=.09). Based on evaluation of 4565 longitudinal measurements of hemoglobin (median, 7 per infant), the rate of NEC was significantly increased among VLBW infants with severe anemia in a given week compared with those who did not have severe anemia (adjusted cause-specific hazard ratio, 5.99 [95% CI, 2.00-18.0]; P=.001).

Conclusions and Relevance.—Among VLBW infants, severe anemia, but not RBC transfusion, was associated with an increased risk of NEC. Further studies are needed to evaluate whether preventing severe anemia is more important than minimizing RBC transfusion.

▶ Over the past decade, there has been an increasing concern that necrotizing enterocolitis (NEC) in preterm infants is caused by blood transfusions. This has led to interesting practices, such as withholding enteral feedings for varying periods of time before and after transfusions. As described in this article, the majority of the previous studies that have shown this relationship have been retrospective comparisons and meta-analyses of these have even strengthened the concept that many cases of NEC are caused by blood transfusions. Is this another case of "garbage-in, garbage-out" meta-analysis?

This study by Patel and colleagues evaluated 598 infants using a prospective design with a priori sample size determination using multivariate regression models. They evaluated blood transfusion or significant anemia as antecedents to NEC and showed that severe anemia, but not blood transfusions, was strongly associated with the development of NEC.

This is an important study because it not only disputes a dogma that has developed over the past decade in neonatal intensive care, but also has important clinical therapeutic implications. The main implication is that we should prevent anemia in these infants. By doing this, we may also decrease the incidence of NEC and the necessity for blood transfusions.

Another question this raises is what is the mechanism of anemia-associated NEC? Is this a perfusion problem, or is it due to another mechanism, such as low iron stores causing alterations in the intestinal microbiota with altered host intestinal mucosal interaction and inflammation, or increased susceptibility to intestinal damage with the anemia.

J. Neu, MD

Identifying Barriers to Initiating Minimal Enteral Feedings in Very Low-Birth-Weight Infants: A Mixed Methods Approach

Malhotra Y, Nzegwu N, Harrington J, et al (Montefiore Med Ctr, Bronx, NY; Brigham and Women's Hosp, Boston, MA; Columbia Univ Med Ctr, NY; et al)
Am J Perinatol 33:47-56, 2015

Objective.—This study aims to elicit physician and nursing perceptions about initiation of minimal enteral feedings (MEF) in very low-birth-weight (VLBW) infants.

Study Design.—A three-phase, mixed methods study including a quantitative chart review of 37 VLBW infants, followed by 26 qualitative observations of morning rounds, 26 interviews of neonatal intensive care unit (NICU) medical team members, tailored interventions based on the identified barriers to MEF, and finally a postintervention chart audit of 50 VLBW infants.

Results.—The main barriers to initiation of MEF were failure to appreciate the differences between the goals of MEF versus nutritive feedings, inconsistent definition of "sick" infant, indomethacin for intraventricular hemorrhage prophylaxis, awaiting mother's own milk, complicated feeding protocols/algorithms for feeding intolerance, and lack of buy-in from nurses/nurse practitioners. The compliance with early initiation of MEF per the feeding guidelines rose from 25 to 92% after our interventions.

Conclusion.—Understanding the complex interplay of provider, system and patientbased factors that interfere with initiation of MEF may enable NICUs to develop consensus guidelines and targeted interventions and to achieve timely initiation of nonnutritive feedings.

▶ Neonatal intensive care units (NICU) overall have a poor record of providing both enteral and parenteral nutrition for low birth weight infants. This often results in extrauterine growth delays but, more importantly, may enhance the odds of short-term morbidities such as surgical necrotizing enterocolitis (NEC) and late-onset sepsis and long-term neurodevelopmental delays. Some of us can remember the days when it was common for preterms to have enteral feedings withheld for not only days, but weeks. During this time, parenteral nutrition was provided but in relatively small amounts, not nearly providing what these babies would be receiving had they remained in utero. This iatrogenic enteral starvation has been due primarily to our fear of NEC. Over the past couple of decades, numerous studies have shown that early provision of enteral feedings does not increase the odds of NEC. Despite this, the dogmas remain, and it is taking a long time for us to change our old ingrained bad habits. This article illustrates just how difficult it is for some NICUs to change. With a stepwise approach, it has taken several years to develop a set of guidelines that are a definite step toward progress but required careful and tedious team consensus building. Many of the measures taken in these guidelines are based on what the medical and nursing teams would be able to accept rather than based on evidence. Although these measures are a definite step forward, there are many questions that need to be raised. For example:

1. Why do routine gastric residual measurements after minimal enteral feedings are reached?
2. Why is it necessary to provide minimal enteral feedings shortly after birth and not use a standard approach that is designed to provide full enteral feedings within about a week? Deviations from this standard should be justified by the medical team.
3. What is the rationale for not providing some enteral feedings even if the baby has oxygen requirements > 60 mm Hg?
4. What is the rationale for not providing enteral feedings if the Hct is < 35 and the baby is receiving a blood transfusion?

I applaud this group for making progress in their NICU's feeding guidelines. It is probably not necessary to use a complex systematic approach for making such progress in all NICUs, but the general principles that involve team discussions, education using the best evidence available, and the courage to make changes that are contrary to the existing dogma that starves babies and actually may be causing harm will be a major advance in the care of preterm babies in the NICU.

J. Neu, MD

Factors Determining Optimal Fatty Acid Absorption in Preterm Infants

Martin CR, Cheesman A, Brown J, et al (Beth Israel Deaconess Med Ctr, Boston, MA)

J Pediatr Gastroenterol Nutr 62:130-136, 2016

Objectives.—The aim of the present study was to quantify absorption coefficients of specific fatty acids in preterm infants as a function of diet, formula or breast milk (BM), and postnatal age; to identify the fatty acid structural characteristics that determine optimal fatty acid absorption.

Methods.—Fatty acids from dietary and fecal samples were extracted and quantified by gas chromatography-mass spectroscopy. Fatty acid absorption coefficients (FA-CFAs) were calculated by comparing the total amount of fatty acids supplied by the diet to the amount quantified in the total fecal output during a 3-day period.

Results.—A total of 18 infants (BM 8, formula 10) were studied at 2 weeks of age, and 20 infants (BM 10, formula 10) were studied at

6 weeks of age. FA-CFAs decreased with increasing carbon length in formula-fed infants at 2 and 6 weeks. Results were similar but less in magnitude in BM-fed infants at 2 weeks with no difference at 6 weeks.

Conclusions.—Preterm infants fed formula demonstrated lower FA-CFAs as a function of increasing carbon length. This is consistent with limited pancreatic lipase production and with lipase being present in BM but not in formula. The fact that this pattern was seen in BM-fed infants at 2 weeks but not 6 weeks of age suggests that intestinal immaturity may also play a role in impaired fatty acid absorption. These data highlight principles that need to be considered to optimize delivery and absorption of dietary long-chain polyunsaturated fatty acids in preterm infants.

▶ It has been known for several decades that preterm infants have difficulty with digestion and absorption of certain lipids and carbohydrates. However, few recent studies evaluated the digestive absorptive capability of the preterm infant to digest and absorb lipids. Several factors are involved in the physiology of the lipid digestion and absorption, and these include the various lipases that are found in human milk but not in formula. Lingual, gastric, and pancreatic lipases also are involved in breaking the triglyceride bonds. Pancreatic lipase activity is known to be relatively low in preterm infants, and this may lead to suboptimal lipid hydrolysis. Another factor is the presence of bile acids, which are produced by the liver and used in the gastrointestinal lumen for emulsification of fat globules. These bile acids are then reabsorbed in the ileum of the small intestine. It is known that bile acids are not required for medium-chain or short-chain lipid emulsification. There are lipases present in unpasteurized human milk and are highly active but are lost in the pasteurization process for banked donor milk.

This study provides interesting new information that focuses on fat digestion and absorption at 2 weeks and 6 weeks after birth in preterm infants born between 28 to 30 weeks gestational age. The coefficient of the fat absorption between milk derived from the babies' own mothers and formula was not different at either 2 or 6 weeks. However, when evaluating individual lipids, chain length appeared to be of importance, with the longer-chain fatty acids not being as well digested or absorbed. A similar phenomenon was seen with docosahexaenoic (DHA) and arachidonic acids (AA) in which they were not as well digested and absorbed in the formula-fed infants. The lipase activity in human milk is speculated to play a significant role in this phenomenon. The role of bile acids was not studied in this investigation. The authors concluded that even adding the DHA and AA to formula may not be an effective strategy without also optimizing lipolysis.

This study has interesting implications in terms of formula feeding with the added DHA and AA and donor milk feeding. Preterm infants are generally not provided with significant quantities of enteral feedings in the first 1 to 2 weeks after birth, and the current intravenous lipid emulsion most commonly provided in the United States does not contain significant quantities of these very long-chain polyunsaturated fatty acids. Hence, even if these infants are given their own mother's milk that contains significant quantities of active lipase, these infants still have a deficiency of these long-chain fatty acids. The findings from this study suggest that strategies are required to provide these long-chain fatty acids to preterm infants as well as providing or stimulating the enzymes and other mechanisms required for their appropriate digestion, absorption, and processing.

J. Neu, MD

A dose response randomised controlled trial of docosahexaenoic acid (DHA) in preterm infants

Collins CT, Sullivan TR, McPhee AJ, et al (The Univ of Adelaide, South Australia, Australia; South Australian Health and Med Res Inst, Adelaide, South Australia, Australia; et al)

Prostaglandins Leukot Essent Fatty Acids 99:1-6, 2015

Thirty one infants born less than 30 weeks' gestational age were randomised to receive either 40 ($n = 11$), 80 ($n = 9$) or 120 ($n = 11$) mg/kg/day of docosahexaenoic acid (DHA) respectively as an emulsion, via the feeding tube, commenced within 4 days of the first enteral feed. Twenty three infants were enroled in non-randomised reference groups; $n = 11$ who had no supplementary DHA and $n = 12$ who had maternal DHA supplementation. All levels of DHA in the emulsion were well tolerated with no effect on number of days of interrupted feeds or days to full enteral feeds. DHA levels in diets were directly related to blood DHA levels but were unrelated to arachidonic acid (AA) levels. All randomised groups and the maternal supplementation reference group prevented the drop in DHA levels at study end that was evident in infants not receiving supplementation. Australian New Zealand Clinical Trials Registry: ACTRN12610000382077.

▶ Multiple animal and human clinical data support the role of docosahexaenoic acid (DHA) in optimizing infant health. However, to date, nutritional interventions with DHA have failed to consistently demonstrate health benefit in large clinical cohorts. Many reasons contribute to this lack of translation, such as unknown target dose, unknown timing of delivery, and unknown duration of delivery. Over the years, Maria Makrides and her colleagues have contributed substantial data that have incrementally refined our knowledge of DHA across the spectrum of pregnancy into early childhood.

In this study, different dosages of DHA were provided as a fractionated tuna oil product (thus also containing eicosapentaenoic acid [EPA]), in a cohort of premature infants less than 33 weeks of gestation. In a dose-dependent manner, there was a positive correlation in the increase in DHA and EPA levels with increasing DHA dosing. However, only the highest dosing group at 120 mg/k/day prevented the postnatal decline in DHA observed in preterm infants by 7 days of age. Additionally, although not statistically significant, there was a negative, dose-dependent correlation of decreasing arachidonic acid (AA) levels with increasing DHA delivery. Most importantly, enteral administration was well tolerated.

This study and others consistently demonstrate several axioms in fish oil administration (enteral or parenteral) in preterm infants: (1) DHA levels will increase, and the increase is in a positive correlation with total dose; (2) fish oils also have EPA and thus EPA will substantially increase in tandem; and (3) an increase in omega 3 delivery will result in a decrease in omega 6 levels (AA) due to physiologic mechanisms that tightly regulate the balance of fatty acids. These axioms are critical to understand because each fatty acid has biological effects that are emitted not only through absolute levels but also as a ratio of levels to one another.

Providing a single fatty acid as a therapy is unlikely to yield maximal health benefits without addressing the developmental needs for AA and without understanding the effects of elevated EPA levels. Additional studies with precise, incremental dosing of multiple fatty acids coupled with measurements of longitudinal fatty acid levels and other regulatory compensatory mechanisms will get us closer to understanding long-chain polyunsaturated fatty acids delivery to maximize health benefit while minimizing the potential trade-offs.

C. Martin, MD

Intermittent Bolus or Semicontinuous Feeding for Preterm Infants?

Rövekamp-Abels LWW, Hogewind-Schoonenboom JE, de Wijs-Meijler DPM, et al (Sophia Children's Hosp, Rotterdam, The Netherlands; Emma Children's Hosp, Amsterdam, The Netherlands)

J Pediatr Gastroenterol Nutr 61:659-664, 2015

Objectives.—The aim of the present study was to assess the clinical benefits and risks of semicontinuous (CON) versus intermittent nasogastric tube feeding in low-birth-weight infants.

Methods.—Infants with a birth weight <1750 g and gestational age <32 weeks were stratified according to birth weight and assigned to either CON or intermittent bolus (BOL) feeding. The primary endpoint was days to full enteral feeding (defined as $120\ mL \cdot kg^{-1} \cdot day^{-1}$). We also collected data on feeding tolerance, weight gain, respiratory support, and complications (sepsis, necrotising enterocolitis, and death).

Results.—There was no difference between the 2 groups (CON n = 121, BOL n = 125) in days to reach full enteral feeding—7 (5–10) versus 6 (5–8) days, respectively, with a difference 1 (−0.05 to 2.1). Mean daily gastric residual volumes, however, were significantly lower in the BOL group (4.8 vs 3.9 mL/day, difference 0.9 mL/day [0.1–1.7]), as was the total number of patients with feeding interruptions (76 vs 59, difference 16% [3%–28%]).

Conclusions. Bolus and continuous feeding are equally suitable feeding strategies for preterm neonates. BOL feeding, however, may be preferable.

▶ This study partially addresses a commonly asked question about the relative merits of bolus versus continuous feedings in very low birthweight infants. A Cochrane review evaluating this question in babies less than 1500 g birth weight concluded that the evidence was inadequate to make a recommendation; hence, this study evaluated a large number of infants admitted to the Erasmus Neonatal Intensive Care Unit in Rotterdam, the Netherlands, over a 2-year period. The babies were fed using a protocol that advanced these infants to full feedings over a period of about 1 week. Intermittent bolus feedings were provided every 3 hours and "continuous" feedings were provided using an open syringe that was resupplied every 15 minutes. No differences in days to full feeds (primary outcome), feeding tolerance as measure by gastric residuals, weight gain, or need for respiratory support was seen between the 2 groups. There were no differences in adverse outcomes such as necrotizing enterocolitis. The authors concluded that both of these methods are equally suitable for preterm infants; however, it was thought that in their setting, bolus feeding might be preferable because it is more convenient for the parents to be involved.

Of interest is the fact that these infants achieved full enteral feedings (both groups) as rapidly as they did, usually in about 6 days. This speaks positively for having a relatively "aggressive" feeding protocol that is followed closely by the staff. There are also some infants who are on bolus feedings and exhibit symptoms such as a high number of oxygen desaturation episodes and apneic and bradycardia spells that are changed from bolus to continuous feedings that seem to respond positively. However, the period after these infants go back to their original form of feeding has not been systematically studied to determine whether their symptoms reappear. One other consideration not mentioned in this article is that most babies subsequently go on to some form of bolus feeding, and starting them on this method rather than continuous mitigates the need to make the switch.

J. Neu, MD

Longitudinal Study of Cytokine Expression, Lipid Profile and Neuronal Growth Factors in Human Breast Milk from Term and Preterm Deliveries

Collado MC, Santaella M, Mira-Pascual L, et al (Inst of Agrochemistry and Food Technology-Spanish Natl Res Council (IATA-CSIC), Valencia, Spain; Univ of Murcia, Spain; et al)

Nutrients 7:8577-8591, 2015

Breast milk (BM) is considered as a reference for infant nutrition. The role of bioactive components, such as cytokines, hormones, growth factors (GFs) and fatty acids (FAs) is poorly known, but they might be implicated in immune response development. The aim of this study was to identify the lipid profile and the spectrum of cytokines and neuronal GF in BM samples and analyse the influence of gestational age and lactation time on these components. This study used a longitudinal prospective method for the characterization of cytokines, FAs and GFs global profiles in 120 BM samples from 40 healthy mothers (20 preterm and 20 term) collected as colostrum, transitional and mature milk. The cytokines were analysed by protein array (Ray Bio® Human Cytokine Array G6. Ray Biotech, Inc. Norcross, GA, USA) and the FAs were analysed by gas chromatography. The FA profile was similar between the term and the preterm BM samples. Omega-3-α-linoleic and docosahexaenoic acid (DHA) and omega-6-linoleic acid were the most abundant in the term and preterm samples during lactation. Omega-3 ETA and omega-3 EPA we observed exclusively in the preterm samples. The cytokine profile showed a different trend based on gestational age. A significantly higher expression of neurotrophic factors was found in the mature preterm milk samples as compared to the mature term samples. Our study is the first to identify the influence and interactions of perinatal factors on cytokine, GFs and FAs in human milk.

▶ Knowing what nutrition and accompanying immunonutrients to deliver, when, and how remains one of the greatest challenges in neonatology. One way to view this problem is to understand what the preterm infant would have been getting if able to remain in utero (analysis of amniotic fluid) or if able to feed in sufficient quantities soon after birth (analysis of preterm human milk).

This study performed a comprehensive analysis on the presence of cytokines, lipids (the highest macronutrient component in human milk), and neuronal growth factors in preterm versus term human milk. Compared with mature term milk, mature preterm milk had a higher omega 6 to omega 3 ratio emphasizing the importance omega 6 in preterm infant development. Mature preterm milk had higher concentrations of cytokines and neuronal growth factors studied compared with mature term milk. Notable neurotropic and growth factors with at least a 2-fold increase in mature preterm milk included brain-derived neurotrophic factor, glial cell–derived neurotrophic factor, neurotrophin-3, angiogenin, bone morphogenetic protein 4, epidermal growth factor, insulin-like growth factor-1 and insulin-like growth factor-binding protein 1. Cytokines overexpressed in mature preterm milk compared with mature term milk included eotaxin, fractalkine, monocyte-chemoattractant protein-1, macrophage colony-stimulating factor, MIP-3-α, and pulmonary and activation-regulated cytokine.

Each of these human milk–derived bioactive factors are potential targets to understand neonatal development and disease pathophysiology, and to develop new therapies.

C. Martin, MD

Manifestations of Cow's-Milk Protein Intolerance in Preterm Infants

Cordova J, Sriram S, Patton T, et al (Univ of Chicago, IL)

J Pediatr Gastroenterol Nutr 62:140-144, 2016

Objectives.—Cow's-milk protein intolerance (CMPI) is poorly recognized in preterm infants. This study examined the clinical events that preceded the diagnosis of CMPI in preterm infants.

Methods.—This was a retrospective study of infants in a level-III neonatal intensive care unit of those who received parenteral nutrition (PN) support during a 12-month period. Parameters assessed included birth weight (g), diagnosis, duration and frequency on PN, type of enteral feeds at initiation, and achievement of enteral autonomy. CMPI was diagnosed based on persistent feeding intolerance that resolved after change of feeds from intact protein to a protein hydrolysate or crystalline amino acid formula.

Results.—Three hundred forty-eight infants with birth weight (median/range) 1618 g (425–5110) received PN. Fifty-one (14%) infants required multiple courses of PN, and 19 of 348 (5%) were diagnosed with CMPI. The requirement for multiple courses on PN versus single course was associated with a high likelihood of CMPI: 14 of 51 versus 5 of 297, $P < 0.001$. Nine of the 14 infants identified with CMPI were initially diagnosed with necrotizing enterocolitis (NEC) after a median duration of 22 days (19–57) on intact protein feeds. After recovery from NEC, they had persistent feeding intolerance including recurrence of "NEC-like illness" ($N = 3$) that resolved after change of feeds to a protein hydrolysate or crystalline amino acid formula.

Conclusions.—The requirement for multiple courses of PN because of persistent feeding intolerance after recovery from NEC and recurrence of "NEC-like illness" may be a manifestation of CMPI in preterm infants.

▶ The belief that necrotizing enterocolitis is associated with and potentially can be caused by exposure to cow's milk–based proprietary formulas is the converse of the belief that exclusive human milk feeding may be protective. The mechanism of this association remains uncertain, however. Using an operational definition of cow's milk protein intolerance (CMPI) in a retrospective analysis, these authors describe a surprisingly high 5% incidence among newborn infants who received at least 1 course of parenteral nutrition in their unit. There is potential for circularity in this reasoning, because CMPI was diagnosed based on resolution of feeding intolerance after adoption of extensively hydrolyzed or elemental formula feedings, which may not have been necessary. Nonetheless, recurrence of feeding problems, including frank NEC in 3 cases, until that change in feeding was made suggests that these observations should be taken seriously. Whether exquisite sensitivity to dietary proteins is the primary cause of an NEC-like illness or NEC predisposes to development of such sensitivity with refeeding following recovery, recurrent episodes of apparent NEC or persistent feeding intolerance may be signs of unrecognized CMPI. A trial of an extensively hydrolyzed or elemental amino acid formula in this setting may be both diagnostic and therapeutic. If successful, resumption of feeding with a cow's milk–based formula should be deferred and undertaken only with close monitoring for signs of persistent CMPI because the reaction can be catastrophic.

W. E. Benitz, MD

Impact of Early Sodium Supplementation on Hyponatremia and Growth in Premature Infants: A Randomized Controlled Trial

Isemann B, Mueller EW, Narendran V, et al (Univ of Cincinnati Med Ctr, OH; Cincinnati Children's Hosp Med Ctr, OH)

JPEN J Parenter Enteral Nutr 40:342-349, 2016

Background.—We tested the hypothesis that sodium supplementation in early preterm infants prevents late-onset hyponatremia and improves growth without increasing common morbidities during birth hospitalization.

Materials and Methods.—This was a randomized, masked controlled trial of 4 mEq/kg/d of sodium (intervention) versus sterile water (placebo) from days-of-life 7 to 35 in infants born at <32 weeks corrected gestational age. The primary outcome was weight gain in the first 6 weeks of life. Secondary outcomes included weekly serum sodium concentrations, growth in body length and head circumference, and complications of prematurity during birth hospitalization.

Results.—Fifty-three infants with an average corrected gestational age of 28.5 ± 2.4 weeks were randomized. Infants receiving the intervention had fewer ($P = .012$) reports of serum sodium concentrations <135 mmol/L and greater velocity of weight gain during the study period, mean (SD) 26.9 (3.1) vs 22.9 (4.7) g/kg/day, $P = .012$. At 6 weeks of age, infants <28 weeks' gestation who received sodium supplementation had greater percentage weight change from birth, mean (SD) 193% (22%) vs 173% (10%), $P = .041$, and maintained fetal reference birth percentile for body weight more often ($P = .002$) compared with infants receiving placebo. Growth in length and head circumference was not significantly different between study arms. No increase in common prematurity-related morbidities was detected in infants who received supplemental sodium chloride.

Conclusion.—Sodium supplementation of enteral feedings in very premature infants averts hyponatremia and enhances weight gain.

▶ There are many reasons why preterm infants might become hyponatremic and need sodium supplementation. First, the full complement of nephrons is not attained until 32 to 34 weeks' gestational age (GA). Also, their renal function is characterized by a diminished ability to reabsorb water and respond to mineralocorticoids. There is also a high excretion of filtered sodium. Furthermore, perinatal complications leading to acute kidney injury are common and affect tubular function. Additionally, the use of medications such as diuretics, indomethacin, and amphotericin B are common factors leading to sodium and potassium imbalances in this age group. Another group of infants with severe sodium disturbances are those with congenital adrenal hyperplasia and Bartter syndrome.

Hence compared with term newborns, preterm infants have increased sodium requirements. It is well known that feeding mother's milk to preterm decreases the incidence of infection and necrotizing enterocolitis and improves neurodevelopmental outcome but, at the same time, may decrease ponderal and linear growth. The goal of mimicking intrauterine remains elusive but with aggressive early enteral nutrition, increased protein supplementation and appropriate fortification of human milk growth parameters are vastly improved compared with 2 decades ago. Add sodium supplementation to selective infants to this list.

Although sodium is measured on a regular basis, there has been a paucity of data on the benefits of sodium supplementation. The Cincinnati group has provided valuable information on the benefits of sodium supplementation in preterm infants. They noted that sodium is important for growth, yet fortified human milk and commercial formulas often fail to provide the 3 to 7 mEq/kg/d current sodium intake recommendations for preterm infants during the first few months of birth hospitalization. Preterm infants supplemented with sodium had better weight gain with no differences in head circumference or length. The limitation of the study is the small sample size, but the intervention is simple and inexpensive, and the increased weight gain, on the order of 80 g over the 6-week study period compared with the nonsupplemented group translates into shorter stay, diminished costs, and avoidance of hospital-related problems.

A. A. Fanaroff, MD

Neonatal Acute Liver Failure

Taylor SA, Whitington PF (Northwestern Univ, Chicago, IL)
Liver Transplant 22:677-685, 2016

Neonatal acute liver failure (NALF) is a rare disease about which there is little published data; however, NALF is an extremely important condition as it is distinct from acute liver failure seen in older children and adults. First, unlike acute liver failure in older patients, NALF can be diagnosed in an infant with cirrhosis. This is due to the fetal-neonatal continuum of liver disease, or the principle that neonatal liver failure may be the result of a liver disease that began in utero. Further differences exist in the mechanism of disease, diagnostic principles, and the common etiologies of NALF when compared with pediatric and adult acute liver failure. This review will address many of the distinguishing features of NALF and focus on the most common etiologies of NALF, including gestational alloimmune liver disease (GALD), the most common cause of NALF. Additionally, this review will provide insight into the pathogenesis, diagnosis, and treatment of this rare condition (Table 1).

▶ This is a review article on a rare topic. However, because it is also a wonderful teaching and learning resource, it has been included in the 2016 YEAR BOOK.

TABLE 1.—Presenting Clinical Findings in NALF Based on Etiology

	GALD-NH	Viral Infection	HLH	Mitochondrial Hepatopathy
Age at presentation	Usually at birth and almost always < 3 days	Typically 5-14 days	Variable, sometimes at birth	Variable, often first weeks to months of life
Premature birth	Most (70%-90%)	Usual population incidence	Uncommon	Uncommon
History of maternal sibling death	Common	Almost never	Uncommon	25% risk in full siblings
Oligohydramnios	Most (70%-90%)	Rare	Rare	Uncommon (polyhydramnios seen)
Intrauterine growth restriction	Most (70%-90%)	Rare	Rare	Possible (20%-30%)
Multiorgan involvement	Renal tubular dysplasia	Common in HSV especially brain	Bone marrow	Central nervous system and heart
Ascites	Common (40%-60%)	Rare	Uncommon	Uncommon
Patent ductus venosus	Most (70%-90%)	Never	Never	Never
Hepatomegaly	Uncommon (10%-20%)	Common	Common	Common
Splenomegaly	Uncommon (10%-20%)	Common though often mild	Common	Uncommon
Hypoglycemia	Usual	Common	Common	Usual
Coagulopathy	Profound (INR, 4-10)	Moderate to profound	Moderate to profound	Moderate to profound
Metabolic acidosis	No	No	No	Yes
Cholestasis	Not at birth; increasing afterward	Minimal at presentation	Moderate to severe	Moderate
ALT	Typically low or normal and almost always < 100 IU/L	Typically high and often > 1000 IU/L	Typically high and often > 1000 IU/L	Typically high and often 100-500 IU/L
Ferritin	Almost always > 800 ng/mL and < 7000	Often very high (>20,000 ng/mL)	Very high (>20,000 ng/mL)	Variable elevation
Alpha-fetoprotein	Almost always high (> 80,000 ng/mL in term neonate); typically > 300,000 ng/mL	Almost always normal (< 80,000 ng/mL in term neonate)	Almost always normal (< 80,000 ng/mL in term neonate)	Variable elevation
Lactate:pyruvate molar ratio and ketone body ratios	Normal	Normal	Normal	Abnormal

Reprinted from Taylor SA, Whitington PF. Neonatal acute liver failure. *Liver Transplant.* 2016;22:677-685, with permission from American Association for the Study of Liver Diseases.

Of note the authors are the leaders and most experienced clinicians in the field of children's hepatic disorder, with special knowledge and experience in neonatal disorders. They share their experience and thoughts in an orderly fashion. I have used a number of their words because the abstract is limited and omits these important facts and associations.

The terminology can be confusing, so we must first familiarize ourselves with their acronyms: acute liver failure (ALF), neonatal acute liver failure (NALF), pediatric acute liver failure (PALF), neonatal hemochromatosis (NH), gestational autoimmune liver disease (GALD), and hemophagocytic syndrome (HLH).

Taylor and Whitington note that "Because GALD always presents in the newborn, typically at birth, it can further be assumed that these were cases of NALF. GALD appears to be the single most common disease causing NALF. Importantly, GALD and NH are not synonyms. GALD is a cause of NH, and NH is a symptom of GALD. NH proven to be due to GALD can be referred to as GALD-NH."

"Four etiologies, GALD-NH, viral infection (mainly herpes), HLH, and mitochondrial hepatopathy, comprise nearly all cases of NALF. The varying clinical features of these are presented in Table 1. Just a few variables reasonably clearly separate them: age at onset, evidence of fetal insult, presence of a patent ductus venosus, hepatomegaly, alanine aminotransferase (ALT) level, ferritin level, alpha-fetoprotein level, and persistent metabolic acidosis.

"By going through this simple checklist, one can rapidly decide on an approach to a definitive diagnosis. An aberrant finding not typical of these diseases should lead in an alternate direction. For example, if a NALF patient were to have metabolic acidosis and the lactate level was high, mitochondrial disease should be considered. Likewise, genetic cholestasis might be considered in a NALF patient with significant cholestasis. The tendency, unfortunately, is to attempt to rule out every known cause of infant liver disease in these patients by exhaustive and expensive testing. Genetic diagnosis is not relevant in these patients because of the time it takes to get results back, and many diseases that are prominent causes of cholestatic disease, such as alpha-1-antitrypsin deficiency, just do not cause ALF." In light of the ability to do whole gene sequencing in 26 hours, the authors might want to revise this paragraph.

Neonatal hemochromatosis (NH) is a rare, often fatal disorder characterized by liver failure and hepatic and extra-hepatic iron overload. Clinical manifestations can occur in utero or immediately after birth. Gestational alloimmune liver disease (GALD) has been established as the cause of fetal liver injury resulting in nearly all cases of NH. In GALD, a women is exposed to a fetal antigen that she does not recognize as "self" and subsequently begins to produce immunoglobulin G antibodies that are directed against fetal hepatocytes.[1,2] These antibodies bind to fetal liver antigen and activate the terminal complement cascade resulting in hepatocyte injury and death. GALD can cause congenital cirrhosis or acute liver failure with and without iron overload and siderosis. Practitioners should consider GALD in cases of fetal demise, stillbirth, and neonatal acute liver failure. Identification of infants with GALD is important because treatment is available and effective for subsequent pregnancies. Treatment with immunoglobulins and exchange transfusions has radically changed the prognosis without liver transplant. Also the preventive use of immunoglobulin in pregnant women with a past history of neonatal hemochromatosis, thus decreasing the rate of disease recurrence up to 70%.[3] The combination of double volume exchange transfusion and intravenous immunoglobulin therapy has obviated the need for liver transplantation in many neonates with GALD.

A. A. Fanaroff, MD

References

1. Jimenez-Rivera C, Gupta A, Feberova J, de Nanassy JA, Boland MP. Successful treatment of neonatal hemochromatosis as gestational alloimmune liver disease with intravenous immunoglobulin. *J Neonatal Perinatal Med.* 2014;7:301-304.
2. Feldman AG, Whitington PF. Neonatal hemochromatosis. *J Clin Exp Hepatol.* 2013;3:313-320.
3. Molera Busoms C, Quintero Bernabeu J, Martín de Carpi J. Neonatal hemochromatosis: another entity that is no longer orphan. Advances in thediagnosis and management of the main cause of neonatal acute liver failure. *An Pediatr (Barc).* 2015;83:218.e1-3.

Prenatal Perfluoroalkyl Substance Exposure and Child Adiposity at 8 Years of Age: The HOME Study

Braun JM, Chen A, Romano ME, et al (Brown Univ, Providence, RI; Univ of Cincinnati, OH; et al)

Obesity 24:231-237, 2016

Objective.—To examine relationships between prenatal perfluoroalkyl substance (PFAS) exposure and adiposity in children born to women who lived downstream from a fluoropolymer manufacturing plant.

Methods.—Data are from a prospective cohort in Cincinnati, Ohio (HOME Study). Perfluorooctanoic (PFOA), perfluorooctane sulfonic (PFOS), perfluorononanoic (PFNA), and perfluorohexane sulfonic (PFHxS) acids were measured in prenatal serum samples. Differences were measured in body mass index *z*-scores (BMI), waist circumference, and body fat at 8 years of age ($n = 204$) and BMI between 2-8 years of age ($n = 285$) according to PFAS concentrations.

Results.—Children born to women in the top two PFOA terciles had greater adiposity at 8 years than children in the 1st tercile. For example, waist circumference (cm) was higher among children in the 2nd (4.3; 95% CI: 1.7, 6.9) and 3rd tercile (2.2; 95% CI: −0.5, 4.9) compared to children in the 1st tercile. Children in the top two PFOA terciles also had greater BMI gains from 2 to 8 years compared to children in the 1st tercile ($P < 0.05$). PFOS, PFNA, and PFHxS were not associated with adiposity.

Conclusions.—In this cohort, higher prenatal serum PFOA concentrations were associated with greater adiposity at 8 years and a more rapid increase in BMI between 2-8 years.

▶ Braun and colleagues performed a prospective cohort study of 204 mother–infant pairs in Cincinnati, OH, to analyze the association of maternal exposure to 4 perfluoroalkyl substances (PFAS) including perfluorooctanoic (PFOA), perfluorooctane sulfonic (PFOS), perfluorononanoic (PFNA), and perfluorohexane sulfonic (PFHxS) acids and offspring adiposity at 8 years of age. PFAS are often used in nonstick cookware, food containers, and home textiles and may be obesogenic. Biomonitoring studies have demonstrated ubiquitous exposure to these substances in the United States. Rodent and in vitro studies have shown that PFAS exposure may impair glucose tolerance and cause obesity. In this study, children born to women with higher PFOA levels had higher adiposity as measured by waist circumference and body mass index. The importance of this study lies in the recognition that persistent environmental chemicals may contribute to childhood obesity and potentially other multifactorial chronic conditions. Replication in other cohorts and exploration into the mechanisms through which humans are adversely affected are important next steps.

H. H. Burris, MD, MPH

Temporal Association Between Reflux-like Behaviors and Gastroesophageal Reflux in Preterm and Term Infants

Funderburk A, Nawab U, Abraham S, et al (Thomas Jefferson Univ/Nemours, Philadelphia, PA)

J Pediatr Gastroenterol Nutr 62:556-561, 2016

Objectives.—Multichannel intraluminal impedance studies (MII-pH) have become the criterion standard for the diagnosis of gastroesophageal reflux (GER). Several clinical signs and symptoms that are attributed to GER during infancy may not be related to true reflux. Our objective was to correlate the observed reflux-like behaviors to reflux events on MII-pH studies.

Methods.—This is a retrospective study on infants being evaluated for GER with MII. During the MII-pH study, the infants were observed for clinical behaviors. Symptom Index (SI), symptom sensitivity index (SSI), and symptom association probability were used to correlate symptoms with reflux events.

Results.—Of 58 infants (40 preterm, 18 term) included in the study, only 6 infants (10%) had an abnormal MII-pH study. Irritability (32 infants), bradycardia (20), and desaturation (18) were the common signs and symptoms. A total of 2142 (755 acidic and 1386 nonacidic) reflux episodes and 953 clinical reflux behaviors were recorded. The incidence and pattern of GER was similar in preterm and term infants. There was no significant difference in GER episodes and acid exposure in preterm infants fed orally or via nasogastric tube. The symptom association probability was abnormal in only 6 (19%), 1 (5%), and 5 (28%) infants with irritability, bradycardia, and desaturation, respectively.

Conclusions.—The prevalence of GER as detected by MII-pH was low (10%) in symptomatic preterm and term infants. The incidence and

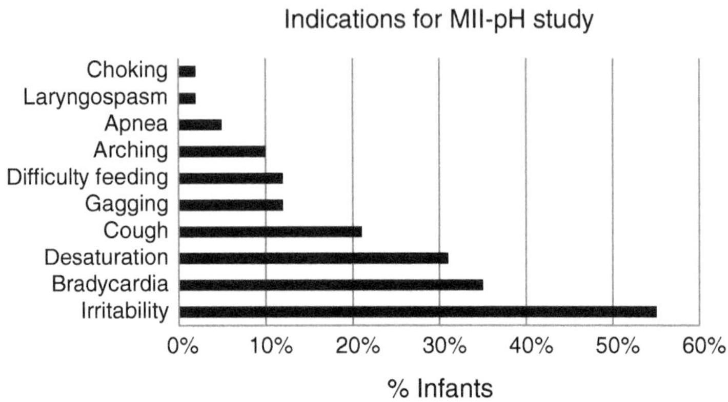

FIGURE 1.—Indications for MII-pH study in the study population expressed in percentage (some infants had more than 1 indication for MII-pH study). MII-pH = multichannel intraluminal impedance study. (Reprinted from Funderburk A, Nawab U, Abraham S, et al. Temporal association between reflux-like behaviors and gastroesophageal reflux in preterm and term infants. *J Pediatr Gastroenterol Nutr.* 2016;62:556-561, with permission from European Society for Pediatric Gastroenterology Hepatology, and Nutrition and North American Society for Pediatric Gastroenterology, Hepatology, and Nutrition.)

pattern of GER was similar in preterm and term infants. The majority of suspected clinical reflux behaviors did not correlate with reflux events (Fig 1).

▶ Apnea of prematurity and gastroesophageal reflux (GER) are both common occurrences in preterm infants and widely perceived to be causally related. Medications used to treat clinical signs thought to be from GER, such as apnea, bradycardia, or feeding intolerance, are among the most commonly prescribed medications in neonatal intensive care units in the United States, despite the lack of evidence of safety and efficacy in this population. In the neonatal "Choosing wisely" article by Ho et al, number one on the list of conditions that are overdiagnosed and treated unnecessary is GER. "Avoid routine use of antireflux medications for treatment of symptomatic gastro-esophageal reflux disease (GERD) or for treatment of apnea and desaturation in preterm infants" is the recommendation.[1]

Funderburk's findings strongly support that recommendation. The multichannel intraluminal impedance with pH probe (MII-pH), used by Funderburk, has advantages over a pH study because it not only detects both acidic and nonacidic refluxate but can also differentiate antegrade (swallow) from retrograde (true GER) flow; measure the height of refluxate; determine whether refluxate is liquid, gas, or mixed; and also assess symptom association. From this report, we learn that only 10% of term and preterm infants have reflux, and there is no difference in the pattern or prevalence. The presence of a nasogastric tube does not affect the rate of reflux, and there is minimal correlation between the so-called major symptoms of reflux (ie, irritability, desaturations, and bradycardia) with MII-pH evidence of reflux. The majority of suspected clinical reflux behaviors do not correlate with reflux events. Fig 1 shows the various symptoms for which the probe was initiated. Gagging was the only symptom with positive correlation in more than 50% of infants. Arching and feeding difficulty, while commonly attributed to GERD, had poor temporal correlation with reflux events in this study. From the literature, acid suppression may reduce the number of acid reflux events but does not change the number of episodes of reflux. Thickening feeds and position change may modify the incidence of GER. In contrast, pharmacotherapy, including acid suppression therapy, may have adverse effects, including sepsis, and should only be used in infants with clear evidence of clinical benefit.

Because this is a single-center retrospective study the results may not be extrapolated to the general population. However, this is a relatively large sample size and included preterm infants fed orally as well as per nasogastric tube. The take-home message remains that reflux is uncommon, as are symptoms due to reflux, thus only by establishing a relationship between the symptoms and reflux can the use of medications be justified.

A. A. Fanaroff, MD

Reference

1. Ho T, Dukhovny D, Zupancic JA, Goldmann DA, Horbar JD, Pursley DM. Choosing wisely in newborn medicine: five opportunities to increase value. *Pediatrics*. 2015;136:e482-e489.

10 Hematology and Bilirubin

Assessment of G6PD screening program in premature infants in a NICU

Lam R, Li H, Nock ML (Oregon Health and Science Univ, Portland; Case Western Reserve Univ, Cleveland, OH; Univ Hosps Case Med Center Rainbow Babies and Children's Hosp, Cleveland, OH)

J Perinatol 35:1027-1029, 2015

Objective.—Targeted screening for glucose-6-phosphate dehydrogenase deficiency (G6PDdef) using fluorescent spot test (FST) is done in our newborn nursery (NN) and now in our NICU. Premature infants have higher G6PD levels than term infants. FST may result in under diagnosis of G6PDdef in preterms. We sought to determine if FST is appropriate for diagnosis of G6PDdef at <35 weeks and assess screening in NICU.

Study Design.—Retrospective chart review of male, inborn infants < 35 weeks in NICU from 2008 to 2011. Difference in G6PDdef incidence <5% between NN and NICU was acceptable for equivalence.

Results.—Out of 679 subjects, 442 were screened for G6PDdef and 11.3% had abnormal results. Binomial testing comparing 11.3% (95% confidence interval (CI) 8.5 to 14.6) incidence of G6PDdef in NICU and reported incidence in NN (11%) demonstrated no difference. 12.2% of Black/African American males were not screened.

Conclusion.—FST is appropriate for screening all at-risk newborns. A number of at-risk premature males were not screened.

▶ Identification of infants with glucose-6-phosphate dehydrogenase (G6PD) deficiency to prevent severe neonatal hyperbilirubinemia has been the hallmark guideline for risk assessment and interventions by the American Academy of Pediatrics (AAP) and other expert groups.[1,2] The disproportionate occurrence of severe hyperbilirubinemia and kernicterus in G6PD-deficient neonates has been characterized by diverse and sometimes unpredictable clinical manifestations of increased bilirubin production that could be confounded by delayed or decreased bilirubin elimination. The report by Lam et al serves to highlight 3 issues that are relevant to screening of newborns of all gestational ages and deserve further scrutiny for equitable, practical, and affordable implementation. First, regardless of neonatal maturity, the current incidence of G6PD deficiency appears to be uniform when relying solely on self-declared maternal race. Reliance on neonatal racial profile alone is problematic because of inherent inequities and the changing racial profiles of US citizens to being highly multi-ethnic. Thus, the identification process needs to be universal. Second, screening through quantitative enzyme assays alone will only identify hemizygous males and homozygous females, but not the moderately affected hemizygous females.[2] Thus, enzyme-based screening should integrate the phenotypic manifestations of the quantitative enzyme deficiency to the severity of the hyperbilirubinemia (ie, hour-specific, percentile risk zones). Selective genotyping would be limited for hemizygous females, who will have lower than expected enzyme levels.[2] Lastly, measurements of concurrent increased bilirubin production in newborns with G6PD deficiency as well as that triggered by "favism" can selectively identify phenotypic manifestations of hemolysis. Novel technologies, such as a point-of-care quantitative G6PD enzyme assay[3] and noninvasive hemolysis identification by exhaled carbon monoxide determinations,[4] can provide a universal integrated algorithmic treatment approach. This would include universal risk assessment for hyperbilirubinemia followed by hemolysis identification and point-of-care quantitative enzyme measurement, together with selective genotyping of at-risk female newborns.

Lam et al provide the evidentiary basis to expand the inquiry for a spectrum of the complex neonatal manifestations of G6PD deficiency that could have long-term consequences in adulthood, such as hematological, infectious, pharmacological safety, and neurological morbidities. Self-knowledge and parental education are key and protective interventions that may help ameliorate or eliminate any potential life-long complications.[5] It is time for all babies born in the United States, rather than just babies born at Cleveland's University Hospitals Case Medical Center, to be systematically screened for one of the most common genetic disorders.

V. K. Bhutani, MD

References

1. American Academy of Pediatrics. Management of hyperbilirubinemia in the newborn infant 35 or more weeks of gestation. *Pediatrics*. 2004;114:297-316.
2. Watchko JF, Kaplan M, Stark AR, Stevenson DK, Bhutani VK. Should we screen newborns for glucose-6-phosphate dehydrogenase deficiency in the United States? *J Perinatol*. 2013;33:499-504.
3. Bhutani VK, Wong RJ, Vreman HJ, Stevenson DKfor the Jaundice Multinational Study Group. Bilirubin production and hour-specific bilirubin levels. *J Perinatol*. 2015;35:735-738.
4. Bhutani VK, Kaplan M, Glader B, Cotten M, Kleinert J, Pamula V. Point-of-care quantitative measure of glucose-6-phosphate dehydrogenase enzyme deficiency. *Pediatrics*. 2015;136:e1268-e1275.
5. Kaplan M, Hammerman C, Bhutani VK. Parental education and the WHO neonatal G-6-PD screening program: a quarter century later. *J Perinatol*. 2015;35: 779-784.

Point-of-Care Quantitative Measure of Glucose-6-Phosphate Dehydrogenase Enzyme Deficiency

Bhutani VK, Kaplan M, Glader B, et al (Stanford Univ School of Medicine, CA; Faculty of Medicine of the Hebrew Univ, Jerusalem, Israel; et al)

Pediatrics 136:e1268-e1275, 2015

Background and Objectives.—Widespread newborn screening on a point-of-care basis could prevent bilirubin neurotoxicity in newborns with glucose-6-phosphate dehydrogenase (G6PD) deficiency. We evaluated a quantitative G6PD assay on a digital microfluidic platform by comparing its performance with standard clinical methods.

Methods.—G6PD activity was measured quantitatively by using digital microfluidic fluorescence and the gold standard fluorescence biochemical test on a convenience sample of 98 discarded blood samples. Twenty-four samples were designated as G6PD deficient.

Results.—Mean ± SD G6PD activity for normal samples using the digital microfluidic method and the standard method, respectively, was 9.7 ± 2.8 and 11.1 ± 3.0 U/g hemoglobin (Hb), respectively; for G6PD-deficient samples, it was 0.8 ± 0.7 and 1.4 ± 0.9 U/g Hb. Bland-Altman analysis determined a mean difference of −0.96 ± 1.8 U/g Hb between the digital microfluidic fluorescence results and the standard biochemical test results. The lower and upper limits for the digital microfluidic platform were 4.5 to 19.5 U/g Hb for normal samples and 0.2 to 3.7 U/g Hb for G6PD-deficient samples. The lower and upper limits for the Stanford method were 5.5 to 20.7 U/g Hb for normal samples and 0.1 to 2.8 U/g Hb for G6PD-deficient samples. The measured activity discriminated between G6PD-deficient samples and normal samples with no overlap.

Conclusions.—Pending further validation, a digital microfluidics platform could be an accurate point-of-care screening tool for rapid newborn G6PD screening.

▶ Glucose-6-phosphate dehydrogenase deficiency (G6PDd) is the most common enzymatic defect in the world, estimated to affect about 400 million people.[1] Point-of-care testing for this X-linked disorder is of great interest and has been pursued mostly to safely administer antimalarial therapies because some of these medications can induce significant hemolysis in those with G6PDd.[2,3] Current screening is typically by the qualitative fluorescent spot test (FST), but this test detects only those with severe deficiency and thus will identify those with severe deficiency such as hemizygous males and homozygous females, but not those with intermediate G6PD levels as may be encountered in affected heterozygous females with unequal lyonization.[4,5] The gold standard for diagnosis of G6PDd is quantitative enzyme activity determination; however, it requires a skilled laboratory setting that is not available to many.[5]

In newborn infants, G6PDd can cause severe hyperbilirubinemia and kernicterus, even in countries historically without high prevalence of the disease because of modern ease of travel, intermarriage, and migration.[6,7] The World Health Organization has recommended screening newborns for G6PDd using cord blood wherever it affects > 3% to 5% of males.[6] Newborn screening has been adopted in some countries with high prevalence.[6] Recently, Nkhoma et al estimated the prevalence in the United States at 4% to 7%.[1] Some screening has been instituted in the United States. Washington, DC, and Pennsylvania perform testing for a few known G6PDd mutations as part of their state newborn screening programs; however, results are typically not available when an infant is at highest risk for severe hyperbilirubinemia.[7] In Cleveland, we currently test male newborns with the FST, which gives results before birth hospitalization discharge,[8] but has the limitations described above. Experts in the field of neonatal hyperbilirubinemia have recently began the discussion of testing newborns in the United States, favoring universal screening of all newborns that provides results before birth hospitalization discharge to allow for parental education, assessment of hyperbilirubinemia, and determination and arrangement of appropriate follow-up.[6,7] This would require the availability of quantitative enzyme activity testing in all birth hospitals with a quick turnaround time, thus an easy-to-use, portable, point-of-care test would be ideal.

Digital microfluidics allows for active fluid handling with computerized droplet manipulation and the performance of all steps of different types of assays, such as immunoassays, enzyme assays, chemistry assays, and DNA amplification and extraction on the same platform.[9,10] The authors used a digital microfluidic analyzer employing electrowetting for all droplet operations and waste disposal to perform G6PDd assays. This study demonstrated the ability of the digital microfluidics analyzer to determine G6PDd by quantitative enzyme assay and this technology could be the answer for universal newborn screening for the disorder. The authors envision a digital microfluidics "hyperbilirubinemia chip" for point-of-care assessment of G6PDd, bilirubin level, Gilbert syndrome (which is associated with G6PDd-related hyperbilirubinemia), and other tests that would allow for identifying newborns at risk for severe hyperbilirubinemia before discharge after birth. Digital microfluidics has already shown potential in newborn screening for lysosomal storage diseases,[11] and chips could be developed for multiplex testing for the disorders included in state newborn screening programs. Perhaps the G6PD quantitative enzyme assay could be incorporated into a "newborn screen chip" such that all newborn screening could be accomplished during birth hospitalization, giving results that could be acted on much faster than current state screening allows.

M. L. Nock, MD

References

1. Nkhoma ET, Poole C, Vannappagari V, et al. The global prevalence of glucose-6-phosphate dehydrogenase deficiency: a systematic review and meta-analysis. *Blood Cells Mol Dis.* 2009;42:267-278.
2. Roca-Feltrer A, Khim N, Kim S, et al. Field trial evaluation of the performances of point-of-care tests for screeing in G6PD deficiency in Cambodia. *PLoS One.* 2014;9:e116143.
3. Satyagraha AW, Sadhewa A, Elvira R, et al. Assessment of point-of-care diagnostics for G6PD deficiency in malaria endemic rural eastern Indonesia. *PLoS NegL Trop Dis.* 2016;10:e0004457.
4. Wong FL, Boo NY, Ainoon O, et al. Comparison of detection of glucose-6-phosphate dehydrogenase deficiency using fluorescent spot test, enzyme assay,

and molecular method for prediction of severe neonatal hyperbilirubinaemia. *Singapore Med J*. 2009;50:62-67.
5. LaRue N, Kahn M, Murray M, et al. comparison of quantitative and qualitative tests for glucose-6-phosphate dehydrogenase deficiency. *Am J Trop Med Hyg*. 2014;91:854-861.
6. Kaplan M, Hammerman C. The need for neonatal glucose-6-phosphate dehydrogenase screening: a global perspective. *J Perinatol*. 2009;29:S46-S52.
7. Watchko J, Kaplan M, Stark AR, et al. Should we screen newborns for glucose-6-phosphate dehydrogenase deficiency in the United States? *J Perinatol*. 2013;33: 499-504.
8. Nock ML, Johnson EM, Krugman RR, et al. Implementation and analysis of a pilot in-hospital newborn screening program for glucose-6-phosphate dehydrogenase deficiency in the United States. *J Perinatol*. 2011;31:112-117.
9. Sista R, Hua Z, Thwar P, et al. Development of a digital microfluidic platform for point of care testing. *Lab Chip*. 2008;8:2091-2104.
10. Millington DS, Sista R, Eckhardt A, et al. Digital microfluidics: a future technology in the newborn screening laboratory? *Semin Perinatol*. 2010;34:163-169.
11. Sista RS, Wang T, Wu N, et al. Multiplex newborn screening for Pompe, Fabry, Hunter, Gaucher, and Hurler Diseases using a digital microfluidic platform. *Clin Chim Acta*. 2013;424:12-18.

Bilirubin Concentrations in Jaundiced Neonates with Conjunctival Icterus

Azzuqa A, Watchko JF (Univ of Pittsburgh School of Medicine, PA)
J Pediatr 167:840-844, 2015

Objectives.—To assess the total serum bilirubin (TSB) levels at which conjunctival icterus is observed in neonates of ≥34 weeks gestation during the first week of life.

Study Design.—Two convenience samples of neonates were examined for conjunctival icterus within 4 hours of TSB measurements. A concurrent assessment of cephalopedal cutaneous icterus was performed and the TSB characterized using the Bhutani hour-specific risk zone nomogram.

Results.—Two hundred forty neonates were studied of which 76 had conjunctival icterus. Conjunctival icterus was always accompanied by cutaneous jaundice to at least the chest and more often than not a TSB >14.9 mg/dL (255 umol/L) consistently in the 76th%-95th% to >95th% range on the Bhutani nomogram. Only a few infants with TSB in the range of 10-14.9 mg/dL (171-255 umol/L) had conjunctival icterus.

Conclusions.—Conjunctival icterus was observed in a subset of jaundiced neonates and associated with elevated hour-specific TSB levels frequently >95th% on the Bhutani nomogram. Conjunctival icterus is a sign of clinically relevant hyperbilirubinemia that merits a TSB measurement and evaluation of the infant.

▶ In adults, the earliest clinical diagnosis of jaundice is almost always made by inspecting the patient's eyes, and the eyes of adults with total serum bilirubin (TSB) levels as low as 2.5 to 4 mg/dL will acquire a yellow hue. Similar eye coloration can also be seen in newborn infants but, as documented by both of these studies, mostly at significantly higher bilirubin levels. Why are the eyes of jaundiced individuals yellow? For years, the deposition of bilirubin in the eye has been referred to in textbooks and journals as "scleral icterus," but, contrary to popular belief, this eye color is primarily the result of bilirubin deposition in the conjunctiva, not the sclera,[1,2] a fact of which I was blissfully unaware until educated by my colleague, Jon Watchko, who was engaged in the study discussed in this commentary.

Azzuqa and Watchko studied 2 cohorts of 120 term and late preterm infants admitted to their neonatal intensive care unit with TSB levels ≥10 mg/dL. When the examiners were blinded (the second cohort), 31 of 36 (86%) infants with conjunctival icterus had TSBs ≥15 mg/dL, while only 5 of 76 (7%) of those with TSBs 10.0 to 14.9 mg/dL had conjunctival icterus. They concluded that "conjunctival icterus is a sign of clinically relevant hyperbilirubinemia that merits a TSB measurement and evaluation of the infant."

The study by Maisels et al came to a somewhat different conclusion, but the populations studied and the study design were also different Azzuqa and Watchko studied a selected infant population, some of whom were readmitted for hyperbilirubinemia. The examiners knew, ab initio, that every infant had a TSB of at least 10 mg/dL. In the Maisel et al[3] study, infants were not seen because they were jaundiced. They were part of a large and unsolicited population of healthy newborn infants seen for routine follow-up after hospital discharge in 5 pediatric office practices and a hospital-based clinic, where transcutaneous (TcB, not serum) bilirubin levels were routinely obtained. They were assessed for the presence or absence of conjunctival icterus by pediatricians or pediatric residents, all of whom were blinded to the TcB level. Although infants with conjunctival icterus tended to have higher TcB values than those without conjunctival icterus, only 41% of infants with conjunctival icterus had a TcB ≥13 mg/dL, and 20% had a TcB ≥15 mg/dL, but 20% had a TcB <10 mg/dL. Only 4.5% of infants with no conjunctival icterus had a TcB ≥13 mg/dL, and only 1.8% had a TcB ≥15 mg/dL. These investigators concluded that "in the absence of other clinical or laboratory indications, the presence of conjunctival icterus does not imply the need to measure the transcutaneous bilirubin or serum bilirubin level, but the absence of conjunctival icterus helps to rule out significant hyperbilirubinemia."

The reasons for the lack of agreement in these 2 studies is not readily explained. Factors that might have contributed to these findings include the differences in the study populations, the reason for assessing the presence or absence of conjunctival icterus, and the difference in the type of bilirubin measurement (serum vs transcutaneous). Nevertheless, both studies agree that the absence of conjunctival icterus is a very good negative predictor of significant jaundice in a 3- to 4-day-old otherwise healthy newborn, an observation that should be helpful to the practicing pediatrician. Whether every newborn with conjunctival icterus requires a measurement of the TcB or TSB is a matter for further investigation.

M. J. Maisels, MD, DSc

References

1. Kuiper JJ. Conjunctival icterus. *Ann Intern Med.* 2001;134:345-346.
2. Tripathi RC, Sidrys LA. 'Conjunctival icterus,' not 'scleral icterus'. *JAMA.* 1979; 242:2558.
3. Maisels MJ, Coffey MP, Gendelman B, et al. Diagnosing jaundice by eye—outpatient assessment of conjunctival icterus in the newborn. *J Pediatr.* 2016;172: 212-214.e1.

Bilirubin Concentrations in Jaundiced Neonates with Conjunctival Icterus

Azzuqa A, Watchko JF (Univ of Pittsburgh School of Medicine, PA)

J Pediatr 167:840-844, 2015

Objectives.—To assess the total serum bilirubin (TSB) levels at which conjunctival icterus is observed in neonates of ≥34 weeks gestation during the first week of life.

Study Design.—Two convenience samples of neonates were examined for conjunctival icterus within 4 hours of TSB measurements. A concurrent assessment of cephalopedal cutaneous icterus was performed and the TSB characterized using the Bhutani hour-specific risk zone nomogram.

Results.—Two hundred forty neonates were studied of which 76 had conjunctival icterus. Conjunctival icterus was always accompanied by cutaneous jaundice to at least the chest and more often than not a TSB >14.9 mg/dL (255 umol/L) consistently in the 76th%-95th% to >95th% range on the Bhutani nomogram. Only a few infants with TSB in the range of 10-14.9 mg/dL (171-255 umol/L) had conjunctival icterus.

Conclusions.—Conjunctival icterus was observed in a subset of jaundiced neonates and associated with elevated hour-specific TSB levels frequently >95th% on the Bhutani nomogram. Conjunctival icterus is a sign of clinically relevant hyperbilirubinemia that merits a TSB measurement and evaluation of the infant. (Fig 2).

► Neonatal jaundice has been a subject of discussion in the medical literature for centuries. As early as 1724, Johann Juncker drew a distinction between "true jaundice" and "the icteric tinge which may be observed in infants, immediately after birth."[1] Much has changed with respect to the recognition and management of jaundice in the last 300 years, yet, those of us who see newborns in clinical practice still wrestle with the same essential question. Which infants have jaundice in excess of that which is physiologic?

Pediatricians have long observed that newborns primarily manifest jaundice via discoloration of the skin. Clinical experience tells us and this study confirms that while conjunctival icterus is present in some infants, it is never the first sign of hyperbilirubinemia, the way it is in older children. As the authors point out, the classic description of head-to-toe neonatal jaundice progression published by Kramer[2] doesn't even mention the appearance of the conjunctiva. Interesting!

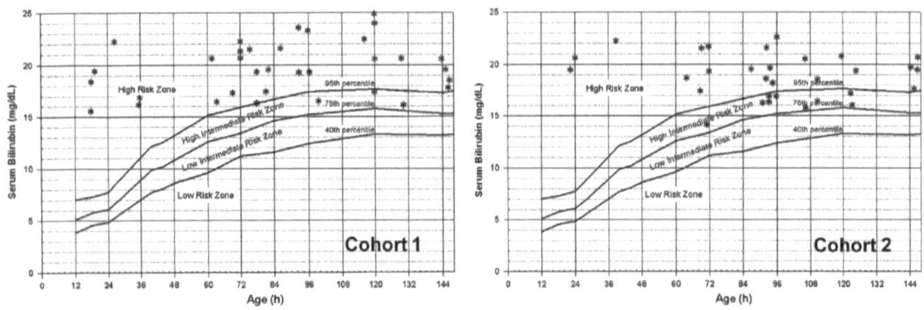

FIGURE 2.—Plot of TSB levels in infants with conjunctival icterus as a function of hour-specific percentile risk zone on the Bhutani nomogram in cohort 1 and cohort 2. *Represents an individual neonate with conjunctival icterus; those in cohort 2 represent concordant exams. (Reprinted from Azzuqa A, Watchko JF. Bilirubin concentrations in jaundiced neonates with conjunctival icterus. *J Pediatr.* 2015;167:840-844, with permission from Elsevier.)

The temptation in our current era of universal hyperbilirubinemia screening via serum or transcutaneous bilirubin measurements is to rely so heavily on these objective data that we almost disregard the appearance of the baby. But unless we are making repeated serial measurements routinely, we still are faced with the problem of how to decide which babies are jaundiced enough to need follow-up testing.

Thankfully, this study reminds us that a careful physical examination of the entire baby can still provide helpful information. By collecting some data on the relationship between total serum bilirubin (TSB) levels and conjunctival icterus, Azzuqa and Watchko have finally given us an evidence-based reason to believe the widely accepted notion that infants with yellow eyes generally have jaundice that is worse than those without. The presence of a strong correlation between conjunctival icterus and TSB levels greater than the 75th percentile on the Bhutani nomogram (Fig 2) makes this finding useful in clinical practice, with a couple of notable exceptions: First, because conjunctival icterus was primarily noted when the TSB level was in the mid-teens or above, this finding would likely be absent in very young babies (<48 hours old) even if the TSB level was well greater than the 95th percentile. Second, because some babies without any conjunctival icterus had TSB levels as high as 20 or 21, we must not let the absence of conjunctival icterus deter us from further evaluation when other information suggests it is justified.

The study by Maisels et al[3] mentioned in this article also finds a general connection between higher bilirubin levels and the presence of conjunctival icterus. In contrast to this study, Maisels et al[3] made transcutaneous bilirubin measurements on an outpatient cohort of infants 3 to 10 days old and found conjunctival icterus present in 17% of infants with transcutaneous bilirubin levels less than 10 mg/dL and 73% of infants with levels 10 to 14.9 mg/dL. Obviously, conjunctival icterus was not a very useful indicator of significant hyperbilirubinemia in their patients, as most babies with moderately elevated bilirubin levels exhibited it. I do think it's worth noting that these assessments were made in infants coming to the clinic for any reason, even if jaundice was not a clinical concern. It makes me wonder if conjunctival icterus has a somewhat different time course for appearance and resolution than dermal icterus does. Might it be that conjunctival icterus is a late-to-appear and last-to-disappear sign?

Just as the benefits (and pitfalls) of using a visual assessment for jaundice have been debated,[4-7] I'm sure the same will be true of the visual assessment of conjunctival icterus. There is bound to be some disagreement on the utility of this clinical sign. After all, the recognition of physical findings is dependent on the eye of the observer, something inextricably influenced by experience, history, and suboptimal room lighting.

At least we now know that the yellow discoloration we see in the whites of the eyes is most correctly referred to as *conjunctival icterus*, not *scleral icterus*. As someone who has frequently used the more popular (but incorrect) term, I've made a note of it.

J. Aby, MD

References

1. Gartner LM. Neonatal jaundice a selected retrospective. In: Smith GF, Vidyasagar D, editors. Historical Review and Recent Advances in Neonatal and Perinatal Medicine. 1980. http://www.neonatology.org.
2. Kramer LI. Advancement of dermal icterus in the jaundiced newborn. *Amer J Dis Child*. 1969;118:454-458.
3. Maisels MJ, Coffey MP, Gendelman B, et al. Diagnosing jaundice by eye – outpatient assessment of conjunctival icterus in the newborn. *J Pediatr*. 2016;172: 212-214.e1.
4. Manzar S. Cephalo-caudal progression of jaundice: a reliable, non-invasive clinical method to assess the degree of neonatal hyperbilirubinemia. *J Trop Pediatr*. 1999; 45:312-313.
5. Riskin A, Tamir A, Kugelman A, Hemo M, Bader D. Is visual assessment of jaundice reliable as a screening tool to detect significant neonatal hyperbilirubinemia? *J Pediatr*. 2008;152:782-787.
6. Kaplan M, Shchors I, Algur N, Bromiker R, Schimmel MS, Hammerman C. Visual screening versus transcutaneous bilirubinometry for predischarge jaundice assessment. *Acta Paediatr*. 2008;97:759-763.
7. Keren R, Tremont K, Luan X, Cnaan A. Visual assessment of jaundice in term and late preterm infants. *Arch Dis Child Fetal Neo Ed*. 2009;94:F317-F322.

Early formation of bilirubin isomers during phototherapy for neonatal jaundice: effects of single vs. double fluorescent lamps vs. photodiodes

Mreihil K, Madsen P, Nakstad B, et al (Akershus Univ Hosp, Lørenskog, Norway; Aalborg Univ Hosp, Denmark; et al)

Pediatr Res 78:56-62, 2015

Background.—In neonatal jaundice, phototherapy converts bilirubin to more polar photoisomers which can be excreted without conjugation. We measured changes in the concentration of bilirubin *Z,E*-photoisomer during the first 4 h of intensive phototherapy using single fluorescent lights as a reference, compared to double fluorescent lights, and a single unit of photodiodes.

Methods.—Neonates ($N = 42$; birth weight: 1,200–4,690 g; gestational age: 28–42 wk) were studied during phototherapy. Infants were randomized to: (i) single, or (ii) double fluorescent phototherapy; or (iii) single unit photodiodes. Irradiance was measured. Serum bilirubin (by cooximetry) and *Z,E* bilirubin (by high-pressure liquid chromatography) were measured at 0,15, 30, 60, 120, and 240 min after the start of phototherapy. Data were analyzed with a linear mixed model.

Results.—There was a highly significant increase of *Z,E*-bilirubin over time ($P < 0.0001$), starting at 15 min. Photoisomers reached ~25% of total bilirubin concentration after 4 h. However, there were no significant differences between the three randomized groups in spite of significantly higher irradiance using double fluorescent lights vs. single fluorescent or photodiodes.

Conclusion.—Formation of bilirubin photoisomers is rapid, and occurs early during intensive phototherapy for neonatal jaundice. The rate and level of photoisomerization was not influenced by irradiance and light source.

▶ One might have thought that because phototherapy for the newborn was first described in 1958,[1] we should, by now, have worked out how it works and where it works. It turns out, thanks to our colleagues in Norway and Denmark, that there is still much work to be done. It is certainly well established that, in vivo, a combination of configurational (4Z,15E; 4E,15Z;4E,15E) and structural (Z-lumirubin; E-lumirubin) isomers are formed rapidly when the lights are turned on. The difference between these 2 groups of isomers, however, is that although the 4Z,15E isomer constitutes about 20% to 30% of the total unconjugated bilirubin during phototherapy, it is cleared very slowly from the circulation (T½ of ~15 hours) and can therefore play only a small role (if any) in the well-documented elimination of bilirubin by phototherapy. It is nevertheless surprising to find that increasing the irradiance (in this case, by using 2 lights above the infant at an angle of about 30–40 degrees) does not increase the concentration of 4Z,15E photoisomers.

We know from substantial clinical experience and from earlier data[2,3] that double phototherapy (lights above and below the infant) lowers bilirubin levels more rapidly than single phototherapy, but the irradiance used in these studies was relatively low. In the study by Mreihil et al, serum bilirubin levels were only measured 4 hours after the initiation of phototherapy, and although with increasing irradiance, there was a significant decrease in the bilirubin levels, the differences were small. Note, however, that these results cannot be compared directly with studies in which lights are placed both above and below the infant. Although irradiance delivered both from above and to the flanks was significantly higher, with lights above and below, phototherapy is probably delivered to a larger surface area and is therefore expected to be more effective.

Mreihil et al did not measure any of the other configurational photoisomers, nor did they measure lumirubin, long postulated to be the major isomer responsible for the bilirubin lowering effects of phototherapy.[4,5] Some 3 decades ago, Costarino et al[5] showed that doubling the irradiance delivered to premature infants from 6 to 12 μW/cm²/nm, increased the proportion of lumirubin in the serum from 0.7% to 1.3%. Most recently, in an abstract presented in May 2016 at the Pediatric Academic Societies meeting in Baltimore,[6] the same group of Danish and Norwegian investigators documented, once again, that high irradiance double phototherapy (lights above and below) is significantly more effective than single phototherapy in lowering the bilirubin levels, but they did not provide any data on the production of isomers, including lumirubin.

The other question addressed by Mreihil et al is where phototherapy works. We know that phototherapy bleaches the yellow color in the skin of the newborn infant and must therefore convert the bilirubin in the skin and subcutaneous tissues to colorless derivatives, but does this contribute to the lowering of the serum bilirubin level? There are now several studies that suggest this is not the case. First, it has been shown repeatedly that rotating the infant from prone to supine or supine to prone has no effect on the rate at which the bilirubin level is lowered.[7-10] Thus, exposing skin and subcutaneous tissues that are still yellow (and presumably contain more bilirubin than skin that has already been bleached) has no effect on the decrease in serum bilirubin levels. This can only mean that although phototherapy does convert bilirubin in the skin to colorless derivatives, this has no effect on lowering the serum bilirubin level. Second, Donneborg et al[8] have shown that bilirubin is converted to photoisomers at the same rate in both yellow and blanched skin. Finally, these groups have shown that photoisomers are detectable in the blood within 15 minutes after starting phototherapy.[11] All of this evidence suggests that the primary site responsible for the bilirubin-lowering effect of phototherapy is the blood in the superficial capillaries and not the skin.

So we now know that phototherapy lowers the serum bilirubin by acting on the blood in the superficial capillaries, but we need additional measurements of the rate of formation of lumirubin in response to increasing irradiance to fully understand the mechanism of this remarkable therapy. Perhaps our Danish and Norwegian colleagues are already working on this.

M. J. Maisels, MD, DSc

References

1. Cremer RJ, Perryman PW, Richards DH. Influence of light on the hyperbilirubinemia of infants. *Lancet.* 1958;1:1094-1097.
2. Holtrop PC, Madison K, Maisels MJ. A clinical trial of fiberoptic phototherapy vs conventional phototherapy. *Am J Dis Child.* 1992;146:235-237.
3. Tan KL. The pattern of bilirubin response to phototherapy for neonatal hyperbilirubinemia. *Pediatr Res.* 1982;16:670-674.
4. Maisels MJ, McDonagh AF. Phototherapy for neonatal jaundice. *N Engl J Med.* 2008;358:920-928.
5. Costarino AT, Ennever JF, Baumgart S, Speck WT, Paul M, Polin RA. Bilirubin photoisomerization in premature neonates under low- and high-dose phototherapy. *Pediatrics.* 1985;75:519-522.
6. Donneborg ML, Vandborg PK, Hansen BM, Ebbesen F. Intensive phototherapy, double versus single in treatment of neonatal hyperbilirubinemia using light emitting diodes. *E-PAS.* 2016:1523-1609.
7. Chen C-M, Liu S-H, Lai C-C, Hwayg C-C, Hsu H-H. Changing position does not improve the efficacy of conventional phototherapy. *Acta Paediatr Taiwan.* 2002; 43:255-258.

8. Donneborg ML, Knudsen KB, Ebbesen F. Effect of infants' position on serum bilirubin level during conventional phototherapy. *Acta Paediatr.* 2010;99: 1131-1134.
9. Mohammadzadeh A, Bostani Z, Jafarnejad F, Mazloom R. Supine versus turning position on bilirubin level during phototerapy in healthy term jaundiced neonates. *Saudi Med J.* 2004;25:2051-2052.
10. Shinwell ES, Sciaky Y, Karplus M. Effect of position changing on bilirubin levels during phototherapy. *J Perinatol.* 2002;22:226-229.
11. Mreihil K, McDonagh A, Nakstad B, Hansen TWR. Early isomerization of bilirubin in phototherapy of neonatal jaundice. *Pediatr Res.* 2010;67:656-659.

Jaundice, phototherapy and DNA damage in full-term neonates

Ramy N, Ghany EA, Alsharany W, et al (Cairo Univ, Egypt; Ain Shams Univ, Cairo, Egypt; et al)
J Perinatol 36:132-136, 2016

Objective.—Phototherapy is the standard therapeutic approach for neonatal hyperbilirubinemia. Oxidative effects of phototherapy may have potential harms, including DNA damage. Unconjugated bilirubin (UCB) might also possess antigenotoxic potential. Intensive phototherapy is more efficacious than conventional phototherapy in treating hyperbilirubinemia. This study aimed to assess the impact of hyperbilirubinemia and the two different types of phototherapy on DNA damage in peripheral blood mononuclear cells of neonates.

Study Design.—The study was conducted on term neonates with nonhemolytic hyperbilirubinemia and control healthy neonates. Genotoxicity was assessed using single-cell gel electrophoresis (Comet assay) in peripheral mononuclear cells. Blood samples were obtained at enrollment in all infants and after intensive or conventional phototherapy in jaundiced infants.

Result.—DNA damage did not significantly differ between jaundiced and non-jaundiced neonates (11.4 ± 8.7 and 10.9 ± 8.3 arbitrary units (AU), respectively, $P = 0.58$). It increased significantly after exposure to phototherapy compared with prephototherapy values (45.6 ± 14.7 vs 11.4 ± 8.7 AU, respectively, $P < 0.001$). The duration of phototherapy correlated positively with markers of DNA damage ($r = 0.86$, $P < 0.001$); however, the intensity of used light did not significantly impact genotoxicity.

Conclusion.—Hyperbilirubinemia does not influence DNA damage, whereas both conventional and intensive phototherapy are associated with DNA damage in term infants with hyperbilirubinemia (Figs 1 and 2).

▶ The title of this article immediately caught my attention because it brought me back to my residency training nearly 40 years ago when Professor Jerry O'Dell did not want us to use phototherapy in jaundiced babies because of several concerns including the possibility of chromosomal breakage. We did a lot of exchange transfusions in those days. Furthermore, even though this was a

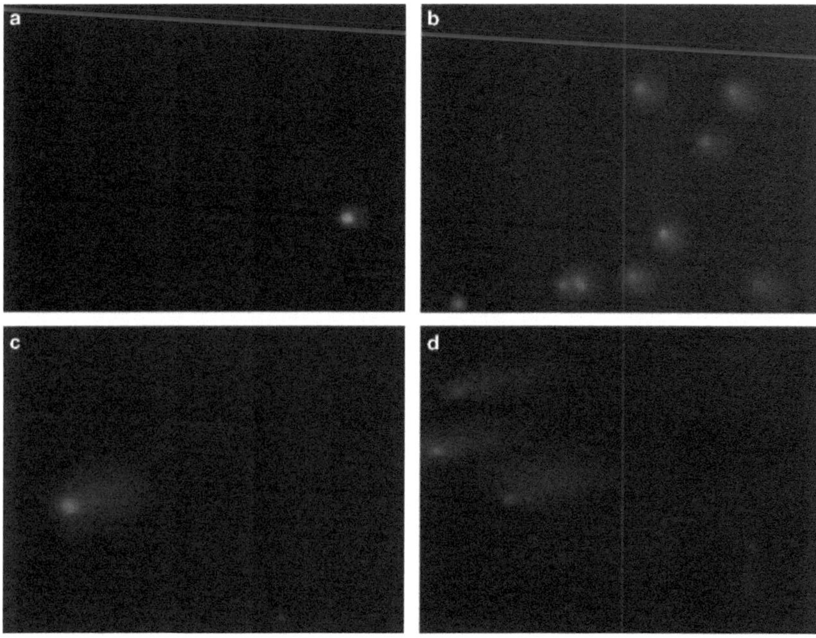

FIGURE 1.—Visual analysis. Images of peripheral blood mononuclear cells showing different classes of DNA damage using visual scoring ((a): score=1, (b): score=2, (c): score=3, and (d): score=4). (Reprinted from Ramy N, Ghany EA, Alsharany W, et al. Jaundice, phototherapy and DNA damage in full-term neonates. *J Perinatol.* 2016;36:132-136, with permission from Nature America, Inc.)

concern, little evidence was ever produced that Professor O'Dell's concern was valid. Of course, phototherapy is one of the most common interventions used in neonatal intensive care over the past several decades.

This article cites some recent in vitro and animal studies showing that phototherapy can "induce DNA strand breaks, sister chromatid exchange and mutations." In this study, the authors employed a widely used method, the "comet assay"[1] to evaluate genotoxicity in peripheral blood mononuclear cells derived from infants with and without hyperbilirubinemia and in those in whom phototherapy was applied or not. Images of 4 classes of DNA damage using a scoring system that uses this electrophoretic method of DNA analysis is seen in Fig 1.

Hyperbilirubinemia itself did not alter the DNA damage score, but phototherapy (conventional or intensive) both significantly increased the damage score (Fig 2). Of interest is that the genotoxicity did not appear to be affected by the intensity of the phototherapy. The authors mention a few limitations of their study including the fact that the control group was tested for DNA damage only once. Furthermore, the issue of safety, with few studies suggesting adverse effects being reported in the literature.

Nevertheless, we use a lot of prophylactic phototherapy in neonatal intensive care, especially in very preterm infants. This study resurrects the concern

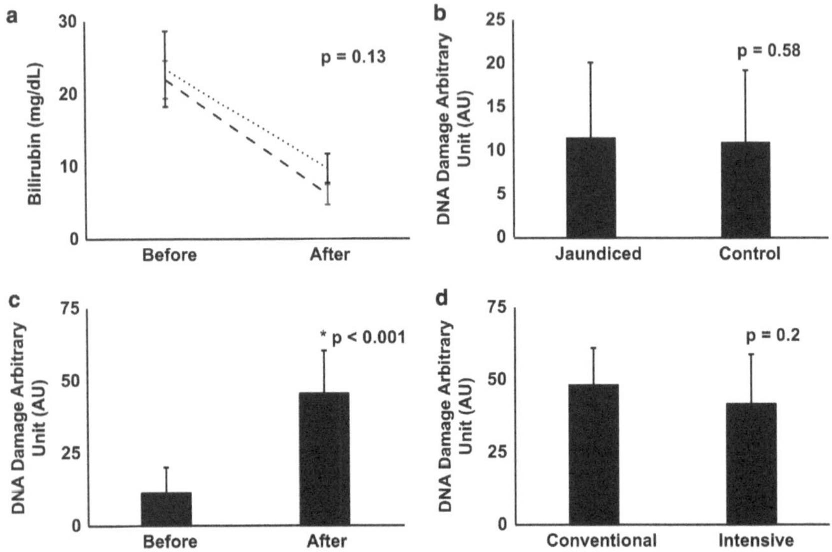

FIGURE 2.—. Bilirubin concentrations and frequency of DNA damage in the study population. (a) Bilirubin concentrations before and after phototherapy in the intensive group (......) and the conventional group (——), (b) DNA damage in cases vs controls ($n = 76$), (c) significant DNA damage in cases after exposure to phototherapy ($n = 36$) and (d) DNA damage in cases after receiving conventional and intensive phototherapy ($n = 36$). (Reprinted from Ramy N, Ghany EA, Alsharany W, et al. Jaundice, phototherapy and DNA damage in full-term neonates. *J Perinatol.* 2016;36:132-136, with permission from Nature America, Inc.)

that I learned several decades ago and begs the question of how we can best address the rational use of phototherapy in our neonatal intensive care population.

J. Neu, MD

Reference

1. Collins AR. The comet assay: a heavenly method! *Mutagenesis.* 2015;30:1-4.

Effect of Ursodeoxycholic Acid on Indirect Hyperbilirubinemia in Neonates Treated With Phototherapy

Honar N, Ghashghaei Saadi E, Saki F, et al (Shiraz Univ of Med Sciences, Iran; et al)

J Pediatr Gastroenterol Nutr 62:97-100, 2016

Background.—Hyperbilirubinemia is a common neonatal problem. The present study aimed to investigate the effect of ursodeoxycholic acid in reducing indirect hyperbilirubinemia of infants under phototherapy.

Methods.—This double-blind randomized clinical trial was conducted on neonates with jaundice, who had received phototherapy in the hospitals affiliated with the Shiraz University of Medical Sciences in 2013. A total of 80 neonates were enrolled in the study and were randomly divided into 2 groups. The intervention group (n = 40) with indirect hyperbilirubinemia received 10 $mg \cdot kg^{-1} \cdot day^{-1}$ divided every 12 hours Ursobil (capsule 300 mg) in addition to phototherapy, whereas the control group (n = 40) received only phototherapy. Total bilirubin levels were measured every 12 hours until reaching <10 mg/dL, and then phototherapy was disrupted. The duration of phototherapy was measured. The 2 groups were compared regarding total bilirubin levels at different time points and duration of phototherapy using the generalized estimating equation (GEE) test.

Results.—The mean of total bilirubin in the intervention group was 12 ± 1.6, 10 ± 1.1, and 9.8 ± 0.2 mg/dL 12, 24, and 48 hours after the beginning of phototherapy, respectively. On the contrary, these measures were 14.4 ± 1.3, 12.5 ± 1.4, and 10.1 ± 1.1 mg/dL in the control group, respectively, ($P < 0.05$). The mean time required for phototherapy to decrease the bilirubin level to <10 mg/dL was 15.5 ± 6 and 44.6 ± 13.3 hours in the case and the control group, respectively, ($P = 0.001$).

Conclusions.—Ursodeoxycholic acid had additive effect with phototherapy in neonates with indirect hyperbilirubinemia. This drug also reduced the time period needed for phototherapy and, consequently, decreased the hospitalization period.

▶ Phototherapy converts indirect bilirubin to isomers that can be excreted in the bile or urine without the need for conjugation and the ability of phototherapy to decrease the serum bilirubin level depends both on the rate of formation of these isomers as well as the rapidity with which they can be cleared. Ursodeoxycholic acid (UDCA) is known to stimulate bile flow and lowers conjugated bilirubin levels in various cholestatic conditions, so it seems reasonable to expect that an agent that increases bile flow might also help to decrease indirect serum bilirubin levels in infants who are receiving phototherapy. Although not previously studied in infants in a controlled fashion, the use of UDCA has been recommended as a means of optimizing bile flow in infants and children with Crigler-Najjar disease who are receiving phototherapy in response to an exacerbation of their hyperbilirubinemia.[1]

In this study, Honar and colleagues randomly assigned 80 jaundiced infants who were receiving phototherapy for the treatment of their nonhemolytic hyperbilirubinemia, to receive, in addition, either UDCA (study group) or a placebo (controls). When the study group was compared with the control subjects, the bilirubin levels at 12, 24, and 48 hours after initiation of phototherapy were significantly lower, and the time required for phototherapy to reduce the bilirubin to a level below 10 mg/dL was, on average, 29 hours less. The strengths of the study include the randomized, controlled, study design and the blinding of the participating clinicians.

One might question, however, the need for phototherapy in infants who were, on average, more than 3½ days old and, in the absence of hemolytic disease, would not have met the American Academy of Pediatrics guidelines for the use of phototherapy. Although both groups received similar phototherapy treatment, none received what would be considered intensive phototherapy, nor do we have any measurements of the irradiance delivered to these infants. The mean duration of phototherapy in the study group was 15.5 ± 6 hours, a duration of phototherapy that is very similar to that provided to 3- to 5-day-old infants readmitted to our institution with significantly higher bilirubin levels. We do, of course, provide intensive phototherapy with an irradiance of at least 30 μW/cm^2/nm above and a fiberoptic LED blanket below the infant, and we discontinue phototherapy when the bilirubin level is < 14 mg/dL. Nevertheless, the use of more irradiance delivered to a greater surface area can achieve results that are similar to those obtained in the UDCA infants in this study.

On the other hand, because UDCA is a drug that is well tolerated and has a good safety profile, its use might well be considered in limited-resource countries where both equipment and electricity are not readily available. In this situation, either supplementing phototherapy with UDCA or using UDCA to avoid the need for phototherapy is an intervention that certainly deserves consideration.[2]

Although phototherapy has long been considered safe, detailed, long-term follow-up studies of infants who have received phototherapy are limited, and numerous short-term adverse effects of this therapy are well documented.[3] But we also need considerably more data on the use and safety of UDCA in the newborn before we can consider its wider use as a means of preventing or treating hyperbilirubinemia.

M. J. Maisels, MD, DSc

References

1. Strauss KA, Robinson DL, Vreman HJ, Puffenberger EG, Hart G, Morton DH. Management of hyperbilirubinemia and prevention of kernicterus in 20 patients with Crigler-Najjar disease. *Eur J Pediatr.* 2006;165:306-319.
2. Slusher TM, Olusanya BO, Vreman HJ, et al. A randomized trial of phototherapy with filtered sunlight in african neonates. *N Engl J Med.* 2015;373:1115-1124.
3. Maisels MJ. Sister Jean Ward, phototherapy, and jaundice: a unique human and photochemical interaction. *J Perinatol.* 2015;35:671-675.

Follow-up of extreme neonatal hyperbilirubinemia in 5- to 10-year-old children: a Danish population-based study

Vandborg PK, Hansen BM, Greisen G, et al (Aalborg Univ Hosp, Aalborg, Denmark; Copenhagen Univ Hosp, Denmark)

Dev Med Child Neurol 57:378-384, 2015

Aim.—To investigate whether infants with neonatal hyperbilirubinaemia but without intermediate or advanced bilirubin encephalopathy develop long-term sequelae, with impairment of motor development, executive function, or hearing.

Method.—This nested double-cohort study included 167 exposed children (107 males, 60 females) born in Denmark 2000 to 2005 at gestational age ≥35 weeks with a total serum bilirubin ≥450 μmol/L (26.3 mg/dL) and 163 age-, sex-, and gestational age-matched unexposed children (103 males, 60 females). The children were examined at a mean age of 7.7 years (SD 1.7 y) using the Movement Assessment Battery for Children-Second Edition (MABC-2), pure tone audiometry, and the Behavioural Regulation Inventory of Executive Function (BRIEF) questionnaire.

Results.—The follow-up rate was 70% of the eligible infants in the exposed group and 45% in the unexposed group. Mean difference was −0.2 (95% confidence interval [CI] −1.1 to 0.8) in adjusted standard score for MABC-2 and 0.3 (95% CI −2.9 to 3.5) in adjusted BRIEF executive composite standard score. No children had significant hearing impairment or a diagnosis of cerebral palsy, attention-deficit-hyperactive disorder, or autism spectrum disorder recorded in national registries.

Interpretation.—No evidence was found of an increased risk of deficits in motor development, executive function, or hearing in children with extreme hyperbilirubinaemia who did not have intermediate or advanced bilirubin encephalopathy.

▶ This important population-based study provides data on 167 children who, as neonates born between 2000 and 2005, with gestational ages ≥35 weeks, had total serum bilirubin levels of ≥450 μmol/L (26.2 mg/dL) but minimal or absent symptoms of acute bilirubin encephalopathy (they showed only lethargy, poor sucking, or hypotonia). These children were then examined at a mean age of 7.7 ± 1.7 years and compared with matched, unexposed children.

In their commentary on this study, Newman and Kuzniewicz[1] point out the advantages of the nested, double-cohort design used when effects of a rare exposure on health outcomes are sought. They note that the advantage of "nesting this double cohort study within a larger cohort" allows a comparison of participants with nonparticipants. The investigators found no children in either group with cerebral palsy, attention-deficit/hyperactivity disorder, or autism. They also found no difference between the groups with regard to hearing, including pure tone audiometry, and no differences in the scores obtained with the Movement Assessment Battery for Children second edition (MABC-2), a standardized test for motor difficulties or an 86-item questionnaire completed by parents for the assessment of executive function in children aged 5 to 18 years.

These results are doubly reassuring. First, they confirm recent reports that kernicterus is a rare condition and, in the absence of prematurity and/or significant comorbidities, is unlikely to occur at total serum bilirubin levels < 600 μmol/L (35 mg/dL)[2,3]; and second the results confirm that nonextreme hyperbilirubinemia in otherwise healthy neonates is unlikely to have long-term subtle, deleterious consequences. These observations also suggest the need for a reassessment of current recommendations for the use of phototherapy and exchange transfusions, issues that are currently being addressed by the

American Academy of Pediatrics Subcommittee on Hyperbilirubinemia—but don't hold your breath. These decisions require much thought and time.

M. J. Maisels, MD, DSc

References

1. Newman TB, Kuzniewicz MW. Follow up of extreme neonatal hyperbilirubinemia: more reassuring results from Denmark. *Dev Med Child Neurol.* 2015;57: 314-315.
2. Ebbesen F, Bjerre JV, Vandborg PK. Relation between serum bilirubin levels > 450 μmol/L and bilirubin encephalopathy; a Danish population-based study. *Acta Paediatr.* 2012;101:384-389.
3. Kuzniewicz MW, Wickremasinghe AC, Wu YW, et al. Incidence, etiology, and outcomes of hazardous hyperbilirubinemia in newborns. *Pediatrics.* 2014;134: 504-509.

Preschool Assessment of Preterm Infants Treated With Darbepoetin and Erythropoietin

Ohls RK, Cannon DC, Phillips J, et al (Univ of New Mexico, Albuquerque; et al)
Pediatrics 137:e20153859, 2016

Background.—We previously reported improved neurodevelopmental outcomes at 2 years among infants treated with the erythropoiesis-stimulating agents (ESAs) darbepoetin alfa (darbepoetin) or erythropoietin. Here we characterize 4-year outcomes.

Methods.—Former preterm infants randomly assigned to receive darbepoetin (10 μg/kg, once per week), erythropoietin (400 U/kg, 3 times/week), or placebo through 35 weeks' postconceptual age were evaluated at 3.5 to 4 years of age. For comparison, healthy children formerly delivered full term (term controls [TCs]) were also recruited. All participants were assessed by using measures of full-scale IQ (FSIQ) and general language from the Wechsler Preschool and Primary Scale of Intelligence, Third Edition, and an overall measure of executive function, on the basis of tests evaluating inhibitory control and spatial working memory. Rates of neurodevelopmental impairment were compared across groups.

Results.—Multivariate analysis of variance compared children randomly assigned to ESAs ($n = 39$), placebo ($n = 14$), and TCs ($n = 24$). FSIQ and performance IQ were significantly higher in the ESA group than in the placebo group (FSIQ: 91.1 ± 17.5 vs 79.2 ± 18.5, $P = .036$; performance IQ: 93.0 ± 17.0 vs 79.5 ± 19.5, $P = .018$). Follow-up analyses revealed that the children receiving ESAs performed better than those who received placebo on executive function tasks. The ESA group's performance was below that of TCs, but the results did not reach significance on executive function. The incidence of neurodevelopmental impairment was greater in the placebo group than in the ESA group.

Conclusions.—ESA-treated infants had better cognitive outcomes and less developmental impairment at 3.5 to 4 years of age compared with placebo-treated infants. ESAs show promise in improving long-term cognitive outcomes of infants born prematurely.

► Neurodevelopmental challenges including cerebral palsy, intellectual disability, and attention deficits are common in children born extremely preterm. Erythropoiesis-stimulating agents (ESAs) increase oligodendrogenesis and decrease inflammation, oxidative injury, and apoptosis. Retrospective studies in children born preterm exposed to erythropoietin have suggested significant neurologic benefits, and several randomized controlled trials are ongoing. The latest follow-up to date was recently published by researchers from New Mexico and Utah. This group enrolled 99 infants born at less than 32 weeks gestational age to erythropoietin 3 times weekly, darbepoetin once weekly, or placebo. Prior publications have demonstrated the safety of the regimens used, significant improvement in cognitive scores measured at 18 to 22 months by the Bayley Scales of Infant Development III, and a lower incidence of cerebral palsy. Follow-up of more than half of these children at 3.5 to 4 years of age revealed higher full-scale IQ (91 vs 79, $P = .036$) and performance IQ (93 vs 80, $P = .018$) among children randomized to ESAs than among children in the control group measured by the Wechsler Preschool and Primary Scale of Intelligence (3rd edition). Additional benefits included superior executive function and a lower incidence of mild cerebral palsy.

Benefits at preschool age from a neuroprotective therapy initiated in the newborn period are extremely enticing. Additionally, this trial lends further support to the notion that darbepoetin administered once weekly provides equivalent benefits to erythropoietin administered multiple times per week. The initially small sample size and substantial attrition over time are limitations that temper enthusiasm to some degree. It should be noted that the small number of children remaining in the placebo group have IQs well below those reported in previous randomized controlled trials examining similar populations of preterm-born children. Much larger ongoing trials of erythropoietin in Switzerland and the United States have the potential to fully evaluate benefits and potential adverse effects. The authors of this study have already shifted their focus to 5.5- to 6-year testing and magnetic resonance imaging, as they continue to lead in the study of those incredibly promising interventions.

C. McPherson, PharmD

Vitamin K prophylaxis for prevention of Vitamin K deficiency bleeding: A systematic review

Sankar MJ, Chandrasekaran A, Kumar P, et al (All India Inst of Med Sciences, New Delhi)

J Perinatol 36:S29-S34, 2016

We conducted a systematic review to evaluate the burden of late vitamin K deficiency bleeding (VKDB) and the effect of vitamin K prophylaxis on the incidence of VKDB. We searched MEDLINE and other electronic databases, and included all observational studies including population surveys as well as randomized controlled trials (RCT). The median (interquartile range) burden of late VKDB was 35 (10.5 to 80) per 100 000 live births in infants who had not received prophylaxis at birth; the burden was much higher in low- and middle-income countries as compared with high-income countries-80 (72 to 80) vs 8.8 (5.8 to 17.8) per 100 000 live births. Two randomized trials evaluated the effect of intramuscular (IM) prophylaxis on the risk of classical VKDB. Although one trial reported a significant reduction in the incidence of any bleeding (relative risk (RR) 0.73, 95% confidence interval (CI) 0.56 to 0.96) and moderate to severe bleeding (RR 0.19, 0.08 to 0.46; number needed to treat (NNT) 74, 47 to 177), the other trial demonstrated a significant reduction in the risk of secondary bleeding after circumcision in male neonates (RR 0.18, CI 0.08 to 0.42; NNT 9, 6 to 15). No RCTs evaluated the effect of vitamin K prophylaxis on late VKDB. Data from four surveillance studies indicate that the use of IM/subcutaneous vitamin K prophylaxis could significantly reduce the risk of late VKDB when compared with no prophylaxis (pooled RR 0.02; 95% CI 0.00 to 0.10). When compared with IM prophylaxis, a single oral dose of vitamin K increased the risk of VKDB (RR 24.5; 95% CI 7.4 to 81.0) but multiple oral doses did not (RR 3.64; CI 0.82 to 16.3). There is low-quality evidence from observational studies that routine IM administration of 1 mg of vitamin K at birth reduces the incidence of late VKDB during infancy. Given the high risk of mortality and morbidity in infants with late VKDB, it seems appropriate to administer IM vitamin K prophylaxis to all neonates at birth. Future studies should compare the efficacy and safety of multiple oral doses with IM vitamin K and also evaluate the optimal dose of vitamin K in preterm neonates (Table 2).

▶ There is no reason in 2016 and beyond for newborns to suffer from vitamin K–deficient hemorrhagic disease of the newborn unless they have biliary atresia or hepatitis. The administration of prophylactic intramuscular vitamin K effectively prevents what can be a devastating disorder. Nonetheless, given that prophylactic vitamin K has been a routine part of care in most countries since the American Academy of Pediatrics report in 1961,[1] after scouring the literature, the authors had difficulty finding all the supporting evidence they required to back up the preceding statements. It is nonetheless gratifying that the World Health Organization, after a noncommitment to routine vitamin K administration in 2005,[2] recanted and recommended prophylactic vitamin K in 2013.[3]

TABLE 2.—Median Burden of Late VKDB in Different Settings

Setting	Median Incidence (per 100 000 Live Births)	Interquartile Range
Overall[a]	35	10.5–80
LMICs	80	72–80
High-income countries	8.8	5.8–17.8

Abbreviations: LMICs, low- and middle-income countries; VKDB, vitamin K deficiency bleeding.
[a]Irrespective of the country and prophylaxis status.
Reprinted from Sankar MJ, Chandrasekaran A, Kumar P, et al. Vitamin K prophylaxis for prevention of Vitamin K deficiency bleeding: a systematic review. *J Perinatol*. 2016;36:S29-S34, with permission from Nature America, Inc.

The 2 major objectives of this review were to evaluate (1) the burden of vitamin K deficiency bleeding (VKDB) by estimating the incidence of late VKDB in infants who did not receive vitamin K prophylaxis at birth and (2) the effect of vitamin K prophylaxis on the incidence of classical and late VKDB in neonates and infants up to 1 year of age.

The authors retrieved a total of 883 citations, of which 722 were excluded after screening the title/abstract. Of the remaining 161 citations, 15 were found to be eligible for inclusion in the review. Almost all of the studies listed were surveillance studies in which different hospitals were requested to report on cases of hemorrhage disease of the newborn admitted during the study period.

Table 2 summarizes the estimated burden of late VKDB in different settings. The median interquartile range burden in the absence of any prophylaxis is 35 (10.5–80.0) per 100 000 live births; the median burden in low/middle-income and high-income countries is 80 (72–80) and 8.8 (5.8–17.8) per 100 000 live births, respectively. There was a significant reduction in the incidence of secondary bleeding after circumcision in neonates who received vitamin K prophylaxis (relative risk 0.18, 0.08–0.42; number needed to treat 9, range 6–15).

Although vitamin K given intramuscularly may be traumatic, the effects are rarely significant. The dose of 1 mg is far in excess of needs but to date after more than 55 years, there is no convincing evidence of harm. Oral vitamin K is effective but requires additional doses and follow-up, which in many countries is impractical if not impossible.

So the old-fashioned IM vitamin K will retain its place in the history of triumphs in neonatology.

A. A. Fanaroff, MD

References

1. American Academy of Pediatrics, Committee on Nutrition. Vitamin K compounds and the water soluble analogues. *Pediatrics*. 1961;28:7.
2. WHO. *Pocket Book of Hospital Care for Children: Guidelines for the management of Common Illnesses with Limited Resources*. Geneva, Switzerland: WHO; 2005.
3. WHO. Pocket Book of Hospital Care for Children: Guidelines for the Management of Common Illnesses.

11 Renal, Metabolism, and Endocrine Disorders

Neonatal Glycemia and Neurodevelopmental Outcomes at 2 Years

McKinlay CJD, for the CHYLD Study Group (Univ of Auckland, New Zealand; et al)

N Engl J Med 373:1507-1518, 2015

Background.—Neonatal hypoglycemia is common and can cause neurologic impairment, but evidence supporting thresholds for intervention is limited.

Methods.—We performed a prospective cohort study involving 528 neonates with a gestational age of at least 35 weeks who were considered to be at risk for hypoglycemia; all were treated to maintain a blood glucose concentration of at least 47 mg per deciliter (2.6 mmol per liter). We intermittently measured blood glucose for up to 7 days. We continuously monitored interstitial glucose concentrations, which were masked to clinical staff. Assessment at 2 years included Bayley Scales of Infant Development III and tests of executive and visual function.

Results.—Of 614 children, 528 were eligible, and 404 (77% of eligible children) were assessed; 216 children (53%) had neonatal hypoglycemia (blood glucose concentration, <47 mg per deciliter). Hypoglycemia, when treated to maintain a blood glucose concentration of at least 47 mg per deciliter, was not associated with an increased risk of the primary outcomes of neurosensory impairment (risk ratio, 0.95; 95% confidence interval [CI], 0.75 to 1.20; P = 0.67) and processing difficulty, defined as an executive-function score or motion coherence threshold that was more than 1.5 SD from the mean (risk ratio, 0.92; 95% CI, 0.56 to 1.51; P = 0.74). Risks were not increased among children with unrecognized hypoglycemia (a low interstitial glucose concentration only). The lowest blood glucose concentration, number of hypoglycemic episodes and events, and negative interstitial increment (area above the interstitial glucose concentration curve and below 47 mg per deciliter) also did not predict the outcome.

Conclusions.—In this cohort, neonatal hypoglycemia was not associated with an adverse neurologic outcome when treatment was provided to maintain a blood glucose concentration of at least 47 mg per deciliter. (Funded by the Eunice Kennedy Shriver National Institute of Child Health and Human Development and others.)

▶ The Children with Hypoglycemia and their Later Development (CHYLD) studies have added a lot of information about the effects of neonatal hypoglycemia on developmental outcomes. This year, they reported on 614 term and late preterm children born at risk using the same categories as the American Academy of Pediatrics Committee on the Fetus and Newborn statement.[1]

The hypothesis of this CHYLD study was that the neuropsychological development of 2-year-old children is related to the severity, duration, and frequency of low plasma glucose levels in the neonatal period. This study also included continuous glucose monitoring that did not influence clinical care because it was masked from the clinicians. The patient population included those without hypoglycemia (<47 mg/dL), with treated and untreated hypoglycemia. The children in the publication were assessed at 2 years of age and some preliminary data on the 4.5-year follow-up was presented at the 2016 Pediatric Academic Societies meeting.[2]

McKinley et al screened and treated all the at-risk infants with the aim of keeping plasma concentration of glucose >47 mg/dL. Surprisingly, there were long and undetected periods of interstitial glucose concentrations <47 mg/dL. Additionally, high or unstable glucose concentrations were observed and associated themselves with worse developmental outcomes. A "U-shaped curve describes the potential morbidity with both low and elevated plasma glucose levels.

More than half of the at-risk infants were diagnosed with hypoglycemia when using 47 mg/dL as the definition for neonatal hypoglycemia. Almost 1 in 4 had hypoglycemic episodes not detected with intermittent blood sampling. Twenty-five percent of those undetected episodes lasted more than 5 hours in the first week of life.

Neurosensory impairment or processing difficulty at 2 years of age did not differ among the 5 groupings studied, including a reference group never having a level <47 mg/dL, any episode of hypoglycemia, >3 episodes of hypoglycemia, or >3 days of hypoglycemia or severe hypoglycemia. There was no relationship between neonatal hypoglycemia and neurodevelopmental outcome at 2 years of age.

The authors also looked at undetected episodes of hypoglycemia and outcome at 2 years of age. Again, 108 with no events vs 33 who had at least 1 episode of <47 mg/dL showed no difference in neurosensory impairment or processing difficulty.

Finally, data on the 4.5-year follow-up demonstrated an increase in executive function difficulty in the infants who had suffered more than 1 episode of hypoglycemia only on continuous monitoring versus no episodes of hypoglycemia, 13% versus 3%, respectively. Further follow-up will be necessary to appreciate the full scope of outcomes with age.

The authors conclude that a margin of safety is required when setting a threshold for intervention in neonatal hypoglycemia. However, the definition of clinically significant hypoglycemia remains among the most confused and contentious issues in neonatal medicine.[3] More than 50 years ago, Cornblath et al recognized that low blood glucose levels in small for gestational age infants and preterm infants were associated with seizures.[4] It became clear that symptomatic hypoglycemia could lead to long-term neurologic deficits. Although there is agreement that recurrent severe hypoglycemia causes brain injury, there have been few high-quality studies shedding light on the neurodevelopmental outcomes related to transient neonatal hypoglycemia.[5]

Four other important studies use the neurodevelopmental approach to address hypoglycemia. In 1988, a study influenced neonatal care around the world. It concluded that a glucose concentration < 47 mg/dL was the threshold that would reliably predict outcomes.[6] The study evaluated glucose levels drawn daily initially, then weekly until discharge on 661 infants weighing less than 1850 g at birth who were enrolled in a nutrition study looking at the effect of early diets on cognitive outcomes. They used statistical strategies to determine a threshold value that reliably predicted an adverse outcome. They found that the number of days that these infants experienced moderate hypoglycemia (< 47 mg/dL) was strongly related to reduced scores for mental and motor development at 18 months' corrected age, even after adjustment for a wide range of factors known to influence development.[7] There were several study weaknesses. Sicker infants had more frequent determinations of blood glucose, and hypoglycemia was not really the focus of this prospective controlled feeding trial. In fact, some infants were permitted to have plasma glucose levels < 20 mg/dL for as long as 3 to 7 days without intervention. Only the first glucose value of the day was used in the analyses.[7] This value of 47 mg/dL was used worldwide and applied even to term appropriate for gestational age, healthy neonates as the gold standard and critical threshold defining hypoglycemia and risk of brain injury. However, less dramatic differences were found when the children were 7 to 8 years of age.[7]

Another study, also performed in the United Kingdom, published almost 25 years later, found no evidence to support that recurrent low blood glucose levels of < 45 mg/dL pose a hazard to preterm infants.[8] In this randomized controlled trial, which included infants less than 32 weeks' gestation who had blood glucose levels measured daily for the first 10 days of life, there were no differences in developmental outcomes at 2 years of age. At 15 years of age, outcomes (including full-scale intelligence quotient, behavioral and emotional outcomes, and adaptation to daily living as adolescents) were nearly identical between controls and those with blood glucose concentrations < 45 mg/dL on at least 3 days of the first 10 days of life.[8]

A recent study from Arkansas suggests an association between transient newborn hypoglycemia and fourth-grade achievement test proficiency.[9] This cohort had nearly 1400 largely late preterm and term infants, all of whom had glucose screening (within the first 3 hours of life) and identified infants who had a glucose level below 35, 40, or 45 mg/dL, followed by a second value above those cutoffs. They reported on the relationship between a single initial low glucose concentration and subsequent academic performance.[8] The glucose testing was done by the standard glucose oxidase method. Using data collected from fourth-grade school examinations from across the state of Arkansas, they found that a single episode of hypoglycemia, defined by a level < 40 mg/dL soon after birth followed by a second level above that cutoff was associated with a 50% reduction in the odds of achieving proficiency in literacy and numeracy at age 10 years.[9] Similar findings for < 35 mg/dL and for < 45 mg/dL were also shown. In total, 10% of the cohort experienced a glucose level < 40 mg/dL. The population included all infants born at the study center over a 12-month period not only those considered to be at risk.

Finally, 75 healthy term large for gestational age infants born to nondiabetic mothers had screening of glucose levels at 1, 3, and 5 hours after birth.[10] Intravenous glucose was provided for severe or symptomatic hypoglycemia.[11] Patients development and behavior was examined at 4 years of age. There were no significant differences between children with normoglycemia and hypoglycemia < 40 mg/dL at 1 hour or < 45 mg/dL subsequently.[10] There were no differences in any of the test scores between hypoglycemic children who had and who had not been treated with intravenous glucose.[10]

It is clear that 47 mg/dL is not the critical threshold for injury from low glucose levels. In fact, a value < 47 mg/dL is more important after 48 hours than it is the first 48 hours. Continuous glucose monitoring demonstrates that despite aggressive treatment, infants identified with hypoglycemia experience up to 5 hours of hypoglycemia. All agree that there needs to be a considerable margin of safety in setting thresholds. Current practice is based largely on expert opinion, which for almost 50 years hasn't agreed on whether transient low glucose concentrations in healthy neonates is a normal physiologic variation or a marker of aberrant metabolism with risk of injurious neuroglycopenia.[11-13]

D. H. Adamkin, MD

References

1. Committee on Fetus and Newborn, Adamkin DH. Clinical report-postnatal glucose homeostasis in late-term and preterm infants. *Pediatrics*. 2011;127:575.
2. McKinley, et al. *Undetected Hypoglycemia and Outcome at 4.5 Years*. Baltimore, MD: Pediatric Research; 2016:753916.
3. Adamkin DH. Metabolic screening and postnatal glucose homeostasis in the newborn. *Pediatr Clin North Am*. 2015;62:385-409.
4. Cornblath M, Odell GB, Levin E. Symptomatic Neonatal hypoglycemia associated toxemia of pregnancy. *J Pediatr.* 1959;55:545-562.
5. Simmons R, Stanley C. Neonatal Hypoglycemia Studies: is there a sweet story of success yet? *N Engl J Med*. 2015;373:16.
6. Lucas A, Morley R, Cole TJ. Adverse neurodevelopmental outcome of moderate neonatal hypoglycemia. *BMJ*. 1988;297:1304-1308.
7. Lucas A, Morley R, Cole TJ. Randomized trial of early diet in preterm babies and later intelligence quotient. *BMJ*. 1998;318:195.
8. Tin W, Brunskill G, Kelly T, Fritz S. 15 year follow-up of recurrent "hypoglycemia: in preterm infants". *Pediatrics*. 2012;130:1497-1503.
9. Kaiser JR, Bai S, Gibson N, et al. Association between transient newborn hypoglycemia and fourth-grade achievement test proficiency: a population-based study. *JAMA Pediatr.* 2015;169:913-921.
10. Brand PLP, Molenaar NLD, Kaaijk WS. Neurodevelopmental outcome of hypoglycemia in healthy, large for gestational age, term newborns. *Arch Dis Child*. 2005;90:78-81.

11. McKinley JD, Harding JE. Revisiting traditional hypoglycemia only time will tell. *JAMA Pediatr.* 2015;169:10.
12. Boluyt N, van Kempen A, Offringa M. Neurodevelopment after neonatal hypoglycemia. *Pediatrics.* 2006;117:2231-2243.
13. Stanley CA, Rozance PJ, Thornton PS, et al. Re-evaluating "transitional neonatal hypoglycemia". *J Pediatr.* 2015;166:1520-1525.

Neonatal Glycemia and Neurodevelopmental Outcomes at 2 Years

McKinlay CJD, for the CHYLD Study Group (Univ of Auckland, New Zealand)

N Engl J Med 373:1507-1518, 2015

Background.—Neonatal hypoglycemia is common and can cause neurologic impairment, but evidence supporting thresholds for intervention is limited.

Methods.—We performed a prospective cohort study involving 528 neonates with a gestational age of at least 35 weeks who were considered to be at risk for hypoglycemia; all were treated to maintain a blood glucose concentration of at least 47 mg per deciliter (2.6 mmol per liter). We intermittently measured blood glucose for up to 7 days. We continuously monitored interstitial glucose concentrations, which were masked to clinical staff. Assessment at 2 years included Bayley Scales of Infant Development III and tests of executive and visual function.

Results.—Of 614 children, 528 were eligible, and 404 (77% of eligible children) were assessed; 216 children (53%) had neonatal hypoglycemia (blood glucose concentration, <47 mg per deciliter). Hypoglycemia, when treated to maintain a blood glucose concentration of at least 47 mg per deciliter, was not associated with an increased risk of the primary outcomes of neurosensory impairment (risk ratio, 0.95; 95% confidence interval [CI], 0.75 to 1.20; $P = 0.67$) and processing difficulty, defined as an executive-function score or motion coherence threshold that was more than 1.5 SD from the mean (risk ratio, 0.92; 95% CI, 0.56 to 1.51; $P = 0.74$). Risks were not increased among children with unrecognized hypoglycemia (a low interstitial glucose concentration only). The lowest blood glucose concentration, number of hypoglycemic episodes and events, and negative interstitial increment (area above the interstitial glucose concentration curve and below 47 mg per deciliter) also did not predict the outcome.

Conclusions.—In this cohort, neonatal hypoglycemia was not associated with an adverse neurologic outcome when treatment was provided to maintain a blood glucose concentration of at least 47 mg per deciliter. (Funded by the Eunice Kennedy Shriver National Institute of Child Health and Human Development and others.)

▶ Hypoglycemia is a common metabolic problem in neonatal medicine, and maintaining glucose homeostasis is one of the important physiologic events during fetal-to-neonatal transition. Although frequently observed transient low blood glucose levels in the majority of healthy newborns are the reflections of normal metabolic adaptation during this transition, there has been a genuine concern that prolonged or recurrent low blood glucose levels in newborn infants at a high risk of hypoglycemia may result in acute systemic effects and long-term neurologic consequences. Hence, it is not surprising that the caregivers get obsessed with the numbers and figures felt to be a "cutoff" for its definition.

There has been much controversy about the "functional" definition of neonatal hypoglycemia, a blood glucose level below which the risk of long term neurodevelopmental consequences would be imposed. The systematic review of all the available data until 2006 by Boluyt et al concluded that none of the 18 eligible studies they identified provided a valid estimate of neonatal hypoglycemia on neurodevelopment.[1] However, there has been widespread acceptance for nearly 30 years that a blood glucose level of 47 mg/dL (2.6 mmol/L) should be used to define neonatal hypoglycemia, profoundly influenced by the important observational data from babies with birth weight <1850 grams, reported by Lucas et al in 1988, that the number of days on which moderate hypoglycemia (glucose concentration <2.6 mmol/L or <47 mg/dL) occurred was strongly related to reduced mental and motor development at 18 months of age, even after adjustment for a wide range of factors known to influence development.[2] It was not long before clinicians were extrapolating this retrospective observational data from preterm babies and assuming that all newborn babies could be equally at risk from similar blood glucose levels, even when they seemed normal on clinical examination.[3] More recently published data from the prospectively planned, 15-year follow-up study comparing the outcomes of preterms (<32 weeks' gestation) with "hypoglycemia" and the matched controls found no evidence to support the belief that recurrent low blood glucose levels of <2.6 mmol/L or <47 mg/dL posed a hazard to preterm babies.[4]

A prospective cohort study by McKinlay and his colleagues has made an important contribution to the literature and debate in defining and managing hypoglycemia in late preterm and term infants who are at risk. The investigators used the widely accepted blood glucose level of <47 mg/dL to define neonatal hypoglycemia and concluded that it was not associated with an adverse neurologic outcome when treatment was provided with an aim to maintain that level. The method of measuring the masked interstitial glucose concentrations continuously in addition to the routine practice of intermittent blood glucose measurements is unique and has strengthened the study. This method has provided additional important information that nearly a quarter of infants in this study had low blood glucose levels that were not detected by intermittent monitoring, highlighting the limitations of previous observational studies that attempted to correlate blood glucose levels and neurodevelopmental outcomes, and also highlighting the high risk of "sampling bias" in the retrospective observational study by Lucas et al.[2] The other strength of this study is a comprehensive assessment of the skills that are most likely to be affected by neonatal hypoglycemia. One unexpected finding of this study is the association of cognitive delay with higher glucose concentrations. The authors should be given credit for not overanalyzing this observation, but this finding has raised the potential harmful effect of overzealous and rapid correction of hypoglycemia in otherwise "asymptomatic" newborn infants.

Much progress has been made in our understanding of the causes and mechanisms of glucose homeostasis in the early postnatal life. However, the definition of hypoglycemia for newborns at high risk remains elusive. It is most important that we accept the knowledge gaps[5] and develop a collaborative research agenda to address the questions surrounding the management of neonatal hypoglycemia.

W. Tin, FRCPCH

References

1. Boyult N, van Kempen A, Offringa M. Neurodevelopment after neonatal hypoglycemia: a systematic review and design of an optimal future study. *Pediatrics.* 2006; 117:2231-2243.
2. Lucas A, Morley R, Cole TJ. Adverse neurodevelopmental outcome of moderate neonatal hypoglycaemia. *BMJ.* 1988;317:1481-1487.
3. Cornblath M, Schwartz R, Aynsley-Green A, et al. Hypoglycemia in infancy: the need for rational definition. A Ciba Foundation discussion meeting. *Pediatrics.* 1990;85:834-837.
4. Tin W, Brunskill G, Kelly T, et al. 15 Year follow-up of recurrent "hypoglycemia" in preterm infants. *Pediatrics.* 2012;130:e1497-e1503.
5. Hay WW, Raju TNK, Higgins RD, et al. Knowledge gaps and research needs for understanding and treating neonatal hypoglycemia: workshop report from Eunice Kennedy Shriver National Institute of Child Health and Human Development. *J Pediatr.* 2009;155:612-617.

Neonatal Glycemia and Neurodevelopmental Outcomes at 2 Years

McKinlay CJD, for the CHYLD Study Group (Univ of Auckland, New Zealand; et al)

N Engl J Med 373:1507-1518, 2015

Background.—Neonatal hypoglycemia is common and can cause neurologic impairment, but evidence supporting thresholds for intervention is limited.

Methods.—We performed a prospective cohort study involving 528 neonates with a gestational age of at least 35 weeks who were considered to be at risk for hypoglycemia; all were treated to maintain a blood glucose concentration of at least 47 mg per deciliter (2.6 mmol per liter). We intermittently measured blood glucose for up to 7 days. We continuously monitored interstitial glucose concentrations, which were masked to clinical staff. Assessment at 2 years included Bayley Scales of Infant Development III and tests of executive and visual function.

Results.—Of 614 children, 528 were eligible, and 404 (77% of eligible children) were assessed; 216 children (53%) had neonatal hypoglycemia (blood glucose concentration, <47 mg per deciliter). Hypoglycemia, when treated to maintain a blood glucose concentration of at least 47 mg per deciliter, was not associated with an increased risk of the primary outcomes of neurosensory impairment (risk ratio, 0.95; 95% confidence interval [CI], 0.75 to 1.20; P = 0.67) and processing difficulty, defined as an executive-function score or motion coherence threshold that was more than 1.5 SD from the mean (risk ratio, 0.92; 95% CI, 0.56 to 1.51; P = 0.74). Risks were not increased among children with unrecognized hypoglycemia (a low interstitial glucose concentration only). The lowest blood glucose concentration, number of hypoglycemic episodes and events, and negative interstitial increment (area above the interstitial glucose concentration curve and below 47 mg per deciliter) also did not predict the outcome.

Conclusions.—In this cohort, neonatal hypoglycemia was not associated with an adverse neurologic outcome when treatment was provided to maintain a blood glucose concentration of at least 47 mg per deciliter. (Funded by the Eunice Kennedy Shriver National Institute of Child Health and Human Development and others.)

▶ By increasing the serum glucose concentration below which concern is indicated, the recently issued statement on neonatal hypoglycemia from the Pediatric Endocrine Society has broadened catchment of infants who require diagnostic monitoring and intervention.[1] That statement acknowledges that these recommendations place a higher value on diagnostic certainty and a lower value on avoiding discomfort, inconvenience, and cost, with the objective of allowing prompt treatment to decrease risk of brain injury from persistent or recurrent severe hypoglycemia. Fear of the latter largely stems from extrapolation from evidence of the dangers of severe hypoglycemia in older subjects because there are remarkably few empirical data on the matter in neonates. That literature is flawed by its post hoc correlative nature, making it impossible to distinguish brain injury caused by hypoglycemia from hypoglycemia caused by brain injury or to exclude underlying causes (eg, genetic disorders) that may be responsible for both.

This report from New Zealand is an important contribution to our knowledge about this condition. These investigators prospectively evaluated outcomes at age 2 years in at-risk infants managed with the goal of maintaining blood glucose concentrations ≥47 mg/dL during the first 7 days after birth. There were no differences in rates of neurodevelopmental impairment (NDI) between infants who experienced hypoglycemia (blood glucose <47 mg/dL), severe hypoglycemia (blood glucose <36 mg/dL), recurrent hypoglycemia (≥3 episodes), or prolonged hypoglycemia (≥3 days) and those who did not. These observations indicate either that the treatment was effective or that hypoglycemia in the ranges observed was not a significant determinant of long-term neurodevelopment. In addition, interstitial glucose concentrations were continuously monitored but were not used to guide management. Nearly 1 in 4 infants had hypoglycemia that was not detected by intermittent blood glucose monitoring, and a similar proportion of those treated for hypoglycemia had low interstitial glucose concentrations for at least 5 hours. There was no increase in risk of NDI in infants with unrecognized and untreated hypoglycemia. These data suggest that the Pediatric Endocrine Society goals (blood glucose >50 mg/dL for the first 48 to 72 hours and >60 mg/dL thereafter) are too conservative. These authors point out their observation that many at-risk infants have periods of hypoglycemia that are not detected by intermittent testing supports criteria that provide a generous margin of safety, however and advise against lowering the treatment threshold below 47 mg/dL.

The abstract of the article does not describe some additional important observations. While failing to demonstrate an association between NDI and hypoglycemia in the first 7 days after birth, the data did reveal an association with higher glucose levels. Infants with maximum interstitial glucose concentrations >77 mg/dL during the first 12 hours and those with mean blood or interstitial glucose concentrations >70 or >76 mg/dL, respectively, during the first 48 hours had significantly greater risks of neurosensory impairment (NSI); similar effects on processing difficulty were not found. Notably, this association was evident at glucose concentrations that would not generally be considered to constitute hyperglycemia. Hypoglycemic infants who developed NSI had a steeper initial rise in interstitial glucose concentrations and higher concentrations for 12 hours after birth than those who did not. This pattern of higher interstitial glucose concentrations was seen only after treatment with dextrose, and the risk of NSI was related to the highest interstitial glucose concentration observed within 12 hours after the first episode; maximum values above the median were associated with a risk ratio of 1.77 (95% confidence interval, 1.01–3.11; $P = .047$; $n = 100$). Although these observations must be considered preliminary, they raise the question of whether aggressive treatment to increase marginal or low blood glucose levels, especially with rapid or overcorrection, may be associated with worse neurodevelopmental outcomes. Until ongoing trials provide evidence to guide aggressiveness of therapy, we may be well advised to approach infants who qualify for treatment of hypoglycemia with a gentle hand.

W. E. Benitz, MD

Reference

1. Thornton PS, Stanley CA, De Leon DD, et al. Recommendations from the Pediatric Endocrine Society for evaluation and management of persistent hypoglycemia in neonates, infants, and children. *J Pediatr.*. 2015;;167:238-245.

Outcome at 2 Years after Dextrose Gel Treatment for Neonatal Hypoglycemia: Follow-Up of a Randomized Trial

Harris DL, on behalf of the Children with Hypoglycaemia and their Later Development (CHYLD) Study Team (Newborn Intensive Care Unit Waikato District Health Board, Hamilton, New Zealand; et al)

J Pediatr 170:54-59, 2016

Objective.—To determine neurodevelopmental outcome at 2 years' corrected age in children randomized to treatment with dextrose gel or placebo for hypoglycemia soon after birth (The Sugar Babies Study).

Study Design.—This was a follow-up study of 184 children with hypoglycemia (<2.6 mM [47 mg/dL]) in the first 48 hours and randomized to either dextrose (90/118, 76%) or placebo gel (94/119, 79%). Assessments were performed at Kahikatea House, Hamilton, New Zealand, and included neurologic function and general health (pediatrician assessed), cognitive, language, behavior, and motor skills (Bayley Scales of Infant and Toddler Development, Third Edition), executive function (clinical assessment and Behaviour Rating Inventory of Executive Function- Preschool Edition), and vision (clinical examination and global motion perception). Coprimary outcomes were neurosensory impairment (cognitive, language or motor score below −1 SD or cerebral palsy or blind or deaf) and processing difficulty (executive function or global motion perception worse than 1.5 SD from the mean). Statistical tests were two sided with 5% significance level.

Results.—Mean (±SD) birth weight was 3093 ± 803 g and mean gestation was 37.7 ± 1.6 weeks. Sixty-six children (36%) had neurosensory impairment (1 severe, 6 moderate, 59 mild) with similar rates in both groups (dextrose 38% vs placebo 34%, relative risk 1.11, 95% CI 0.75-1.63). Processing difficulty also was similar between groups (dextrose 10% vs placebo 18%, relative risk 0.52, 95% CI 0.23-1.15).

Conclusions.—Dextrose gel is safe for the treatment of neonatal hypoglycemia, but neurosensory impairment is common among these children.

Trial Registration.—Australian New Zealand Clinical Trials Registry: ACTRN 12608000623392.

▶ Neonatal hypoglycemia is a common problem and is associated with brain injury,[1] neurodevelopmental delay,[2,3] visual impairment,[4] and behavioral issues.[5] This study from Harris et al adds another modality for the management of asymptomatic neonatal hypoglycemia.

The study was a follow-up of 184 children with hypoglycemia defined as a glucose <47 mg/dL in the first 48 hours of life. Patients were randomized to either dextrose or placebo gel (Sugar Babies Study). The infants considered to be at risk and followed over the first 48 hours with aggressive treatment to maintain plasma glucose levels above the prescribed definition of hypoglycemia are the same risk groups as the those identified in the American Academy of Pediatrics (AAP) guideline published in 2011 and ratified again in 2016.[6] However, the infants in the Sugar Babies Study were screened more frequently, for a longer duration, and used a higher glucose treatment threshold than the AAP guideline.

Using this threshold for neonatal hypoglycemia, almost half of the at-risk infants were diagnosed as having neonatal hypoglycemia. Feedings were encouraged, and if poor feeding was an issue, then the infant was given expressed breast milk or formula by syringe. The primary outcome of the study was treatment failure, defined as a plasma glucose concentration <47 mg/dL after 2 treatment attempts with the gel.

The study assessed both visual global motion perception and executive function into a single measure that they called "processing difficulty." Both of these assessments target cortical networks that may be susceptible to neonatal hypoglycemia. It is important to understand the tests and the basis for these because the outcome measures for neonatal hypoglycemia used vary from study to study among those that have been cited, suggesting impaired outcomes with transient hypoglycemia and those finding no correlation between outcome and transient hypoglycemia.

Magnetic resonance imaging of the brain in humans suggests that the occipital lobe may be vulnerable to injury caused by neonatal hypoglycemia, and a link between hypoglycemia and visual impairment has been previously reported.[4] There was particular interest in the visual global perception because it involves extrastriate visual areas within the dorsal visual cortical processing stream, which emanates from the occipital lobe.[7,8]

Executive function is a collective term for the skills required to learn and interact with the environment, including working memory, reasoning, task flexibility, and problem solving. These skills involve a network of areas within the brain.[9]

The neurodevelopmental outcomes at 2 years of age were available for 78% of the original hypoglycemic cohort. Rates of neurosensory impairment, processing difficulties, and multiple secondary growth and developmental outcomes were equivalent between the dextrose gel and placebo groups.

The rate of neurosensory impairment at 2 years of age was high at 35% for both groups, control and dextrose gel. Most of the neurosensory impairment was mild, and an overlapping cohort study with hypoglycemia treated below 47 mg/dL was not associated with increase risk of impairment compared with at-risk patients without hypoglycemia.[10]

The truth is that the results of both of these studies, Sugar Babies and the overlapping McKinlay study, will not change the opinions about the best strategy for screening and treating neonatal hypoglycemia. The glucose threshold argument at which treatment should be initiated to avoid neurologic injury will continue.[11] In fact, the Brown and Rozance editorial about dextrose gel concluded that the blood glucose concentration defining hypoglycemia in both studies was arbitrary and did not take into account the glucose levels during the rest of the first week of life. Finally, Brown and Rozance offer the opinion that a glucose <47 mg/dL is likely to be more clinically relevant after the first 3 days of age, when blood glucose concentrations should approach those of a normal adult >70 mg/dL.[11]

Even though Sugar Babies had a "negative" result, the study is useful for health care providers. Short-term outcomes for the at-risk patients showed significant benefit to the dextrose gel as a treatment for asymptomatic hypoglycemia.[1] Infants randomized to dextrose gel had significantly less treatment failure, defined as a glucose <47 mg/dL after 2 treatment attempts with the dextrose gel or placebo. Treatment with the dextrose gel also lowered rates of neonatal intensive care admissions for hypoglycemia, with a number needed to treat of 8. Rebound hypoglycemia within 6 hours (12%) and recurrent hypoglycemia (within 48 hours of birth) in 24% were similar between groups.[12]

The gel appears to be safe and can reduce risks related to treatment of hypoglycemia such as decreased breastfeeding and may also decrease health care costs. Treatment with the gel did not place outcomes in jeopardy compared with more traditional treatment at a follow-up of 2 years of age.[1]

D. H. Adamkin, MD

References

1. Burns CMM, Rutherford MA, Boardman JP, Cowan FM. Patterns of cerebral injury and neurodevelopmental outcomes after symptomatic neonatal hypoglycemia. *Pediatrics*. 2008;122:65-74.
2. Kerstjens JM, Bocca-Tjeertes IF, de winter AF, Reijineveld SA, Bos AF. Neonatal morbidities and developmental delay in moderately preterm-born children. *Pediatrics*. 2012;130:265-272.
3. Lucas A, Morley R, Cole TJ. Adverse neurodevelopmental outcome of moderate neonatal hypoglycemia. *BMJ*. 1988;297:1304-1308.
4. Tam EW, Widjaja E, Blaser SI, MacGregor DL, Satodia P, Moore AM. Occipital lobe injury and cortical visual outcomes after neonatal hypoglycemia. *Pediatrics*. 2008;122:507-512.
5. Stenninger E, Flink R, Eriksson B, Bahlen C. Long term neurological dysfunction and neonatal hypoglycemia after diabetic pregnancy. *Arch Dis Child Fetal Neonatal Ed*. 1988;79:F174-F179.
6. Adamkin DH. Postnatal glucose homeostasis in late-preterm and term infants. *Pediatrics*. 2011;127:575-579.
7. Alkalay AL, Flores-Sarnat HB, Moser FG, Simmons CF. Brain imaging findings in neonatal hypoglycemia: case report and review of 23 cases. *Clin Pediatr (Phila)*. 2005;44:783-790.
8. Braddick OJ, O'Brian JM, Wattam-Bell J, Atkinson J, Hartley T, Turner R. Brain areas sensitive to coherent visual motion. *Perception*. 2001;30:61-72.
9. Collette F, Van der Linden M. Brain imaging of the central executive component of working memory. *Neurosci Biobehav Rev*. 2002;26:105-125.
10. McKinlay CJ, Alsweiler JM, Ansell JM, et al. Neonatal glycemia and neurodevelopmental outcomes at 2 years. *N Engl J Med*. 2015;373:1507-1518.
11. Brown LD, Rozance PJ. A sweet addition for the treatment of neonatal hypoglycemia. *J Pediatr*. 2016;170:10-12.
12. Harris DL, Weston PJ, Signal M, Chase JG, Harding JE. Dextrose gel for neonatal hypoglycemia (the Sugar Babies Study): a randomized, double-blind, placebo-controlled trial. *Lancet*. 2013;382:2077-2083.

Radiographic depiction of intra-abdominal fat in newborns: a marker of infants born to diabetic mothers

Ponrartana S, Goodarzian F, Emadi S, et al (Univ of Southern California, Los Angeles, CA)
J Perinatol 36:389-391, 2016

Objective.—To examine whether the presence of intra-abdominal fat (IAF) in newborns is diagnostic of infants of diabetic mothers (IDMs), and determine whether IAF is merely the consequence of increased body size.

Study Design.—Abdominal radiographs of 277 neonates >34 weeks gestational age (147 male and 130 female) were reviewed to determine the presence of IAF. Unpaired *t*-test and regression analyses were used to examine the influence of gestational age, birth weight, birth length and maternal diabetes on the prevalence and thickness of IAF.

Result.—The prevalence of IAF was higher in IDMs (41.2% vs 13.2%; $P < 0.0001$)—an association that persisted even after accounting for sex, gestational age and weight. Both birth weight and maternal diabetic status

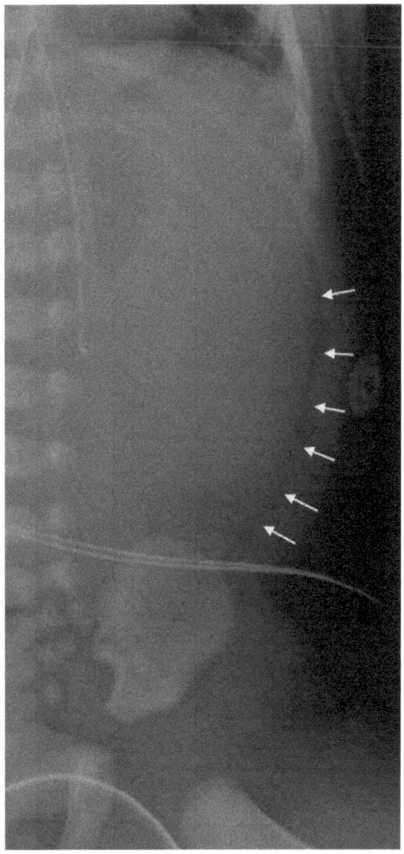

FIGURE 1.—Anterior–posterior abdominal radiograph of a 10-h-old-male infant of diabetic mother. Coned-down view of the left abdomen depicting substantial intra-abdominal fat (white arrows). (Reprinted from Ponrartana S, Goodarzian F, Emadi S, et al. Radiographic depiction of intra-abdominal fat in newborns: a marker of infants born to diabetic mothers. *J Perinatol.* 2016;36:389-391, with permission from Nature America, Inc.)

influenced the amount of IAF. Values of IAF thickness in IDMs were, however, more than threefold greater than those in non-IDMs (2.53 ± 2.08 vs 0.81 ± 0.29 mm; $P < 0.0001$). An IAF thickness >1.5 mm was indicative of an IDM.

Conclusion.—The depiction of IAF in radiographs is significantly more prevalent in IDMs when compared with non-IDMs, regardless of body size. A thickness of IAF >1.5 mm is a marker that should encourage work-up for the physiological, metabolic and congenital complications associated with IDM (Fig 1).

▶ This study compared intra-abdominal fat in newborns who were infants of diabetic mothers (IDMs) to determine radiographically whether intra-abdominal fat is different between these 2 groups and whether the intra-abdominal fat relates to body size in these individuals. Thirty-four IDMs and 243 control infants were evaluated using radiographs similar to that shown in Fig 1. All anterior-posterior abdominal radiographs were independently reviewed by 2 pediatric radiologists to determine the presence or absence of intra-abdominal fat. The intra-abdominal fat thickness in IDMs was approximately 3 times as much as in non IDMs.

Intra-abdominal fat is often considered to be related to metabolic syndrome in adults. The cause of this finding in this study is unclear but likely is due to increased fat production secondary to high levels of insulin. Whether this plays a role in future risk of obesity, diabetesm and cardiovascular disease is not known at this time, but the fact that using plain radiographs to evaluate intra-abdominal fat is exciting and could lead to additional studies that do not require more sophisticated equipment for visceral fat imaging. Future studies using these techniques could be exciting.

J. Neu, MD

Neonatal and early infancy management of prenatally detected hydronephrosis

Swords KA, Peters CA (Children's Natl Health System, Washington, DC)
Arch Dis Child Fetal Neonatal Ed 100:F460-F464, 2015

Hydronephrosis discovered during prenatal ultrasound will often resolve spontaneously; however, it should be evaluated in the postnatal period in a manner commensurate with its risk of renal injury. Early intervention is appropriate in cases of bladder outlet obstruction or the severely obstructed solitary kidney. In most other cases, it is both safe and reasonable to allow the possibility of spontaneous improvement with the intensity of follow-up based on the severity of the hydronephrosis. Clinical decision making should be a shared process between families and caregivers.

► Clinical ambiguity in medical decision making is a common occurrence. The management of many clinical scenarios presses the clinician to use not only best evidence (which is often limited) but also best practice based on clinical experience. The base foundation for this approach is to mitigate the risk for the patient in terms of reducing unnecessary procedures and investigations.

Kelly and Peters provide an excellent review of neonatal and early infancy management of prenatally detected hydronephrosis. Given the frequency and variability in quality of prenatal ultrasonography, defining specific criteria for follow-up and investigation is an important clinical initiative. Indeed, the authors provide a clinical pathway based on the Society for Fetal Urology's prenatal hydronephrosis grading system and management. Although this clinical pathway provides a reasonable and rational approach to infants with prenatally diagnosed hydronephrosis, it does not provide insight into the potential underlying pathology.

The majority of prenatally diagnosed hydronephrosis is unilateral and improves after birth, the authors emphasize that patients with bilateral hydronephrosis and solitary kidneys with more severe hydronephrosis need more immediate attention in terms of specialist referral, laboratory work-up, and medical imaging. Given our emerging understanding of early renal parenchymal damage and long-term renal disability,[1] this review provides a timely and thoughtful approach to management of this often-confusing clinical scenario.

P. D. Brophy, MD, MHCDS

Reference

1. Nogueira PC, Paz IP. Signs and symptoms of developmental abnormalities of the genitourinary tract. *J Pediatr (Rio J)*. 2016;92:S57-S63.

12 Miscellaneous

Choosing Wisely in Newborn Medicine: Five Opportunities to Increase Value

Ho T, Dukhovny D, Zupancic JAF, et al (Beth Israel Deaconess Med Ctr, Boston, MA; et al)

Pediatrics 136:e482-e489, 2015

Background.—The use of unnecessary tests and treatments contributes to health care waste. The "Choosing Wisely" campaign charges medical societies with identifying such items. This report describes the identification of 5 tests and treatments in newborn medicine.

Methods.—A national survey identified candidate tests and treatments. An expert panel of 51 individuals representing 28 perinatal care organizations narrowed the list over 3 rounds of a modified Delphi process. In the final round, the panel was provided with Grading of Recommendation, Assessment, Development and Evaluation (GRADE) literature summaries of the top 12 tests and treatments.

Results.—A total of 1648 candidate tests and 1222 treatments were suggested by 1047 survey respondents. After 3 Delphi rounds, the expert panel achieved consensus on the following top 5 items: (1) avoid routine use of antireflux medications for treatment of symptomatic gastroesophageal reflux disease or for treatment of apnea and desaturation in preterm infants, (2) avoid routine continuation of antibiotic therapy beyond 48 hours for initially asymptomatic infants without evidence of bacterial infection, (3) avoid routine use of pneumograms for predischarge assessment of ongoing and/or prolonged apnea of prematurity, (4) avoid routine daily chest radiographs without an indication for intubated infants, and (5) avoid routine screening term-equivalent or discharge brain MRIs in preterm infants.

Conclusions.—The Choosing Wisely Top Five for newborn medicine highlights tests and treatments that cannot be adequately justified on the basis of efficacy, safety, or cost. This list serves as a starting point for quality improvement efforts to optimize both clinical outcomes and resource utilization in newborn care.

▶ This article does not represent the typical approach to clinical problems. Rather, it addresses the critical roles of evidence-based medicine, patient safety, waste, and cost-savings but, at the same time, enhancing the quality of care.

This article follows the example of the American Board of Internal Medicine Foundation's "Choosing Wisely" campaign, which encourages "physicians, patients, and other healthcare stakeholders to think and talk about medical tests and procedures that may be unnecessary." The American Academy of Pediatrics (AAP) joined the Choosing Wisely campaign in 2013. This article represents the stellar effort from a pediatric subspecialty group. After a comprehensive search for evidence including surveys and literature reviews, they used a sophisticated consensus-building method to make recommendations that enhance inpatient newborn care.

The methodology to determine the 5 neonatal tests that were considered wasteful and not evidence based was complex but is detailed in the article. A panel of 51 experts reduced the initial 2870 suggestions by 1047 survey respondents to the Top Five list. In my opinion, the list was thoughtfully constructed and appropriate. By following these guidelines, patient safety will not be compromised, but costs will be reduced.

Currently, there is gross overuse of antireflux medications. The evidence does not support their use. The apneic or desaturation spells that have been attributed to reflux when carefully monitored actually precede the reflux episodes. Also, overuse of antibiotics has been associated with many harmful outcomes. These include but are not limited to an increase in late-onset infections, necrotizing enterocolitis, and death in both term and preterm infants. Changes in the biome induced by antibiotics may be associated with inflammatory bowel disease. The potential cost savings from reducing exposure to antibiotics in babies who do not have evidence of infection is enormous.

Restricting the use of x-rays, pneumograms, and routine MRIs should not be difficult to implement. There is reason for optimism that the "Choosing Wisely" program will be accepted in the neonatal community as neonatologists are comfortable when guided by "evidence." Neonatology has recently not found magical bullets of the caliber of antenatal corticosteroids, surfactant therapy, continuous positive airway pressure, and hypothermia for hypoxic ischemic encephalopathy. To optimize outcomes, we need to practice safely and as a comprehensive team applying the evidence and guidelines that are available. "Choosing Wisely" takes baby steps forward in these endeavors.

A. A. Fanaroff, MD

A Multifaceted Approach to Improving Outcomes in the NICU: The Pediatrix 100 000 Babies Campaign

Ellsbury DL, Clark RH, Ursprung R, et al (Pediatrix Med Group, Sunrise, FL)
Pediatrics 137:e20150389, 2016

Background and Objective.—Despite advances in neonatal medicine, infants requiring neonatal intensive care continue to experience substantial morbidity and mortality. The purpose of this initiative was to generate large-scale simultaneous improvements in multiple domains of care in a large neonatal network through a program called the "100 000 Babies Campaign."

Methods.—Key drivers of neonatal morbidity and mortality were identified. A system for retrospective morbidity and mortality review was used to identify problem areas for project prioritization. NICU system analysis and staff surveys were used to facilitate reengineering of NICU systems in 5 key driver areas. Electronic health record–based automated data collection and reporting were used. A quality improvement infrastructure using the Kotter organizational change model was developed to support the program.

Results.—From 2007 to 2013, data on 422 877 infants, including a subset with birth weight of 501 to 1500 g (n = 58 555) were analyzed. Key driver processes (human milk feeding, medication use, ventilator days, admission temperature) all improved ($P < .0001$). Mortality, necrotizing enterocolitis, retinopathy of prematurity, bacteremia after 3 days of life, and catheter-associated infection decreased. Survival without significant morbidity (necrotizing enterocolitis, severe intraventricular hemorrhage, severe retinopathy of prematurity, oxygen use at 36 weeks' gestation) improved.

Conclusions.—Implementation of a multifaceted quality improvement program that incorporated organizational change theory and automated electronic health record–based data collection and reporting program resulted in major simultaneous improvements in key neonatal processes and outcomes.

▶ Quality improvement (QI) works. This report by Ellsbury et al demonstrated significant improvement in human milk feeding, medication use, ventilator days, admission temperature, mortality, necrotizing enterocolitis, severe retinopathy of prematurity, and oxygen use at 36 weeks' gestation. They used information from a very large database to identify the key drivers of morbidity and mortality and used an organizational change model to support the QI program. The strength of this project is the availability of enormous numbers (422 877 infants over a 7-year period, with 58 555 with birth weights between 501 and 1500 g) within a single, structured organization. The major weakness was reliance on an electronic health record, which is only as good as the quality and reliability of the inputted data.

What distinguishes this QI endeavor, however, was its focus on changes in the organizational model. In 1999, the Institute of Medicine called for fundamental changes to improve patient safety and the quality of health care in the United States. It suggested that we shift our health care culture from "name and blame" to promotion of patient safety and challenged health care systems to redesign processes and systems to identify and address errors, establish performance standards, and set safety expectations.[1] The authors of the present study are to be congratulated for doing just that. The next challenge will to be to maintain or even exceed what they have accomplished.

S. M. Donn, MD

Reference

1. Kohn LT, Corrigan JM, Donaldson MS, eds.: To Err is Human: Building a Safer Health System. Institute of Medicine (US) Committee on Quality of Health Care in America. Washington, DC: National Academies Press; 2000.

A Multifaceted Approach to Improving Outcomes in the NICU: The Pediatrix 100 000 Babies Campaign

Ellsbury DL, Clark RH, Ursprung R, et al (Pediatrix Med Group, Sunrise, FL)

Pediatrics 137:e20150389, 2016

Background and Objective.—Despite advances in neonatal medicine, infants requiring neonatal intensive care continue to experience substantial morbidity and mortality. The purpose of this initiative was to generate large-scale simultaneous improvements in multiple domains of care in a large neonatal network through a program called the "100, 000 Babies Campaign."

Methods.—Key drivers of neonatal morbidity and mortality were identified. A system for retrospective morbidity and mortality review was used to identify problem areas for project prioritization. NICU system analysis and staff surveys were used to facilitate reengineering of NICU systems in 5 key driver areas. Electronic health record–based automated data collection and reporting were used. A quality improvement infrastructure using the Kotter organizational change model was developed to support the program.

Results.—From 2007 to 2013, data on 422 877 infants, including a subset with birth weight of 501 to 1500 g (n = 58 555) were analyzed. Key driver processes (human milk feeding, medication use, ventilator days, admission temperature) all improved ($P < .0001$). Mortality, necrotizing enterocolitis, retinopathy of prematurity, bacteremia after 3 days of life, and catheter-associated infection decreased. Survival without significant morbidity (necrotizing enterocolitis, severe intraventricular hemorrhage, severe retinopathy of prematurity, oxygen use at 36 weeks' gestation) improved.

Conclusions.—Implementation of a multifaceted quality improvement program that incorporated organizational change theory and automated electronic health record–based data collection and reporting program resulted in major simultaneous improvements in key neonatal processes and outcomes.

▶ After the widespread use of antenatal corticosteroids for preterm births and surfactant, we witnessed a dramatic fall in mortality for infants with a birth weight <1500 g. This has been followed by much slower declines over the past 15 years and almost a plateau in neonatal mortality. There remains wide global disparities with the most outstanding survival for extremely low birth weight reported from Japan and unacceptably high rates still prevalent in the developing countries. The border of viability has progressively dropped and guidelines for the expectant management at the borders of viability been published by many countries.

Taking advantage of their huge database and large number of neonatal units under their control, the Pediatrix group has undertaken and now published an impressive quality improvement program. This is no small achievement, and they are to be complimented and congratulated for what they have achieved.

Indeed, this group has come a long way into the research and education arenas after many years of predominantly clinical service. In this article, the Pediatrix authors describe the processes in detail to accomplish increased survival with decreased short-term morbidity. Their goal was attained so that mortality, necrotizing enterocolitis, retinopathy of prematurity, and infections all decreased. At the same time, survival without the major morbidities (necrotizing enterocolitis, severe intraventricular hemorrhage, severe retinopathy of prematurity, oxygen use at 36 weeks' gestation) improved. The process was long and complicated, but the end justifies the means as there was buy-in to a huge culture change, resulting in restructuring of neonatal intensive care unit care and improved clinical outcomes. The objective must be to sustain and even further improve these outcomes.

A. A. Fanaroff, MD

Effect of early low-dose hydrocortisone on survival without bronchopulmonary dysplasia in extremely preterm infants (PREMILOC): a double-blind, placebo-controlled, multicentre, randomised trial

Baud O, for the PREMILOC trial study group (Université Paris Diderot, France; et al)

Lancet 387:1827-1836, 2016

Background.—Bronchopulmonary dysplasia, a major complication of extreme prematurity, has few treatment options. Postnatal steroid use is controversial, but low-dose hydrocortisone might prevent the harmful effects of inflammation on the developing lung. In this study, we aimed to assess whether low-dose hydrocortisone improved survival without bronchopulmonary dysplasia in extremely preterm infants.

Methods.—In this double-blind, placebo-controlled, randomised trial done at 21 French tertiary-care neonatal intensive care units (NICUs), we randomly assigned (1:1), via a secure study website, extremely preterm infants inborn (born in a maternity ward at the same site as the NICU) at less than 28 weeks of gestation to receive either intravenous low-dose hydrocortisone or placebo during the first 10 postnatal days. Infants randomly assigned to the hydrocortisone group received 1 mg/kg of hydrocortisone hemisuccinate per day divided into two doses per day for 7 days, followed by one dose of 0·5 mg/kg per day for 3 days. Randomisation was stratified by gestational age and all infants were enrolled by 24 h after birth. Study investigators, parents, and patients were masked to treatment allocation. The primary outcome was survival without bronchopulmonary dysplasia at 36 weeks of postmenstrual age. We used a sequential analytical design, based on intention to treat, to avoid prolonging the trial after either efficacy or futility had been established. This trial is registered with ClinicalTrial.gov, number NCT00623740.

Findings.—1072 neonates were screened between May 25, 2008, and Jan 31, 2014, of which 523 were randomly assigned (256 hydrocortisone, 267 placebo). 255 infants on hydrocortisone and 266 on placebo were included in analyses after parents withdrew consent for one child in each group. Of the 255 infants assigned to hydrocortisone, 153 (60%) survived without bronchopulmonary dysplasia, compared with 136 (51%) of 266 infants assigned to placebo (odds ratio [OR] adjusted for gestational age group and interim analyses 1·48, 95% CI 1·02–2·16, $p = 0{\cdot}04$). The number of patients needed to treat to gain one bronchopulmonary dysplasia-free survival was 12 (95% CI 6–200). Sepsis rate was not significantly different in the study population as a whole, but subgroup analyses showed a higher rate only in infants born at 24–25 weeks gestational age who were treated with hydrocortisone (30 [40%] of 83 *vs* 21 [23%] of 90 infants; sub-hazard ratio 1·87, 95% CI 1·09–3·21, $p = 0{\cdot}02$). Other potential adverse events, including notably gastrointestinal perforation, did not differ significantly between groups.

Interpretation.—In extremely preterm infants, the rate of survival without bronchopulmonary dysplasia at 36 weeks of postmenstrual age was significantly increased by prophylactic low-dose hydrocortisone. This strategy, based on a physiological rationale, could lead to substantial improvements in the management of the most premature neonates.

▶ Publication of the largest randomized controlled trial (RCT) of early low-dose hydrocortisone (HC) to prevent BPD comes after a decade-long hiatus in publication of glucocorticoid trials for BPD. In contrast to the only previous large RCT of this therapy (PROPHET study of 360 infants[1]), this study reports that HC therapy resulted in a significant increase in survival without BPD (60% vs 51%, $P = .04$). HC-treated patients were also significantly more likely to be extubated at the end of the treatment period, more likely to wean from supplemental oxygen by 36 weeks' gestation, and less likely to undergo patent ductus arteriosus (PDA) ligation. The rate of death before discharge neared significance for the overall study population (19% vs 25%, $P = .08$) and was significantly lower in the 26- to 27-week gestational age stratum (8% vs 15%). Importantly, there was no increase in spontaneous gastrointestinal perforation in the HC-treated group (5% vs 4%). These findings bring 2 questions to mind: (1) Why are these study results different from the PROPHET study? and (2) Should we now treat extremely preterm infants with early low-dose hydrocortisone?

Why might the results differ? Many factors may have contributed: for example, the mean gestational age of these patients was greater (26.4 vs 25.2 weeks), the time of randomization was earlier (16 vs 32 hours), and previous exposure to HC was an exclusion factor, whereas 8% of HC-treated infants in the PROPHET study were on HC at study start. Caffeine therapy has increased and ventilation strategies have changed during the intervening years, and 20% of these infants were not intubated at study entry. However, 1 major factor is likely to be indomethacin exposure: 75% of the infants in the PROPHET study received indomethacin vs none in the PREMILOC study (ibuprofen was given to 47% of the HC group and 55% of the placebo group). In addition to the adverse synergy of indomethacin and glucocorticoid with regard to spontaneous GI perforation, investigators from the TIPP trial have reported that indomethacin was associated with an increased incidence of bronchopulmonary dysplasia in infants without a PDA.[2]

And should we consider treating extremely preterm infants with early low-dose hydrocortisone? The answer may be a cautious and limited "yes." Both studies found that HC treatment resulted in a significant increase in survival without BPD for chorioamnionitis-exposed infants; the PROPHET study also found HC was associated with a significant decrease in mortality in this group. Although the pathologic diagnosis of histologic chorioamnionitis is not immediately available, intrauterine inflammation/infection is present in about 50% of pregnancies delivering at < 30 weeks' gestation. Deliveries that occur for reasons other than maternal indication, poor fetal growth, or placental insufficiency have a substantial likelihood of antecedent intrauterine inflammation, and such infants may well benefit from early low-dose HC therapy. Neurodevelopmental and growth outcomes of the PROPHET study at 18 to 22 months were reassuring,[3] and we eagerly await the results of the 2-year follow-up of the PREMILOC infants.

K. Watterberg, MD

References

1. Watterberg KL, Gerdes JS, Cole CH, et al. Prophylaxis of early adrenal insufficiency to prevent bronchopulmonary dysplasia: a multicenter trial. *Pediatrics.* 2004;114:1649-1657.
2. Schmidt B, Roberts RS, Fanaroff A, et al. Indomethacin prophylaxis, patent ductus arteriosus, and the risk of bronchopulmonary dysplasia: further analyses from the Trial of Indomethacin Prophylaxis in Preterms (TIPP). *J Pediatr.* 2006;148: 730-734.
3. Watterberg KL, Shaffer ML, Mishefske MJ, et al. Growth and neurodevelopmental outcomes after early low-dose hydrocortisone treatment in extremely low birth weight infants. *Pediatrics.* 2007;120:40-48.

Fetal suprarenal masses—assessing the complementary role of magnetic resonance and ultrasound for diagnosis

Flanagan SM, Rubesova E, Jaramillo D, et al (Univ of Minnesota Med School, Minneapolis; Lucile Packard Children's Hosp, Stanford, CA; The Children's Hosp of Philadelphia, PA)
Pediatr Radiol 46:246-254, 2016

Objective.—To assess the value and complementary roles of fetal MRI and US for characterization and diagnosis of suprarenal masses.

Materials and Methods.—We conducted a multi-institutional retrospective database search for prenatally diagnosed suprarenal masses between 1999 and 2012 and evaluated the roles of prenatal US and fetal MRI for characterization and diagnosis, using postnatal diagnosis or surgical pathology as the reference standard. Prenatal US and fetal MRI were assessed for unique findings of each modality.

Results.—The database yielded 25 fetuses (gestational age 20–37 weeks) with suprarenal masses. Twenty-one fetuses had prenatal

US, 22 had MRI, 17 had both. Postnatal diagnoses included nine subdiaphragmatic extralobar sequestrations, seven adrenal hemorrhages, five neuroblastomas (four metastatic), two lymphatic malformations, one duplex kidney with upper pole cystic dysplasia, and one adrenal hyperplasia. Ultrasound was concordant with MRI for diagnoses in 12/17 (70.6%) cases. Discordant diagnoses between US and MRI included three neuroblastomas and two adrenal hemorrhages. In the three neuroblastomas US was equivocal and MRI was definitive for neuroblastoma, demonstrating heterogeneous, intermediate-signal solid masses and liver metastases. In the two cases of adrenal hemorrhage US was equivocal and MRI was definitive with signal characteristics of hemorrhage. In 2/4 neuroblastomas, Doppler US demonstrated a systemic artery suggesting extralobar sequestration; however MRI signal characteristics correctly diagnosed neuroblastoma. All cases of extralobar sequestration were correctly diagnosed by US and MRI.

Conclusion.—US and MRI both accurately detect suprarenal masses. MRI complements US in equivocal diagnoses and detects additional findings such as liver metastases in neuroblastoma (Table 2).

▶ Adrenal masses in the fetus and newborn are not common but always cause for concern. Purely cystic neuroblastomas are often discovered prenatally. As the main differential diagnosis is adrenal hemorrhage, all would agree that follow-up sonography is warranted after birth.

Surprisingly, there is on occasion complete resolution of the lesion before birth.

Neonatal adrenal hemorrhage, which accounts for the majority of suprarenal masses, is present in 0.2% of newborns. Ten percent of the cases occur bilaterally. It can be associated with birth trauma, large birth weight, or neonatal course complicated by hypoxia and asphyxia, hypotension, or coagulopathy. It may be asymptomatic or may present with flank abdominal mass, anemia, jaundice, or rarely as scrotal bruising or hematoma. The infants may require treatment for shock and hypotension.

Note too that adrenal cystic lesions may be associated with Beckwith-Wiedemann syndrome, and bronchopulmonary sequestration may present as a suprarenal mass. An adrenal abscess in a neonate is another rare condition causing an adrenal mass. The abscess may be drained under ultrasonographic guidance.

Yao et al[1] present a series of 28 patients with adrenal masses encountered over 8 years. They offer some insight into the investigation of these masses including imaging and urine vanillylmandelic acid measurements. They emphasize continued and repeated observation noting that delay in diagnosis for a month will not affect the outcome of a neuroblastoma.

Calisti et al,[2] after a review of 23 neonatal adrenal masses, concluded that there are no clear criteria to differentiate adrenal hemorrhage from neuroblastoma. Whereas the inference of spontaneous regression of the mass is that it is hemorrhage some neuroblastomas will also regress spontaneously. As histology is available only in operated or biopsied cases, "there are not a reliable set of signs for early differentiation and to reduce repeated, invasive investigations."

TABLE 2.—Typical US and MRI Characteristics of Suprarenal Masses

Lesion	US Characteristics	MRI Characteristics
Neuroblastoma	Variable (echogenic, solid, cystic or heterogeneous)	Heterogeneous or high T2 signal intensity (SI)
Extralobar sequestration	Solid, echogenic, "reverse teardrop" appearance	High T2 SI
Adrenal hemorrhage	Cystic or complex with septations	Heterogeneous SI on T1 and T2
Lymphatic malformation	Cystic with septations	High T1, infiltrating the retroperitoneum
Dysplastic duplex kidney	Heterogeneous, echogenic mass with cysts	Cystic changes in the upper pole of a duplex kidney
Adrenal hyperplasia	Bilateral mass-like adrenals	Bilateral, same SI as adrenals

SI signal intensity.

Reprinted from Flanagan SM, Rubesova E, Jaramillo D, et al. Fetal suprarenal masses—assessing the complementary role of magnetic resonance and ultrasound for diagnosis. *Pediatr Radiol.* 2016;46:246-254, with permission from Springer-Verlag Berlin Heidelberg.

Flanagan et al provide valuable insights into the evaluation of fetal suprarenal masses assessing the complementary role of magnetic resonance (MRI) and ultrasound (US) for diagnosis. Table 2 is particularly helpful in summarizing the differences between these 2 modalities. Prenatal US diagnosis was concordant with postnatal diagnosis in 15 of 21 cases, and prenatal MRI diagnosis was concordant with postnatal diagnosis in all cases. Prenatal US and prenatal MRI diagnoses were concordant in 14 of 18 cases; 4 cases had equivocal or discordant diagnoses between MRI, including 3 neuroblastomas and 1 adrenal hemorrhage and US. US and MRI both accurately detect suprarenal masses. MRI complements US for equivocal diagnoses including neuroblastoma, adrenal hemorrhage, and bronchopulmonary sequestration. MRI detects findings that are often missed on US, such as liver metastases. I learned that approximately 10% to 15% of extra lobar sequestrations occur below the diaphragm, and approximately 75% occur on the left side. Unlike extralobar sequestrations, 75% of cases of adrenal hemorrhage occur on the right side.

A. A. Fanaroff, MD

References

1. Yao W, Li K, Xiao X, Zheng S, Chen L. Neonatal suprarenal mass: differential diagnosis and treatment. *J Cancer Res Clin Oncol.* 2013;139:281-286.
2. Calisti A, Oriolo L, Molle P, Miele V, Spagnol L. Neonatal adrenal masses: do we have reliable criteria for differential diagnosis and expectant management? *Minerva Pediatr.* 2012;64:313-318.

Clarifying nipple confusion

Zimmerman E, Thompson K (Northeastern Univ, Boston, MA)
J Perinatol 35:895-899, 2015

Nipple confusion, an infant's difficulty with or preference for one feeding mechanism over another after exposure to artificial nipple(s), has been widely debated. This is in part due to conflicting statements, one by the American Academy of Pediatrics in 2005 suggesting that infants should be given a pacifier to protect against Sudden Infant Death Syndrome, and the other by the World Health Organization in 2009 stating that breastfeeding infants should never be given artificial nipples. Despite the limited and inconsistent evidence, nipple confusion is widely believed by practitioners. Therefore, there is a unique opportunity to examine the evidence surrounding nipple confusion by assessing the research that supports/refutes that bottle feeding/pacifier use impedes breastfeeding efficacy/success/duration. This review examined 14 articles supporting and refuting nipple confusion. These articles were reviewed using the Johns Hopkins Nursing Evidence-Based Practice Rating Scale. Based on our review, we have found emerging evidence to suggest the presence of nipple confusion only as it relates to bottle usage and found very little evidence to support nipple confusion with regards to pacifier use. The primary difficulty in conclusively studying nipple confusion is establishing causality, namely determining whether bottles'/pacifiers' nipples are causing infants to refuse the breast or whether they are simply markers of other maternal/infant characteristics. Future research should focus on prospectively examining the causality of nipple confusion.

▶ "Nipple confusion" is a term that has been very confusing to me. I have experienced situations in the neonatal intensive care unit (NICU) in which babies were kept on prolonged intravenous feedings and/or tube feedings because parents, nurses, and even neonatologists did not want to feed these babies with a bottle that was attached to a nipple. I have been informed that there are NICUs in the United States that have tried to adopt techniques used in India where specialized cups are used to feed infants instead of feeding them with an artificial nipple and a bottle. One of the "10 steps" in the Baby Friendly initiative also strongly discourages use of an artificial nipple.

This article reviews the evidence related to this and comes to the conclusion that the evidence for pacifiers causing "nipple confusion" is insufficient to suggest against usage. In terms of nipple use on bottles for bottle-feeding, they find 6 studies, 2 of which provide no evidence for and 4 studies that provide evidence for nipple confusion. Of interest is that the studies that provide evidence for nipple confusion also associate with babies who are being fed by bottles with nipples who are also in the process of being weaned, babies with preexisting breastfeeding problems who were being provided with nipples, and other confounding factors.

The authors conclude that the evidence for nipple confusion in babies who are occasionally fed a bottle with a nipple is not strong and state that additional studies of causality are needed. I agree. The evidence that would support that an occasional use of a bottle with a nipple will confuse a baby to the point of no longer accepting breastfeeding currently appears very weak at best. Until there is better data to the contrary, I will continue to recommend a bottle over a nasogastric tube or prolonged intravenous nutrition in my NICU babies whose mothers may temporarily be unable to breastfeed their babies.

J. Neu, MD

Congenital Tibial Deficiency: A 37-Year Experience at 1 Institution

Clinton R, Birch JG (Texas Scottish Rite Hosp for Children, Dallas)

J Pediatr Orthop 35:385-390, 2015

Background.—The purpose of this study is to evaluate all cases of tibial deficiency seen at a single institution from 1975 to 2012, to classify these cases by the Jones classification if possible, to evaluate for associated anomalies, and to review the surgical treatments provided to these patients.

Methods.—Ninety-five patients (125 extremities) treated at our institution between 1975 and 2012 with tibial deficiency had complete records allowing for classification and review of full treatment course. These patients' records and imaging were retrospectively reviewed for any associated anomalies, surgical treatment performed, and limb deformity characterized by the Jones classification where possible.

Results.—Seventy-three of 125 limbs (58%) were classified as Jones type 1A, 6 (5%) as type 1B, 18 (14%) as type 2, and 12 (10%) as type 4. Two limbs initially classified radiographically as type 3 deformities subsequently developed a proximal tibia epiphyses and thus did not represent true type 3 deformities. Fourteen limbs (11%) were characterized by global tibial deficiency but with proximal and distal epiphyses and could not be classified according to the Jones classification. Seventy-five of the 95 patients (79%) had associated anomalies. Other lower extremity anomalies were most frequent; however, upper extremity, spine, and visceral anomalies were also noted.

Conclusions.—True type 3 deformity as described by Jones was not seen in our patient population; all patients developed a proximal epiphysis. Therefore, this group may be better served by limb salvage than amputation. Fourteen (11%) limbs, characterized by global tibia shortening relative to the fibula of variable degree, could not be classified according to the Jones classification. We propose adding this group as a new group within the Jones classification, which we call type 5. Finally, in this patient population, the Brown procedure for type 1 tibial deficiency universally failed, confirming results of prior studies.

Level of Evidence.—This is a level IV study, a retrospective review of 95 patients with tibial deficiency from a single institution (Fig 1).

▶ Limb defects may occur in isolation, associated with other anomalies or as part of a syndrome. Some may be drug induced (eg, thalidomide), whereas many in utero are associated with vascular thrombosis. Most neonatologists deal commonly with deformities associated with amniotic bands, polydactyly, syndactyly, and the occasional limb reduction. These anomalies are rare enough that it took 37 years for these authors to accumulate a series of 95 patients and 125 limbs with tibial anomalies. They focus on the Jones classification (Fig 1): type 1A has no tibia present, type 1B has a cartilaginous anlage of proximal tibia not ossified at birth, type 2 has a proximal but no distal tibia, type 3 has a distal tibia with the proximal tibia absent, and type 4 is characterized by diastasis of the distal tibia and fibula. Indeed, they did not encounter any patients with type 3. Three-quarters of the patients had associated anomalies. There has been a suggestion that there is a genetic element to these anomalies,[1] but family history was positive in only 3 of the 95 subjects. We conclude that there is still much to be learned about this rare anomaly. Andrikopoulos et al[2] reported that the prenatal detection rate of isolated fetal limb abnormalities ranges from 4% to 29.5%. To improve these numbers, they routinely imaged both upper and lower extremities, including all long bones, hands, feet, fingers, and toes. The additional time for the scan was less than 5 minutes. They identified 36 of 52 fetuses with isolated fetal limb anomalies, for a detection rate of 69% with no false positives. The authors concluded that "A minimal investment in time for detailed

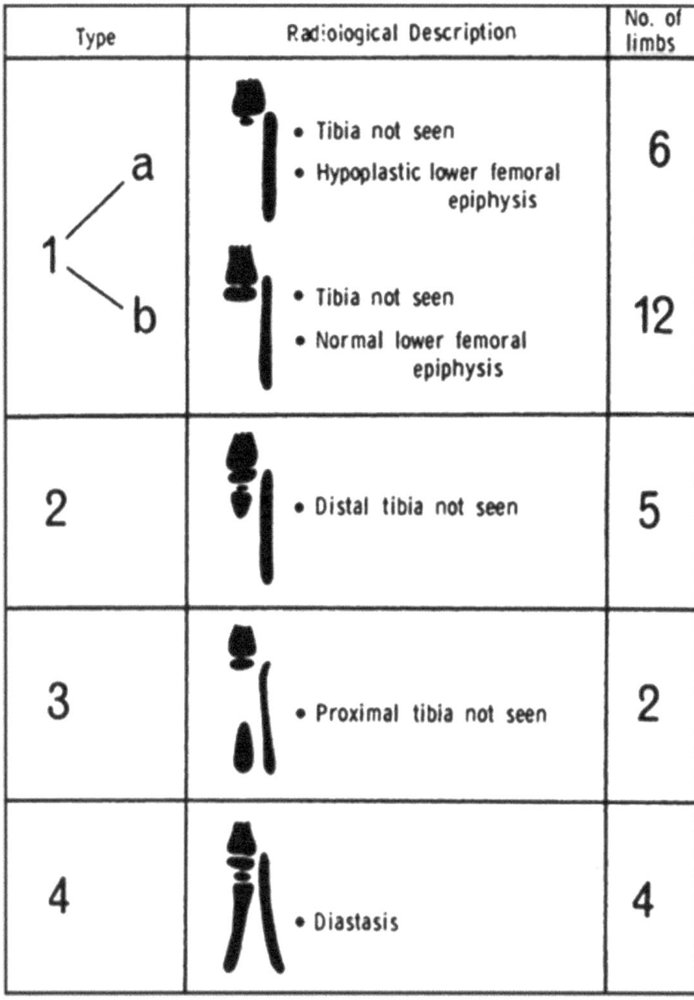

FIGURE 1.—Jones classification of tibial deficiency. Reproduced with permission and copyright © of the British Editorial Society of Bone and Joint Surgery [Jones et al[1]]. *Editor's Note*: Please refer to original journal article for full references. (Reprinted from Clinton R, Birch JG. Congenital tibial deficiency: a 37-year experience at 1 institution. *J Pediatr Orthop*. 2015;35:385-390, with permission from Wolters Kluwer Health, Inc.)

evaluation of fetal limbs more than doubles the previously reported prenatal detection rate."

A. A. Fanaroff, MD

References

1. Cho T-J, Baek GH, Lee H-R, et al. Tibial hemimelia-polydactyly- five-fingered hand syndrome associated with a 404 G > A mutation in a distinct sonic hedgehog cis-regulator (ZRS): a case report. *J Pediatr Orthop B*. 2013;22:219-221.

2. Andrikopoulou M, Vahanian SA, Chavez MR, Murphy J, Hanna N, Vintzileos AM. Improving the ultrasound detection of isolated fetal limb abnormalities. *J Matern Fetal Neonatal Med.* 2016;29:1-4.

Improving the Quality of Radiographs in Neonatal Intensive Care Unit Utilizing Educational Interventions

Gupta AO, Rorke J, Abubakar K (Al DuPont Hosp for Children, Wilmington, Delaware; MedStar Georgetown Univ Hosp, Washington, DC)
Am J Perinatol 32:980-986, 2015

Objective.—We aimed to develop an educational tool to improve the radiograph quality, sustain this improvement overtime, and reduce the number of repeat radiographs.

Study Design.—A three phase quality control study was conducted at a tertiary care NICU. A retrospective data collection (phase1) revealed suboptimal radiograph quality and led to an educational intervention and development of X-ray preparation checklist (primary intervention), followed by a prospective data collection for 4months (phase 2). At the end of phase 2, interim analysis revealed a gradual decline in radiograph quality, which prompted a more comprehensive educational session with constructive feedback to the NICU staff (secondary intervention), followed by another data collection for 6 months (phase 3).

Results.—There was a significant improvement in the quality of radiographs obtained after primary educational intervention (phase 2) compared with phase 1 ($p < 0.001$). During interim analysis after phase 2, radiograph quality declined but still remained significantly better than phase 1. Secondary intervention resulted in significant improvement in radiograph quality to > 95% in all domains of image quality. No radiographs were repeated in phase 3, compared with 5.8% (16/277) in phase 1.

Conclusion.—A structured, collaborated educational intervention successfully improves the radiograph quality and decreases the need for repeat radiographs and radiation exposure in the neonates (Table 2).

▶ I was intrigued by this article for 2 primary reasons. First, it is yet another example that quality improvement (QI), done properly, really works. Second, this is an area of significant importance in the neonatal intensive care unit: exposure of premature (and term) newborns to ionizing radiation. It is easy to lose track of the cumulative dosimetry to which our patients are exposed, and we tend to forget that the most metabolically active cells are the ones that absorb the most radiation. Any measure that can reduce unnecessary exposure would be worthwhile, saving not only radiation exposure but cost and, as a by-product, improving patient safety by producing higher quality images. The metrics used in this project are ones to which we ought to be paying attention, but often don't (such as application of gonadal shielding, not having

TABLE 2.—X-ray Preparation Checklist

1	Verify X-ray order
2	Check patient ID and name
3	Gonadal shield applied
4	Head midline for chest X-rays (CXR)
5	Arms secured to side
6	Chest leads attached to arms/side of the chest
7	Wires moved away from the X-ray field
8	ET tube suction/ventilator tubes out of X-ray field
9	Check ET marking at gum prior to CXR
10	Temp probe moved to side/disconnected
11	Remove gel pads or water heater blankets
12	Nothing on top of incubator within X-ray field

Abbreviations: CXR, chest X-rays; ET, endotracheal.
Reprinted from Gupta AO, Rorke J, Abubakar K. Improving the quality of radiographs in neonatal intensive care unit utilizing educational interventions. *Am J Perinatol*. 2015;32:980-986, with permission from Thieme Medical Publishers, Inc.

obstructive objects in the field of view, proper alignment of the head and neck, etc; see Table 2).

The study also reminds us of another aspect of QI: we can't rest on our laurels. We need to continually reinforce the interventions to avoid the complacency that leads to backsliding.

S. M. Donn, MD

Preterm Versus Term Children: Analysis of Sedation/Anesthesia Adverse Events and Longitudinal Risk

Havidich JE, Beach M, Dierdorf SF, et al (The Dartmouth Inst, Lebanon, NH; Riley Children's Hosp Indianapolis, IN; et al)
Pediatrics 137:e20150463, 2016

Background and Objectives.—Preterm and former preterm children frequently require sedation/ anesthesia for diagnostic and therapeutic procedures. Our objective was to determine the age at which children who are born <37 weeks gestational age are no longer at increased risk for sedation/anesthesia adverse events. Our secondary objective was to describe the nature and incidence of adverse events.

Methods.—This is a prospective observational study of children receiving sedation/anesthesia for diagnostic and/or therapeutic procedures outside of the operating room by the Pediatric Sedation Research Consortium. A total of 57 227 patients 0 to 22 years of age were eligible for this study. All adverse events and descriptive terms were predefined. Logistic regression and locally weighted scatterplot regression were used for analysis.

Results.—Preterm and former preterm children had higher adverse event rates (14.7% vs 8.5%) compared with children born at term. Our analysis revealed a biphasic pattern for the development of adverse sedation/anesthesia events. Airway and respiratory adverse events were most commonly reported. MRI scans were the most commonly performed procedures in both categories of patients.

Conclusions.—Patients born preterm are nearly twice as likely to develop sedation/anesthesia adverse events, and this risk continues up to 23 years of age. We recommend obtaining birth history during the formulation of an anesthetic/sedation plan, with heightened awareness that preterm and former preterm children may be at increased risk. Further prospective studies focusing on the etiology and prevention of adverse events in former preterm patients are warranted.

▶ Preterm infants are at increased risk for the development of adverse events related to sedation/anesthesia for operative procedures. However, it is unknown whether preterm or former preterm children receiving sedation/anesthesia outside of the operating room experience the same adverse events as children born at term. In this observational study, the investigators used data from the Pediatric Sedation Research Consortium (PSRC) to compare the current rate and nature of adverse sedation/anesthesia events through young adulthood for children born preterm to that for children born at term.

Forty-one locations participated in the study, including large children's hospitals, children's hospitals within hospitals, and community hospitals. The participating institutions were self-selected for involvement, and there were no specific selection criteria for participation in the consortium. Preterm was defined as < 37 weeks of gestational age, and subjects older than 22 years were excluded. To determine the effect of postgestational age on outcome a sensitivity analysis was performed in children 0 to 36 months of age.

Of the 57 227 children entered in the database, 685 (1.2%) were preterm. Administration of sedations/anesthetics was most frequently done by pediatric intensivists (59.2%). The most common procedures requiring sedation/anesthesia in the preterm group were magnetic resonance imaging (MRI) scans (57.5%), auditory brainstem response (ABR) testing (7.7%), and upper endoscopy (7.5%). In the term group, the most common procedures performed were MRI scans (41.7%), lumbar puncture (14.7%), and upper endoscopy (6.6%). The most common adverse events reported in the preterm group were oxygen desaturation (4.5%), coughing (3.4%), and airway obstruction (2.9%). In the term group, airway obstruction was the most common adverse event (2.0%), followed by coughing (1.9%) and oxygen desaturation (1.8%). Preterm and former preterm children had a higher risk for adverse events compared with term children (odds ratio 1.93 confidence interval 1.56–2.39) and were at higher risk to develop any adverse event regardless of age. As the investigators indicate in the discussion, a history of prematurity needs to be an essential part of screening prior to the administration of sedations/anesthetics.

L. A. Papile, MD

Rates of Complications After Newborn Circumcision in a Well-Baby Nursery, Special Care Nursery, and Neonatal Intensive Care Unit

Srinivasan M, Hamvas C, Coplen D (Washington Univ School of Medicine/St Louis Children's Hosp, MO)

Clin Pediatr 54:1185-1191, 2015

Objective/Method.—To determine rates of complications after newborn circumcision by performing a retrospective chart review of patients circumcised at a well-baby nursery, neonatal intensive care units (NICU), and special care nursery (SCN) from 2007 to 2012.

Result.—A total of 5129 babies (73%) were circumcised at the well-baby nursery and 1909 babies (27%) at the NICU and SCN. Forty-seven patients (0.67%, 95% CI 0.49% to 0.89%) had circumcision-related complications: 5 (0.07%) patients with acute and 42 (0.6%) with late complications. Babies in the NICU/SCN had increased odds of complication (OR 4.00, 95% CI 2.23 to 7.19) compared with those in well-baby nursery. There were increased odds of complications in babies with Caucasian ethnicity (OR 2.60, 95% CI 1.48 to 4.89) compared with African American babies and in babies with private insurance (OR 4.0, 95% CI 2.1 to 7.5) compared with nonprivate insurance.

Conclusions.—The rates of complications after newborn circumcisions were low. Babies in the NICU/SCN had increased odds of complication.

▶ Srinivasan and colleagues reviewed the complication rate of neonatal circumcision in a total of 7038 infants, of whom 1909 had been circumcised as patients in their neonatal intensive care unit (NICU) or special care nursery (SCN), while 5129 had the procedure performed at in the well baby nursery (WBN). This was a retrospective review of the frequency of complications, and the population studied was considerably smaller than the majority of such studies performed over the past 40+ years. What makes the study unique is that the authors assessed the complication rate in a group of infants who had been "sick" and were hospitalized in either the NICU or SCN, recovered, and were within several days of discharge at the time of the procedure.

They noted an overall complication rate of 0.67% (approximately 7 per 1000 procedures). "Acute" complications (undefined, but occurring within 0–13 days) occurred in 5 infants (0.07% or 7 in 10 000 procedures). These consisted of (1) a small glans laceration not requiring intervention, (2) minimal bleeding 2 days after circumcision that was managed with local pressure, (3) purported bleeding 13 days after the procedure that was not noted by medical personnel and had no intervention, and (4) 2 infants requiring blood transfusion within 24 hours of the procedure because of "excessive bleeding." Forty-two infants (0.6%) had "late" complications, mainly consisting of redundant foreskins or skin bridges requiring minor repair. There was no loss of glans or other tissue, nor were there any deaths. It is not stated in the article, but it appears that all of the infants with "late complications" were managed as outpatients. Overall, circumcised infants that had been hospitalized in the NICU or SCN were 5.2-fold more likely to require an intervention than those who were hospitalized in the WBN.

The circumcision complication rate was 1.5% for the NICU/SCN infants compared with 0.4% in WBN boys. Both infants that required blood transfusion had been NICU/SCN patients.

A couple of thoughts: there are no data concerning the level of expertise of those performing the procedures (residents vs fellows and staff physicians). The complication rate found in this article is "in the neighborhood" of that found in the 2 most recent large studies that have addressed this issue (~0.2% in the latter studies published in Refs[1,2]). Surprisingly, Srinivasan and colleagues did not reference the latter articles, despite patient populations 20- to 50-fold greater than in their review. The major take-home message of this article is that although complications are relatively low among neonates circumcised close to discharge following admission to the NICU or SCN (1.5%), they are more common than in well infants (0.2%–0.5%).

In addition, clinicians should take note that the complication rate after circumcision performed during later childhood or as adults is higher than in those performed during the newborn hospitalization.[3,4] It appears be "safer" to be circumcised at the end of the newborn hospitalization in the WBN or NIC/SCN than having circumcision performed later in life.

T. E. Wiswell, MD

References

1. Wiswell TE, Geschke DW. Risks from circumcision during the first month of life compared with those for uncircumcised boys. *Pediatrics.* 1989;83:1011-1015.
2. *Pediatrics.* 2000;105:246-249.
3. Wiswell TE, Tencer HL, Welch CA, Chamberlain JL. Circumcision in children beyond the neonatal period. *Pediatrics.* 1993;92:791-793.
4. Morris BJ, Waskett JH, Banerjee J. A 'snip' in time: what is the best age to circumcise? *BMC Pediatr.* 2012;12:20.

13 Pharmacology

Medication Use in the Neonatal Intensive Care Unit

Hsieh EM, on Behalf of the Best Pharmaceuticals for Children Act—Pediatric Trials Network (Duke-Natl Univ of Singapore Graduate Med School; et al)

Am J Perinatol 31:811-822, 2014

Objective.—The aim of the article is to provide an update on medication use in infants admitted to the neonatal intensive care unit (NICU) in the United States and examine how use has changed over time.

Study Design.—We performed a retrospective review (2005–2010) of a large prospectively collected administrative database.

Result.—Medications most commonly administered during the study period were ampicillin, gentamicin, caffeine citrate, vancomycin, beractant, furosemide, fentanyl, dopamine, midazolam, and calfactant (56–681 exposures per 1,000 infants). Those with the greatest relative increase in use included azithromycin, sildenafil, and milrinone. Medications with the greatest relative decrease in use included theophylline, metoclopramide, and doxapram.

Conclusion.—Medication use in the NICU has changed substantially over time, and only 35% of the most commonly prescribed medications are Food and Drug Administration – approved in infants.

► In this article, Hsieh et al reported in great detail on medication use in the neonatal intensive care unit (NICU). This study was conducted by investigators of the Pediatric Trials Network on behalf of Best Pharmaceuticals for Children Act (BPCA). The article highlighted the continued lack of safety and efficacy data in neonates based on appropriately designed clinical trials and associated problems. The subsequent increased off-label use of medications in the NICU is described, comparing their data from 2010 to a previous publication from 2005 that used the same database evaluated in the present study.[1]

The first 3 citations in this commentary are some of the few reports that have detailed drug use in NICU. These descriptive publications highlight significant gaps in knowledge regarding medication use in neonates. Most routinely used medications in the NICU are not approved for use in neonates by federal regulatory agencies such as the Federal Drug Administration (FDA), the European Medicines Agency (EMA), or other equivalent authorities around the world. In the United States, federal legislation (BPCA) has led to a significant increase in pediatric studies submitted to the FDA, resulting in new pediatric information in product labeling for new and existing drug molecules. However, approximately 50% of drug labels still have insufficient information on safety, efficacy, or dosing in children, and neonatal information in labeling is even more scarce because neonates comprise a vulnerable subpopulation for which response end points are difficult to define or develop because of continual maturational changes, and clinical research studies in neonates are methodologically more challenging. Given continual challenges of appropriate drug use in the NICU, the potential for medication errors and lack of appropriate dosing data,[2-5] medication use in neonates should be minimized. Drug selection should be based on dosing information on the selected agent. Factors to consider in off-label use of medications should include availability of even lower level of evidence (eg, case series, single patient experiences), experience and comfort level of the practitioner using the agent, and availability of a suitable dosage form that can be safely used in neonates. Expert opinion of clinical pharmacologists should also be sought if such consultative services are available.[6] Use of innovative methods such as data analysis of existing data or producing relevant data from routine use of drugs in NICU, use of residual plasma, serum, or cells to derive pharmacokinetic or pharmacogenomics knowledge as well as well designed pragmatic studies are all avenues to explore neonatal clinical pharmacology data in this extremely vulnerable population. Although some of these research methods are low cost, others may require significant funding. Private-public partnerships to produce drug-dosing data in neonates is highly desirable. This mission can be achieved through government regulations.[7,8] Until further data on appropriate and safe use of medications in neonates are available, caution should be exercised in off-label medications used in this population. First do no harm.

V. Bhatt-Mehta, PharmD, MS (CRDSA), FCCP

References

1. Clark RH, Bloom BT, Spitzer AR, Gerstmann DR. Reported medication use in the neonatal intensive care unit: data from a large national data set. *Pediatrics.* 2006; 117:1979-1987.
2. Laughon MM, Avant D, Tripathi N, et al. Drug labeling and exposure in neonates. *JAMA Pediatr.* 2014;168:130-136.
3. Medication Safety in the Neonatal Intensive care Unit. Position statement. National Association of Neonatal Nurses (NANN). July 2011.
4. Sentinel Event Alert. Issue 39: Preventing Pediatric Medication Errors. The Joint Commission. http://www.jointcommission.org/sentinel_event_alert_issue_39_preventing_pediatric_medication_errors/. Accessed June 2014.
5. Institute of Safe Medication Practice. Medication Safety Alert. Infant's death reinforces need for medications to be dispensed in ready-to-use form. Institute for Safe Medication Practices, 1998. http://www.ismp.org/newsletters/acutecare/articles/19980909_2.asp. Accessed June 2014.
6. Allegaert K, Langhendries JP, van den Anker JN. Do we need neonatal clinical pharmacologists? *Eur J Pediatr.* 2013;172:429-435.
7. Ruggieri L, Giannuzzi V, Baiardi P, et al; on behalf of the GRiP Consortium. Successful private-public funding of paediatric medicines research: lessons from the EU programme to fund research into off-patent medicines. *Eur J Pediatr.* 2015; 174:481-491.
8. Ward RM, Lane RH, Albertine KH. Basic and translational research in neonatal pharmacology. *J Perinatol.* 2006;26:S8-S12.

Gabapentin Use in the Neonatal Intensive Care Unit

Edwards L, DeMeo S, Hornik CD, et al (Duke Univ Med Ctr, Durham, NC; et al)

J Pediatr 169:310-312, 2016

Gabapentin was used for the treatment of term and preterm infants with suspected visceral hyperalgesia caused by a variety of neurologic and gastrointestinal morbidities. Improved feeding tolerance and decreased irritability were seen, as well as decreased usage of opioids and benzodiazepines. Adverse events occurred with abrupt discontinuation of this medication.

▶ In this retrospective case series, the authors report their experience using gabapentin, an analog of gamma-aminobutyric acid, to treat 11 infants who were presumed to have visceral hyperalgesia secondary to neurologic and gastrointestinal morbidities. Apparently, visceral hypersensitivity, defined as increased sensitivity to pain in the visceral system (ie, stomach, intestine, or pancreas), is the holy grail for gastrointestinal investigators and is presumed to be the reason for the development of functional gastrointestinal diseases.[1] Gabapentin is approved for the treatment of neuropathic pain, and there are previous reports of its use in the neonatal population.[2,3] All of the reported infants had a gastrostomy tube or a gastrojejunostomy tube, and 5 of the infants had tracheostomy tubes. The most notable outcome related to the use of benzodiazepines: 3 of the 9 infants who were receiving benzodiazepines were weaned off, and an additional 2 tolerated a lowering of their dose. It is difficult to ascertain from the report if there was any truly beneficial effect regarding feeding tolerance. Adverse events were reported in 5 of the infants, 3 of which were related to abrupt discontinuation of the medication when the infants were put on nothing by mouth. Hopefully, additional studies regarding pharmacokinetics, safety, and efficacy, particularly in preterm infants, are needed before gabapentin therapy gains traction in neonatal medicine.

L. A. Papile, MD

References

1. Camilleri M, Coulie B, Tack JF. Visceral hypersensitivity facts, speculations and challenges. *Gut*. 2001;48:125-131.
2. Haney AL, Garner SS, Cox TH. Gabapentin therapy for pain and irritability in a neurologically impaired infant. *Pharmacotherapy*. 2009;29:997-1001.
3. Behm MO, Kearns GL. Treatment of pain with gabapentin in a neonate. *Pediatrics*. 2001;108:482.

Randomised trial of early neonatal hydrocortisone demonstrates potential undesired effects on neurodevelopment at preschool age

Peltoniemi OM, for The Neonatal Hydrocortisone Working Group (Univ of Oulu, Finland)

Acta Paediatr 105:159-164, 2016

Aim.—We evaluated the neurodevelopment and growth of five- to seven-year-old children who had participated in a randomised trial of early low-dose hydrocortisone treatment to prevent bronchopulmonary dysplasia.

Methods.—The 51 infants in the original study had birthweights of 501–1250 g and gestational ages of 23–30 weeks, required mechanical ventilation during the first 24 hours and received hydrocortisone or a placebo for 10 days. The majority (80%) of the 90% who survived to five- to seven years of age participated in this follow-up study and their growth, neuromotor, cognitive and speech development were evaluated.

Results.—Some neurodevelopment impairment was observed in 61% of the hydrocortisone group and 39% of the placebo group, ranging from minor neurological dysfunction to severe neurological conditions ($p = 0.182$). The mean full-scale intelligence quotient (IQ) was 87.8 (15.3) in the hydrocortisone group and 95.7 (15.0) in the placebo group ($p = 0.135$), and the mean performance IQ was 88.3 (14.5) and 99.1 (14.0) ($p = 0.034$), respectively. A fifth (22%) of the hydrocortisone group required physiotherapy, but none of the placebo group did ($p = 0.034$). The age-standardised growth was comparable between both groups.

Conclusion.—Early hydrocortisone treatment may have undesired effects on neurodevelopment at preschool age, and further safety studies are required.

▶ Following a cluster of reports in the late 1990s of compromised neurodevelopmental outcomes, particularly cerebral palsy, in extremely low birth weight (ELBW) infants treated with dexamethasone in randomized controlled trials, use of dexamethasone in this population rapidly decreased. Within a decade, avoidance of dexamethasone became an indicator of quality of neonatal intensive care. The "siren call"[1] of steroid therapy for prevention or management of bronchopulmonary dysplasia, treatment of hypotension, or correction of hypothalamic-pituitary-adrenal insufficiency has persisted. Its lower potency and endogenous, nonsynthetic origin have made hydrocortisone an attractive alternative, but the indications for and benefits of hydrocortisone in ELBW infants remain controversial. This report provides what may be the first warning of potential adverse developmental effects of hydrocortisone exposure, but these observations must be viewed with caution. This trial was very small, enrolling only a total of 50 subjects, of whom only 36 were available for follow-up. The higher rate of neurodevelopmental impairment in the hydrocortisone group (61%, vs 39% in the control group) was not statistically significant. Of at least 25 outcomes evaluated, statistically significant differences, without adjustment for multiple comparisons, were found for only 2: mean performance

IQ (*P* = .034) and need for physiotherapy (*P* = .034). So far, similar effects have not been apparent in follow-up of nonrandomized exposures to hydrocortisone, and long-term results of other randomized trials have not yet been provided. These authors are correct in recommending collection of additional data to determine whether the trends in their data can be confirmed in larger trials. Until such confirmation is available, it will be premature to raise the alarm and abandon this therapy, as has been largely done with dexamethasone.

W. E. Benitz, MD

Reference

1. Finer NN, Craft A, Vaucher YE, et al. Postnatal steroids: short-term gain, long-term pain? *J Pediatr.* 2000;137:9-13.

A pilot randomized trial of high-dose caffeine therapy in preterm infants

McPherson C, Neil JJ, Tjoeng TH, et al (Brigham and Women's Hosp, Boston, MA; Boston Children's Hospital, Boston, MA; Univ of Hawaii, Honolulu; et al)

Pediatr Res 78:198-204, 2015

Background.—Standard-dose caffeine improves white matter microstructural development assessed by diffusion magnetic resonance imaging (MRI). We hypothesized that early high-dose caffeine would result in further improvement in white matter microstructural development.

Methods.—Seventy-four preterm infants (≤30 wk gestational age) were randomly assigned to either a high (80 mg/kg i.v.) or standard (20 mg/kg i.v.) loading dose of caffeine citrate in the first 24 h of life. MRI and neurobehavioral testing were undertaken at term equivalent age. Infants returned at 2 y of age for developmental testing.

Results.—Clinical characteristics were similar between groups, with the exception of higher maternal age in the high-dose caffeine group. There was an increased incidence of cerebellar hemorrhage in infants randomized to high-dose caffeine (36 vs. 10%, $P = 0.03$). Infants in the high-dose caffeine group also demonstrated more hypertonicity ($P = 0.02$) and more deviant neurologic signs ($P = 0.04$) at term equivalent age. Diffusion measures at term equivalent age and developmental outcomes at 2 y of age did not differ between groups.

Conclusion.—Preterm infants randomized to early high-dose caffeine had a higher incidence of cerebellar injury with subsequent alterations in early motor performance. The results of this pilot trial discourage a larger randomized controlled trial.

▶ If some is good, more is not necessarily better. This report builds on a randomized, controlled trial of high- versus standard-dose caffeine (40 mg/kg once + 10 mg/kg/d vs 10 mg/kg once + 2.5 mg/kg/d, respectively, expressed in quantity of caffeine base) conducted in Australia in the late 1990s.[1] That trial enrolled intubated infants less than 30 weeks of gestation at birth, 24 hours before anticipated extubation. The median age at enrollment was approximately 4 days (interquartile range, approximately 2 to 12 days). Infants in the high-dose group were significantly less likely to require reintubation. In this trial, the same doses were compared, but treatment was initiated within the first 24 hours after birth. Of more than 40 clinical outcomes examined, 3 secondary outcomes were significantly different, including the higher rate of cerebellar hemorrhage in the high-dose group. The conclusions in the abstract are necessarily terse, but those in the Discussion are exemplary in their prudence: "The increased incidence of cerebellar hemorrhage in ... infants randomized to high-dose caffeine indicates that caution should be exercised in considering further exploration of this dosing approach. Notably, this finding and other outcomes reported for this cohort beyond the primary endpoint must be viewed as post hoc. Utilization of high-dose caffeine therapy ... should be carefully considered, given the potential risks. Standard-dose caffeine, as described by the CAP trial, appears to be the best approach to reduce the duration of mechanical ventilation and improve neurodevelopmental outcomes of preterm infants."

W. E. Benitz, MD

Reference

1. Steer P, Flenady V, Shearman A, et al. High dose caffeine citrate for extubation of preterm infants: a randomised controlled trial. *Arch Dis Child Fetal Neonatal Ed.* 2004;89:F499-503.

Association of Early Caffeine Administration and Neonatal Outcomes in Very Preterm Neonates

Lodha A, for the Canadian Neonatal Network (Univ of Calgary, Alberta, Canada; et al)

JAMA Pediatr 169:33-38, 2015

Importance.—Advantages of caffeine for apnea of prematurity have prompted clinicians to use it prophylactically even before apnea.

Objective.—To determine the effect of early initiation of caffeine therapy on neonatal outcomes in very preterm infants born in Canada.

Design, Setting, and Participants.—A retrospective cohort study was conducted. Patients included preterm neonates born at less than 31 weeks' gestation admitted to 29 participating Canadian Neonatal Network neonatal intensive care units between January 1, 2010, and December 31, 2012.

Exposures.—Neonates who received caffeine were divided into 2 groups based on the following timing of caffeine initiation: within the first 2 days after birth (early) and on or after the third day following birth (late).

Main Outcome and Measure.—A composite of death or bronchopulmonary dysplasia.

Results.—Of 5517 eligible neonates, 5101 (92.5%) received caffeine (early: 3806 [74.6%]; late: 1295 [25.4%]). There was no difference in weight or gestational age at birth between the groups. Neonates in the early group had decreased odds of a composite outcome of death or bronchopulmonary dysplasia (adjusted odds ratio [AOR], 0.81; 95% CI, 0.67-0.98) and patent ductus arteriosus (AOR, 0.74; 95% CI, 0.62-0.89). There was no difference between the groups in mortality (AOR, 0.98; 95% CI, 0.70-1.37), necrotizing enterocolitis (AOR, 0.88; 95%CI, 0.65-1.20), severe neurological injury (AOR, 0.80; 95% CI, 0.63-1.01), or severe retinopathy of prematurity (AOR, 0.78; 95% CI, 0.56-1.10).

Conclusions and Relevance.—In very preterm neonates, early (prophylactic) caffeine use was associated with a reduction in the rates of death or bronchopulmonary dysplasia and patent ductus arteriosus. No adverse impact on any other outcomes was observed.

▶ The Caffeine for Apnea of Prematurity (CAP) Trial, conducted between 1999 and 2004 in 2000 infants with birth weights of 500 to 1250 g, demonstrated that treatment with caffeine (10 mg/kg caffeine base followed 2.5 mg/kg daily, beginning within 10 days after birth) resulted in reduced rates of bronchopulmonary dysplasia (oxygen at 36 weeks' postmenstrual age), less medical and surgical treatment to close a patent ductus arteriosus (PDA), and shorter durations of intubation, positive airway pressure, and oxygen supplementation.[1] Follow-up revealed increased survival without neurodevelopmental disability at 18 to 21 months.[2] This difference was no longer evident at 5 years of age,[3] leading some to question the utility of this treatment. It is not known whether those similar outcomes at age 5 years required differential application of early infant development or rehabilitation measures in infants found to have delays or impairments before age 2, so the early benefits of caffeine should not be glibly dismissed.

This report from the Canadian Neonatal Network provides additional evidence of benefit from caffeine treatment. These investigators compared outcomes in preterm infants for whom caffeine was initiated in the first 2 days (early) to those in infants whose treatment started on or after the third day after birth (late). After adjustment for gestational age, antenatal steroid exposure, small for gestational age, site, intubation on day 2, SNAP-II score, and surfactant administration, earlier treatment was associated with decreased odds of the composite outcome of death or bronchopulmonary dysplasia, oxygen use at 36 weeks, PDA diagnosis, and surgical PDA ligation. Although the 2-tailed confidence interval for the odds ratio for severe neurological injury (adjusted odds ratio [OR] = 0.80, 95% confidence interval 0.63–1.01) is not significant at $P < .05$, the 1-tailed upper confidence limit for that adjusted OR is 0.99 (ie, just significant at $P < .05$). The article ends with the requisite suggestion of a randomized controlled trial to more rigorously demonstrate an advantage of earlier initiation of this therapy. However, it seems unlikely that such a trial will be funded and completed. It might be argued that these data, in combination with those from the CAP Trial and other studies, will have to do and are sufficient to support routine use of caffeine in preterm infants, beginning on the first 2 days after birth.

W. E. Benitz, MD

References

1. Schmidt B, Roberts RS, Davis P, et al. Caffeine therapy for apnea of prematurity. *N Engl J Med.* 2006;354:2112-2121.
2. Schmidt B, Roberts RS, Davis P, et al. Long-term effects of caffeine therapy for apnea of prematurity. *N Engl J Med.* 2007;357:1893-1902.
3. Schmidt B, Anderson PJ, Doyle LW, et al. Survival without disability to age 5 years after neonatal caffeine therapy for apnea of prematurity. *JAMA.* 2012;307: 275-282.

Therapeutic drug monitoring in neonates

Pauwels S, Allegaert K (KU Leuven, Belgium)

Arch Dis Child 101:377-381, 2016

Therapeutic drug monitoring (TDM) aims to integrate drug measurement results into clinical decision making. The basic rules apply when using TDM in neonates (aminoglycosides, vancomycin, phenobarbital, digoxin), but additional factors should also be taken into account. First, due to both pharmacokinetic variability and nonpharmacokinetic factors, the correlation between dosage and concentration is poor in neonates, but can be overcome with the use of more complex, validated dosing regimens. Second, the time to reach steady state is prolonged, especially when no loading dose is used. Consequently, the timing of TDM sampling is important in this population. Third, the target concentration may be uncertain (vancomycin) or depend on specific factors (phenobarbital during whole body cooling). Finally, because of differences in matrix composition (eg, protein, bilirubin), assay-related inaccuracies may be different in neonates. We anticipate that complex validated dosing regimens, with subsequent TDM sampling and Bayesian forecasting, are the next step in tailoring pharmacotherapy to individual neonates.

▶ In this article, Pauwels et al discuss considerations in therapeutic drug monitoring (TDM) specific to neonates. Although most of the discussion regarding interindividual variability (such as factors affecting pharmacokinetics [PK] and pharmacodynamics [target range for response; PD]), factors affecting PK/PD, and analytical technique pros and cons are well addressed for neonatal TDM, a few points highlighted by the authors are worthy of comment.

Suggesting that because of "large variability in pharmacokinetics in neonates, therapeutic drug monitoring is more common in these patients, especially as validated dosing regimens are lacking" is true to an extent. Neonatal physiology is very fluid, changing from moment to moment, especially during critical illness and rapid organ maturation. The underlying illness may thus contribute significantly to drug disposition, leading to over- or undertreatment with any therapeutic agent. Because of reduced clearance of most drugs in neonates, especially those undergoing renal elimination, the effect of each therapeutic change may be significantly delayed. Frequent monitoring may not add that much to therapeutic responses, as each change requires achievement of a new steady-state plasma concentration before a full benefit of the change can be realized. However, it may also contribute to an adverse event if treatment decisions are changed too frequently. Thus, clinical judgment is required to determine the timing of TDM, and this must be balanced against excessive phlebotomy and iatrogenic anemia, as well as increased costs of care. In such situations, if the plasma concentration is not in the toxic range (manifested as adverse effects), frequent monitoring may be counterproductive.

Second, only a handful of drugs used in the neonatal population (aminoglycosides, vancomycin, phenobarbital, and digoxin, which is rarely given anymore) are easily amenable to TDM through analytical techniques that allow a rapid, timely turnaround of results that can be used for clinical decision making or where the neonatal physiology does not interfere with results (eg, bilirubin concentrations). TDM is not easily available for the vast majority of the other agents used in routine neonatal practice, including sedatives, analgesics, neuromuscular blocking agents, vasopressors, ibuprofen, and many antimicrobial agents.

Finally, the suggestion of using complex, valid regimens is intriguing. Complex regimens may allow more individualized drug therapies. However, from a practical aspect the prescribing and dispensing under such regimens may increase the risk of medication errors.

Regardless of the reason for using TDM, its frequency of use, or the drugs for which it is used, TDM will only become a meaningful clinical decision making tool if the fundamental understanding of the dose—concentration—effect relationships in neonatal diseases that takes into account the changing physiology and its effect on response is well understood, and true responses, and not surrogate markers, are used to guide therapies.[1]

V. Bhatt-Mehta, PharmD, MS, FCCP

References

1. Khalil F, Läer S. Physiologically based pharmacokinetic modeling: methodology, applications, and limitations with a focus on its role in pediatric drug development. *J Biomed Biotechnol.* 2014;16:1-13.

Achievement of Therapeutic Vancomycin Trough Serum Concentrations with Empiric Dosing in Neonatal Intensive Care Unit Patients

Ringenberg T, Robinson C, Meyers R, et al (The State Univ of New Jersey, Chicago, IL)

Pediatr Infect Dis J 34:742-747, 2015

Background.—The recommended goal serum trough concentration for vancomycin has increased to 10 to 20 mcg/mL, with a higher range of 15 to 20 mcg/mL for serious infections due to methicillin-resistant Staphylococcus aureus in children and adults. Although neonatal references have also recommended these higher target concentrations, dosing recommendations remained unchanged. The objective of this study was to assess the percentage of neonates and young infants achieving a serum trough concentration between 10 and 20 mcg/mL with empiric vancomycin dosing based on Neofax® in a neonatal intensive care unit (NICU) population.

Methods.—A multi-institutional retrospective chart review was conducted to identify NICU patients who received a minimum of three doses of intravenous vancomycin and had at least one appropriately drawn trough. Additional outcomes included the duration of vancomycin therapy, number of dose adjustments required to attain goal trough concentrations, time to goal trough, and incidence of nephrotoxicity and ototoxicity.

Results.—Of the 171 vancomycin serum trough concentrations included in the primary outcome, only 25.1% achieved a goal trough of 10 to 20 mcg/mL with empiric dosing. Only 44.6% of patients achieved the goal trough of 10 to 20 mcg/mL at any time during their vancomycin therapy. The average gestational age was 28.2 ± 4.1 weeks, average postnatal age at start of vancomycin was 34.1 ± 34.6 days, and average weight of the patients at start of vancomycin was 1602 ± 1014.5 g. The average and median total daily dose in those patients who achieved an initial vancomycin trough of 10–20 mcg/mL were 32.4 mg/kg/day and 30 mg/kg/day, respectively.

Conclusion.—Dosing of vancomycin based on Neofax® in NICU patients is insufficient in yielding serum trough concentrations of 10 to 20 mcg/mL. Further studies are needed to evaluate the optimal dosing regimen to achieve higher trough concentrations in this patient population.

▶ For more than 30 years, vancomycin has been used to treat penicillin-resistant infections in neonates, such as those caused by methicillin-resistant *Staphylococcus aureus* (MRSA) and coagulase-negative *Staphylococcus* (CoNS). These years of "experience" combined with recent intensified concerns regarding invasive MRSA infections have resulted in increasing use of vancomycin in many neonatal intensive care units (NICUs).[1] Almost 1 in 10 neonates admitted to a NICU are prescribed vancomycin during their hospitalization, trailing only ampicillin, gentamicin, and caffeine citrate in rate of medication exposure.[2] Yet despite frequent use of vancomycin in neonates, dosing remains a challenge in this population.

Fundamental to the safe and efficacious use of a drug is an understanding of its pharmacokinetics. This understanding is critical in the selection of an appropriate dose to achieve the desired exposure across a patient population. It is well known that a "one-size-fits-all" approach will not be an appropriate drug dosing strategy for neonates. Neonates are a very heterogeneous group, and large variation in vancomycin pharmacokinetics is seen between individual neonates due to differences in size, maturation, and kidney function.[3,4] Current dosing references such as Neofax, Redbook, and LexiComp take into consideration these key predictors in the empiric vancomycin dose selection for a neonate. For example, Neofax uses a dosing table categorized according to a neonate's postmenstrual age and postnatal age to recommend a dose (milligrams/kilograms) and dosing interval. However, dosing tables are inherently limited by the number of dose categories from which to choose. Neofax has only 6 vancomycin dose categories. In addition, large "jumps" in daily dose between adjacent categories may be created. The daily dose for a neonate with a postnatal age of 15 days is 50% higher dose than a neonate with a postnatal age of 14 days. Lastly, the recommended doses in Neofax (and Redbook and LexiComp) were developed to achieve vancomycin trough concentrations of 5 to 10 mcg/mL, the traditional target for CoNS infections. For invasive MRSA infections, higher trough concentrations of 10 to 20 mcg/mL are required to achieve exposures associated with treatment success.[5] Taken together, there is currently a discordance between our current vancomycin dosing strategies in neonates and the desired exposure target.

The study by Ringenberg and colleagues provides useful insight into the current challenges at hand with vancomycin dosing in neonates. They retrospectively examined trough concentrations in 171 neonates who received empiric vancomycin dosing based on Neofax. Only 25.1% of neonates achieved the target trough concentrations of 10 to 20 mcg/mL after empiric dosing, whereas 71.9% of neonates had trough concentrations that were considered low (< 10 mcg/mL). Equally significant is that in their study only 45% of neonates achieved the target trough concentration of 10 to 20 mcg/mL at any time during the course of therapy, even after therapeutic drug monitoring and dose adjustments were performed in an attempt to achieve this target. Clearly an updated approach to vancomycin dosing is needed in neonates to (1) maximize the likelihood that empiric dosing achieves upfront the exposure target of interest and (2) calculate dose adjustments in those not reaching target concentration with empiric dosing. So how do we get there? An innovative approach involves the use of clinical dosing support tools that leverage population pharmacokinetic models and Bayesian estimation methodology. By incorporating specific information about the patient (ie, weight, postmenstrual, and serum creatinine) and drug concentration data as they become available, an individualized dose can be calculated.[6] An exciting prospect is the ability to make these calculations available to clinicians via simple and intuitive user interfaces embedded within the electronic medical record. The technical platform is currently available and need only be implemented and integrated into clinical practice.

A. Frymoyer, MD, FAAP

References

1. Lessa FC, Edwards JR, Fridkin SK, Tenover FC, Horan TC, Gorwitz RJ. Trends in incidence of late-onset methicillin-resistant *Staphylococcus aureus* infection in neonatal intensive care units: data from the National Nosocomial Infections Surveillance System, 1995–2004. *Pediatr Infect Dis J.* 2009;28:577-581.
2. Hsieh EM, Hornik CP, Clark RH, et al. Medication use in the neonatal intensive care unit. *Am J Perinatol.* 2014;31:811-821.
3. Frymoyer A, Hersh AL, El-Komy MH, et al. Association between vancomycin trough concentration and area under the concentration-time curve in neonates. *Antimicrob Agents Chemother.* 2014;58:6454-6461.

4. Capparelli EV, Lane JR, Romanowski GL, et al. The influences of renal function and maturation on vancomycin elimination in newborns and infants. *J Clin Pharmacol.* 2001;41:927-934.
5. Liu C, Bayer A, Cosgrove SE, et al. Clinical practice guidelines by the Infectious Diseases Society of America for the treatment of methicillin-resistant *Staphylococcus aureus* infections in adults and children: executive summary. *Clin Infect Dis.* 2011;52:285-292.
6. Mould DR, D'Haens G, Upton RN. Clinical decision support tools: the evolution of a revolution. *Clin Pharmacol Ther.* 2016;99:405-418.

Using isopropyl alcohol impregnated disinfection caps in the neonatal intensive care unit can cause isopropyl alcohol toxicity

Sauron C, Jouvet P, Pinard G, et al (CHU Sainte-Justine, Montreal, Qubec, Canada)
Acta Paediatr 104:e489-e493, 2015

Aim.—The safety of SwabCap alcohol impregnated disinfection caps was questioned in our unit because of malfunctions in luer access valves. We examined whether SwabCaps affected the integrity of two luer access valves and were associated with alcohol injected into the lines.

Methods.—Our bench test study included seven circuits using SmartSite or CARESITE valves exposed to two environmental temperatures. Passive circuits consisted of a 96-hour contact system using SwabCap without other interventions. Active circuits consisted of nine sham injections during a 24-hour period, with the SwabCap replaced after each injection. The active control circuit used isopropyl alcohol impregnated pads to disinfect valves. Isopropyl alcohol was measured at the extremity of all active circuits by gas chromatography.

Results.—The visual appearance of all SmartSite valves and 67% of the CARESITE valves was changed by SwabCap use. The mean isopropyl alcohol dosages were 52 mmol/L in the SmartSite and 8 mmol/L in the CARESITE at room temperature and 73 and 7 mmol/L, respectively, at 35°C. No alcohol was found in the control circuit.

Conclusion.—The SwabCap altered the valves' appearance and allowed significant amounts of isopropyl alcohol to be injected. It should not be used for neonates without further research.

▶ I was drawn to this article by its title. It turned out to be a bench test in which isopropyl alcohol could be detected downstream of a mock IV circuit in which the luer lock access valves were cleansed with a commercially available device impregnated with isopropyl alcohol. It is, of course, not known whether this can be extrapolated to in vivo use in the neonatal intensive care unit, but it is another example of "environmental toxicity" to which our vulnerable population may be subjected. Moreover, this is virtually an unaccounted variable in clinical trials. Although neonatologists have become very familiar with toxicities of commonly prescribed pharmaceuticals, little is known about other chemicals that may be introduced, including isopropyl alcohol, plasticizers that leach from intravenous catheters and circuits, and other excipients. We would be wise to heed these messages.

S. M. Donn, MD

14 Postnatal Growth and Development/ Follow-up

Greater Early Gains in Fat-Free Mass, but Not Fat Mass, Are Associated with Improved Neurodevelopment at 1 Year Corrected Age for Prematurity in Very Low Birth Weight Preterm Infants

Ramel SE, Gray HL, Christiansen E, et al (Univ of Minnesota, Minneapolis)

J Pediatr 173:108-115, 2016

Objective.—This work investigates the relationship between early body composition changes and neurodevelopment at 1 year age corrected for prematurity (CA).

Study Design.—A prospective, longitudinal study to measure body composition weekly in 34 very low birth weight preterm infants using air displacement plethysmography, beginning when infants stabilized after birth until discharge. Neurodevelopmental testing (Bayley Scales of Infant Development-III) was performed at 12 months CA. Linear mixed effects models were used to obtain inpatient subject-specific changes in fat-free mass (FFM) and fat mass (FM), which were then used as predictors of Bayley subscale scores in subsequent linear regression models, adjusting for potential confounders. Protein and energy provision were calculated for the first week of life.

Results.—Greater FFM gains while inpatient were associated with improved cognitive and motor scores at 12 months CA ($P = .002$ for both). These relationships remained significant when adjusting for birth weight, gestational age, and intraventricular hemorrhage ($P \leq .05$ for both). Similar analysis was performed for FM gains without significant findings. Increased provision of protein and calories during the first week of life was positively associated with FFM gains ($P \leq .01$ for both), but not FM gains ($P \geq .2$ for both), throughout hospitalization.

Conclusions.—Increased FFM gains, but not FM gains, during hospitalization are associated with improved neurodevelopment at 12 months CA. As early FM gains may be associated with long-term risk, more research is needed to develop strategies that optimize FFM gains while minimizing FM gains in very low birth weight preterm infants.

▶ Accruing data from multiple published studies in the neonatal nutrition literature demonstrate the importance of early protein, lipid, and energy delivery (kcals/kg/day) in reducing the risk of acute neonatal morbidities such as bronchopulmonary dysplasia and retinopathy of prematurity and the risk of long-term neurodevelopmental impairment. These conclusions remain intact even after the adjustment for gestational age and severity of illness.

As a community, we have also learned that relying on nutrient calculations plus growth may not be sufficient in assessing for nutritional adequacy. In this study, Ramel et al use body composition testing to longitudinally evaluate the accrual of fat mass and fat-free mass and its impact on neurodevelopment at 12 months corrected age. The authors conclude that gains in fat free mass, not fat mass, are associated with improved long-term developmental outcomes. Importantly, increased early nutritional delivery in protein and total calories was associated with fat-free mass gains versus gains in fat mass, further solidifying the importance of nutritional delivery in the first postnatal week and possibly offering a mechanistic pathway through which early nutrition affects long-term outcomes.

Body composition data, in this case, accrual of fat-free mass versus fat mass, may offer better biomarkers of nutritional adequacy. The challenge now is to firmly establish the nutritional practices that lead to improved fat-free mass in our most critically ill, high-risk preterm infants.

C. Martin, MD

Neurodevelopmental outcome at 2 years of age after general anaesthesia and awake-regional anaesthesia in infancy (GAS): an international multicentre, randomised controlled trial

Davidson AJ, for the GAS consortium (Murdoch Childrens Res Inst, Melbourne, Victoria, Australia)

Lancet 387:239-250, 2016

Background.—Preclinical data suggest that general anaesthetics affect brain development. There is mixed evidence from cohort studies that young children exposed to anaesthesia can have an increased risk of poor neurodevelopmental outcome. We aimed to establish whether general anaesthesia in infancy has any effect on neurodevelopmental outcome. Here we report the secondary outcome of neurodevelopmental outcome at 2 years of age in the General Anaesthesia compared to Spinal anaesthesia (GAS) trial.

Methods.—In this international assessor-masked randomised controlled equivalence trial, we recruited infants younger than 60 weeks postmenstrual age, born at greater than 26 weeks' gestation, and who had inguinal herniorrhaphy, from 28 hospitals in Australia, Italy, the USA, the UK,

Canada, the Netherlands, and New Zealand. Infants were randomly assigned (1:1) to receive either awake-regional anaesthesia or sevoflurane-based general anaesthesia. Web-based randomisation was done in blocks of two or four and stratified by site and gestational age at birth. Infants were excluded if they had existing risk factors for neurological injury. The primary outcome of the trial will be the Wechsler Preschool and Primary Scale of Intelligence Third Edition (WPPSI-III) Full Scale Intelligence Quotient score at age 5 years. The secondary outcome, reported here, is the composite cognitive score of the Bayley Scales of Infant and Toddler Development III, assessed at 2 years. The analysis was as per protocol adjusted for gestational age at birth. A difference in means of five points (1/3 SD) was predefined as the clinical equivalence margin. This trial is registered with ANZCTR, number ACTRN12606000441516 and ClinicalTrials.gov, number NCT00756600.

Findings.—Between Feb 9, 2007, and Jan 31, 2013, 363 infants were randomly assigned to receive awake-regional anaesthesia and 359 to general anaesthesia. Outcome data were available for 238 children in the awake-regional group and 294 in the general anaesthesia group. In the as-per-protocol analysis, the cognitive composite score (mean [SD]) was 98·6 (14·2) in the awake-regional group and 98·2 (14·7) in the general anaesthesia group. There was equivalence in mean between groups (awake-regional minus general anaesthesia 0·169, 95% CI −2·30 to 2·64). The median duration of anaesthesia in the general anaesthesia group was 54 min.

Interpretation.—For this secondary outcome, we found no evidence that just less than 1 h of sevoflurane anaesthesia in infancy increases the risk of adverse neurodevelopmental outcome at 2 years of age compared with awake-regional anaesthesia.

▶ There is mixed evidence from cohort studies that young children exposed to anesthesia can have an increased risk of poor neurodevelopmental outcome. In this international randomized controlled trial, infants younger than 60 weeks postmenstrual age, born at greater than 26 weeks' gestation who had inguinal herniorrhaphy from 28 hospitals in Australia, Italy, the United States, the United Kingdom, Canada, the Netherlands, and New Zealand were recruited. Between February 9, 2007, and January 31, 2013, 363 infants were randomly assigned to receive awake regional anesthesia and 359 to general anesthesia (sevoflurane). Outcome data were available for 238 children in the awake regional group and 294 in the general anesthesia group. The cognitive composite score (mean [SD]) was 98.6 (14.2) in the awake-regional group and 98.2 (14.7) in the general anesthesia group. There was equivalence in mean between groups (awake regional minus general anesthesia 0.169, 95% CI −2.30 to 2.64). The median duration of anesthesia in the general anesthesia group was 54 min. This study found no evidence that just less than 1 h of sevoflurane anesthesia in infancy increases the risk of adverse neurodevelopmental outcome at 2 years of age compared with awake regional anesthesia. The only other factors noted in this study were the increased use of therapy for hypotension in the GA group (17% GA vs 5% regional) and an increased rate of apnea in the GA group in the 12 h after surgery (4% GA vs 2% regional). This study is the strongest evidence to date that <1 h of sevoflurane during early infancy is not associated with neurotoxicity.

T. E. Inder, MD

Personality of adults who were born very preterm

Eryigit-Madzwamuse S, Strauss V, Baumann N, et al (Univ of Brighton, UK; Univ of Oxford, UK; Univ of Warwick, Coventry, UK; et al)

Arch Dis Child Fetal Neonatal Ed 100:F524-F529, 2015

Objectives.—To examine very preterm (gestational age at birth <32 weeks) and/or very low birth weight (birth weight <1500 g: VP/VLBW) adults' personality and risk taking when compared with term controls. To investigate whether differences between VP/VLBW adults and controls remain after taking their general cognitive abilities into account.

Design.—The Bavarian Longitudinal Study is a geographically defined prospective cohort study of neonatal at-risk children born in 1985/1986 in Germany. A total of 200 VP/VLBW and 197 controls completed main outcome measures including broad autism phenotype, personality traits (eg, introversion, neuroticism), and risk taking at 26 years of age.

Results.—When compared with term controls, VP/VLBW adults scored significantly higher in autistic features, introversion and neuroticism but not in conscientiousness and closeness scales. They also reported lower risk taking. Profile analysis showed higher introversion, autistic features and neuroticism and lower risk taking as unique features of VP/VLBW adults ($F_{within\text{-}group} = 0.81$, ns; $F_{between\text{-}group} = 49.56$, $p < 0.001$). These characteristics were found to load onto a single profile factor which was equivalent between the VP/VLBW and control samples ($\chi^2 = 12.49$, df = 7, ns; comparative fit index = 0.98). VP/VLBW birth significantly predicted the profile factor ($\beta = 0.33$, $p < 0.001$) and explained 11% of its variance. Adjusting for general cognitive deficits did not alter the findings.

Conclusions.—VP/VLBW birth poses an important risk for a global withdrawn personality, as indicated by being less socially engaged (introversion), low in taking risks, poor in communication (autistic features) and easily worried (neuroticism). This profile might help to explain the social difficulties VP/VLBW individuals experience in adult roles, such as in peer/partner relationships and career.

▶ Studies evaluating the outcomes of individuals born prematurely in terms of their behavior and personality traits are sparse. It is unclear if such differences in personality characteristics exist, that they may be partially explained by lower intellectual abilities (IQs) of very premature/very low birth weight adults. This study investigated whether very premature/very low birth weight adults differ from full-term controls in terms of personality characteristics and whether personality profiles may be unique. They also evaluated whether various traits seen in very low birth weight premature adults differ from those in full-term controls after controlling for IQ level differences seen between the 2 groups. This study, done in Bavaria, Germany, evaluated 200 individuals who were born very premature/very low birth weight and 197 controls born at full-term gestation.

Some of the descriptive comparisons between the 2 groups showed that those very premature/very low birth weight adults more frequently came from families with low socioeconomic status than full-term counterparts, a factor that also could cause confounding. The results of the evaluations using standard questionnaires showed that there were several behavioral features that differed between these 2 groups. These differences included increased introversion, lower risk taking, increased autistic features, and increased neuroticism. The authors termed this cluster of behavioral differences seen in these very premature/very low birth weight adults as a *socially withdrawn personality*.

The potential etiology for the development of this socially withdrawn personality trait seen in very low birth weight/very premature individuals is of interest. The authors found that these behavioral traits were seen after correcting for IQ. Whether environmental exposures in early life, such as exposure to steroids, high-stress environments, or antibiotics or lack of close contact with their families can? It is obviously difficult to dissect out factors that contributed to this socially withdrawn personality trait seen in these individuals. Nevertheless, the fact that this possibility is now been identified is important. Is it possible to guide parents of the preterm infants in their understanding of these potential problems and give them ways to help their children develop into well-adjusted adults?

J. Neu, MD

Health, Wealth, Social Integration, and Sexuality of Extremely Low-Birth-Weight Prematurely Born Adults in the Fourth Decade of Life

Saigal S, Day KL, Van Lieshout RJ, et al (McMaster Univ, Hamilton, Ontario, Canada)

JAMA Pediatr 170:678-686, 2016

Importance.—Although it has been previously reported that the transition of extremely low-birth-weight survivors (≤1000 g) in their mid-20s was similar to that of normal-birth-weight controls (>2500 g), there was uncertainty as to whether this positive pattern would persist.

Objective.—To compare the social functioning of low-birth-weight prematurely born adults aged 29 to 36 years with that of normal-birth-weight term controls.

Design, Setting, and Participants.—A population-based longitudinal cohort study was conducted in Ontario, Canada, between March 14, 2011, and August 13, 2013, among 100 of 165 low-birth-weight survivors

(60.6%) prematurely born between January 1, 1977, and December 31, 1982, and 89 of 144 sociodemographically matched normal-birth-weight term controls (61.8%) recruited at age 8 years. Neurologic impairments were present in 20 premature participants (20.0%).

Exposures.—Extremely low birth weight.

Main Outcomes and Measures.—Information on health, educational level, employment, social integration, sexuality, and reproduction was obtained through standardized questionnaires completed by the participants.

Results.—Participants included 100 (39 males) extremely low-birth-weight survivors and 89 (33 males) normal-birth-weight term controls. The groups did not differ in the highest educational level achieved or in family and partner relationships. However, a lower proportion of premature adults was employed (odds ratio [OR], 0.37; 95% CI, 0.15 to 0.93) and fewer were employed full time (OR, 0.49; 95% CI, 0.24 to 0.98). The premature group had a mean total personal income of $20 000 less than controls, and more required social assistance (OR, 4.16; 95% CI, 1.13 to 15.33). Compared with the control group, more members of the premature group remained single (OR, 1.95; 95% CI, 1.08 to 3.50), had never had sexual intercourse (OR, 11.30; 95% CI, 2.56 to 49.91), did not have children (OR, 0.52; 95% CI, 0.27 to 0.99), reported more chronic health conditions (β, 1.54; 95% CI, 0.79 to 2.30), had lower self-esteem (β, 8.40; 95% CI, 1.68 to 15.12), and were less likely to have current drug abuse or dependence (OR, 0.29; 95% CI, 0.90 to 0.92) or lifetime alcohol abuse or dependence (OR, 0.30; 95% CI, 0.15 to 0.59). A higher proportion of premature adults without neurosensory impairments identified themselves as nonheterosexual (OR, 4.87; 95% CI, 1.01 to 23.69). After exclusion of individuals with neurosensory impairments, differences in employment, social assistance, marital status, and reproduction were no longer significant.

Conclusions and Relevance.—In the fourth decade of life, extremely low-birth-weight survivors achieved similar educational levels and family and partner relationships, and reported fewer risky behaviors compared with controls. However, they had lower levels of employment, income, and self-esteem, and fewer were married and had children. It is therefore essential that these individuals receive necessary support and continued monitoring throughout life.

▶ In this 4-decade-long follow-up study the investigators report on the social and medical history of former extremely low birth weight infants (ELBW) who are now 29 to 36 years old. Although the attrition rate has steadily increased over the years, the follow-up rate of more than 60% is a remarkable accomplishment and a tribute to the investigators.

In their early 20s, the members of this ELBW cohort did remarkably well in most variables related to transition to adulthood.[1] In contrast, as noted in this report, they have not fared as well in adulthood. Areas of particular concern related to employment; despite a comparable level of education, the employment rate and, when employed, the earning capacity, were lower than for the normal birth weight (NBW) cohort (80.4% vs 91.8%; $26,500 vs $46,500). A higher proportion of the ELBW cohort was single or never married (51.0% vs 34.8%), or if not married, dating (31.3% vs 13.1%); these issues were more prevalent among ELBW women. Although a lower proportion of the ELBW cohort had children (20.0% vs 32.6%), the ELBW women had similar rates of miscarriages and births at less than 37 weeks' gestation compared with women in the NBW cohort. The higher rate of health problems in the ELBW cohort related primarily to vision; this may be a reflection of the lack of treatment for retinopathy of prematurity in the era before cryotherapy. Of note, the rates of asthma, bronchitis, and hypertension were not different between the groups.

The rate of neurosensory impairment in the ELBW cohort was 20%. When these individuals were excluded from the analyses, there was no significant difference in the rates of employment, dating, and marital status and the proportion who had children. However, income discrepancy and chronic health conditions remained significant. Despite the differences, the majority of the ELBW cohort are living independently and contributing to society. As this report illustrates, follow-up studies need to be conducted throughout the life course of ELBW survivors to obtain a better understanding of the ultimate consequences of being born too early.

L. A. Papile, MD

Reference

1. Saigal S, Stoskopf B, Steiner D, et al. Transition of extremely low-birth-weight infants from adolescence to young adulthood: comparison with normal birth-weight controls. *JAMA*. 2006;295:667.

Neonatal Morphine Exposure in Very Preterm Infants—Cerebral Development and Outcomes

Steinhorn R, McPherson C, Anderson PJ, et al (Washington Univ in St. Louis, MO; Brigham and Women's Hosp, Boston, MA; The Univ of Melbourne, Carlton, Australia; et al)

J Pediatr 166:1200-1207, 2015

Objective.—To investigate the association of morphine exposure in very preterm infants with cerebral volumes and neurodevelopmental outcome from birth through middle childhood.

Study Design.—Observational study of very preterm infants in the Victorian Infant Brain Study cohort. A total of 230 infants born <30 weeks' gestational age or <1250 g were recruited from all admissions to the neonatal intensive care unit of the Royal Women's Hospital. Fifty-seven (25%) infants received morphine analgesia during their neonatal intensive care unit stay at the attending physician's discretion. Primary outcomes were regional brain volumes at term and 7 years; neurobehavioral performance at term; and cognitive, motor, emotional, behavioral, communication, and executive function scores at age 2 and 7 years. Linear regressions were used to compare outcomes between participants who did and did not receive morphine.

Results.—At term, preterm infants who received morphine had similar rates of gray matter injury to no-morphine infants, but a trend toward smaller cortical volumes in the orbitofrontal (*P*left = .002, *P*right = .01) and subgenual (*P*left = .01) regions. At 7 years, cortical volumes did not differ between groups. At 2 years, morphine-exposed children were more likely to show behavioral dysregulation (*P* = .007) than no-morphine children, but at 7 years no detrimental impacts of morphine on neurobehavioral outcome were observed.

Conclusions.—Low-dose morphine analgesia received during neonatal intensive care was associated with early alterations in cerebral structure and short-term neurobehavioral problems that did not persist into childhood.

▶ Opioid analgesics such as morphine and fentanyl are administered to critically ill newborn infants in an effort to reduce pain, stress and potentially reduce neurologic injury. However, there are limited data available in regard to long-term neurodevelopmental outcomes of infants exposed to these agents. In this prospective longitudinal cohort study, the authors compared the short- and long-term outcomes of very preterm infants with and without exposure to low-dose morphine. Brain volumes as measured by quantitative magnetic resonance analysis were obtained at term equivalent and 7 years of age; assessment of cognition and behavior was undertaken at 2 years corrected age and 7 years of age.

Infants enrolled in the study were born at < 30 weeks' gestational age or < 1250 g birth weight between July 2001 and December 2003. Infants received morphine analgesia at the attending physician's discretion; no other form of pharmacologic sedation or analgesia, including benzodiazepines, were given, with the exception of intraoperative anesthesia. Fifty-seven (26%) of the 223 infants received morphine; the median cumulative dose was 0.79 mg/kg (interquartile range 0.12–0.95 mg/kg, range 0.1–5.3 mg/kg).

Magnetic resonance imaging data were available for 83% and 51% of the cohort at 2 and 7 years, respectively; 93% and 84% underwent neuropsychological evaluation at 2 and 7 years, respectively. At 2 years' corrected age, brain volumes were similar for the 2 cohorts, but infants exposed to low-dose morphine had region-specific decreases in gray matter volume. At 7 years of age, differences in regional brain volumes were no longer evident. At 2 years of age the morphine and no-morphine groups scored similarly in terms of cognition, motor development, and emotional and social assessment scales, although the parents of the morphine group children reported significantly more dysregulation. Paradoxically, at 7 years of age the morphine group achieved higher scores in areas related to basic educational skills.

The finding that low-dose morphine did not adversely affect the neuropsychological outcomes of very preterm infants in early childhood is encouraging.

However, whether very preterm infants who are exposed to higher cumulative doses will also have a favorable outcome in middle childhood is unknown.

L. A. Papile, MD

Neonatal Morphine Exposure in Very Preterm Infants—Cerebral Development and Outcomes

Steinhorn R, McPherson C, Anderson PJ, et al (Washington Univ in St Louis, MO; Brigham and Women's Hosp, Boston, MA; The Univ of Melbourne, Carlton, Australia; et al)

J Pediatr 166:1200-1207, 2015

Objective.—To investigate the association of morphine exposure in very preterm infants with cerebral volumes and neurodevelopmental outcome from birth through middle childhood.

Study Design.—Observational study of very preterm infants in the Victorian Infant Brain Study cohort. A total of 230 infants born <30 weeks' gestational age or <1250 g were recruited from all admissions to the neonatal intensive care unit of the Royal Women's Hospital. Fifty-seven (25%) infants received morphine analgesia during their neonatal intensive care unit stay at the attending physician's discretion. Primary outcomes were regional brain volumes at term and 7 years; neurobehavioral performance at term; and cognitive, motor, emotional, behavioral, communication, and executive function scores at age 2 and 7 years. Linear regressions were used to compare outcomes between participants who did and did not receive morphine.

Results.—At term, preterm infants who received morphine had similar rates of gray matter injury to no-morphine infants, but a trend toward smaller cortical volumes in the orbitofrontal (Pleft = .002, Pright = .01) and subgenual (Pleft = .01) regions. At 7 years, cortical volumes did not differ between groups. At 2 years, morphine-exposed children were more likely to show behavioral dysregulation (P = .007) than no-morphine children, but at 7 years no detrimental impacts of morphine on neurobehavioral outcome were observed.

Conclusions.—Low-dose morphine analgesia received during neonatal intensive care was associated with early alterations in cerebral structure and short-term neurobehavioral problems that did not persist into childhood.

▶ Opioid analgesics such as morphine and fentanyl are administered to critically ill newborn infants in an effort to reduce pain and stress and potentially reduce neurologic injury. However, limited data are available with regard to long-term neurodevelopmental outcomes of infants exposed to these agents. In this prospective, longitudinal, cohort study, the authors compared the short- and long-term outcomes of very preterm infants with and without exposure to low-dose morphine. Brain volumes as measured by quantitative magnetic resonance analysis were obtained at term equivalent and 7 years of age; assessments of cognition and behavior were undertaken at 2 years corrected age and 7 years of age.

Infants enrolled in the study were born at less than 30 weeks gestational age or less than 1250 g birth weight between July 2001 and December 2003. Infants received morphine analgesia at the attending physician's discretion; no other forms of pharmacologic sedation or analgesia, including benzodiazepines, were given, with the exception of intraoperative anesthesia. Fifty-seven (26%) of the 223 infants received morphine; the median cumulative dose was 0.79 mg/kg (interquartile range, 0.12-0.95 mg/kg; range, 0.1-5.3 mg/kg).

MRI data were available for 83% and 51% of the cohort at 2 and 7 years, respectively; 93% and 84% underwent neuropsychological evaluation at 2 and 7 years, respectively. At 2 years corrected age, brain volumes were similar for the 2 cohorts, but infants exposed to low-dose morphine had region-specific decreases in gray matter volume. At 7 years of age, differences in regional brain volumes were no longer evident. At 2 years of age, the morphine and no-morphine groups scored similarly in terms of cognition, motor development, and emotional and social assessment scales, although the parents of the morphine group reported significantly more dysregulation. Paradoxically, at 7 years of age, the morphine group achieved higher scores in areas related to basic educational skills.

The finding that low-dose morphine did not adversely affect the neuropsychological outcomes of very preterm infants in early childhood is encouraging. However, whether very preterm infants who are exposed to higher cumulative doses will also have a favorable outcome in middle childhood is unknown.

L. A. Papile, MD

Reasons for Rehospitalization in Children Who Had Neonatal Abstinence Syndrome

Uebel H, Wright IM, Burns L, et al (Univ of New South Wales, Kensington, Australia; The Univ of Wollongong, Australia; Univ of New South Wales, Sydney, Australia; et al)

Pediatrics 136:e811-e820, 2015

Background and Objectives.—Neonatal abstinence syndrome (NAS) occurs after in utero exposure to abstract opioids, but outcomes after the postnatal period are unclear. Our objectives were to characterize childhood hospitalization after NAS.

Methods.—Population-based linkage study of births, hospitalization, and death records of all children registered in New South Wales (NSW), Australia, between 2000 and 2011 to a maximum of 13 years. Infants with an *International Statistical Classification of Disease and Related Problems, 10th Edition, Australian Modification*, coding of NAS (P96.1, n = 3842) were compared with 1 018 421 live born infants without an NAS diagnosis.

Results.—Infants with NAS were more likely to be admitted into a nursery (odds ratio 15.6, 95% confidence interval: 14.5–16.8) and be hospitalized longer (10.0 vs 3.0 days). In childhood, they were more likely to be rehospitalized (1.6, 1.5–1.7), die during hospitalization (3.3, 2.1–5.1), and be hospitalized for assaults (15.2, 11.3–20.6), maltreatment (21.0, 14.3–30.9), poisoning (3.6, 2.6–4.8), and mental/behavioral (2.6, 2.1–3.2) and visual (2.9, 2.5-3.5) disorders. Mothers of infants with NAS were more likely to be Indigenous (6.4, 6.0–7.0), have no antenatal care (6.6, 5.9–7.4), and be socioeconomically deprived (1.6, 1.5–1.7). Regression analyses demonstrated that NAS was the most important predictor of admissions for maltreatment (odds ratio 4.5, 95% confidence interval: 3.4–6.1) and mental and behavioral disorders (2.3, 1.9–2.9), even after accounting for prematurity, maternal age, and Indigenous status.

Conclusions.—Children with NAS are more likely to be rehospitalized during childhood for maltreatment, trauma, and mental and behavioral disorders even after accounting for prematurity. This continues to adolescence and emphasizes the critical need for continued support of this vulnerable group after resolution of NAS.

▶ As indicated in this study, infants with neonatal abstinence syndrome (NAS) are at risk for myriad medical and mental conditions throughout childhood. In infancy, NAS was associated with increased risk of hospitalization for maltreatment (neglect, abandonment, physical abuse), accidents (burns, poisonings), trauma, and respiratory infections. In childhood, NAS was associated with an increased risk for mental and behavioral disorders, especially disturbance to attention and activity, and oppositional defiant disorder. Whether the latter conditions were caused by intrauterine substance exposure, parenting influences, or genetic predisposition is unclear. The mothers of this NAS cohort were young, had late prenatal care, and were in the lowest socioeconomic bracket. However intrauterine opioid exposure has been associated with lower brain volumes in human infants and impairs neurogenesis, myelination, and neural longevity in animal models. With proliferation of opioid use among more socially and economically advantaged pregnant women, the demographics of infants with NAS have changed. Long-term tracking of this most recent cohort may be helpful in clarifying the contribution of opioids to alterations in brain development.

L. A. Papile, MD

15 Ethics

Beyond stress: describing the experiences of families during neonatal intensive care

Wraight CL, McCoy J, Meadow W (Univ of Chicago, IL)

Acta Paediatr 104:1012-1017, 2015

Aim.—To determine whether parents of critically ill premature infants feel that neonatal intensive care unit (NICU) therapy is worthwhile, independent of their infant's outcome.

Methods.—The parent(s) of ventilated infants in the NICU were interviewed. Prominent themes were identified within the text of transcribed interviews and the frequency of each theme tabulated.

Results.—The parents of 10 infants were interviewed. All parents experienced stress and understood the uncertain future of their infants. Parents remained optimistic and uniformly expressed that NICU intervention was 'worth it'. No parent described concern about 'torture', 'cruelty' or 'futile care'.

Conclusion.—Although parents experience significant stress while their infant is in the NICU, their emotional experiences are much more broad. They feel confident in their decision to give their child a chance, a responsibility to be informed and to make the best decisions they can and remain hopeful for a good outcome regardless of their child's condition.

▶ Although parents of hospitalized infants often express values and make decisions that appear illogical to their neonatal intensive care unit (NICU) medical providers, little research has been done to formally study parents' opinions and experiences with NICU care. This article sought to address this gap in evidence by exploring attitudes and values expressed by parents of critically ill, hospitalized neonates. In a series of 10 interviews of parents of intubated infants, the authors identified that although parents were aware of the tenuousness of their child's situation, they remained hopeful and optimistic. Additionally, parents experienced stress and fear, particularly related to uncertainty, but often were able to mitigate these feelings with their faith. Parents also described thoughtfully considering their infant's best interest and balancing this against their own hopes for their infant's survival. The interviewed parents expressed that they wanted to feel that all possible options had been provided for their baby, and none felt that their infant's current treatment was futile, unwanted, or causing unnecessary suffering.

This qualitative study had methodological limitations, including very small sample size, nonuniform patient and parent population, and a single coder of the data. Interviews were conducted by 2 individuals who were also providers, which may have reduced parents' willingness to be truthful with their answers, although interviewers were cautious not to approach parents while on service in the unit. Nevertheless, this study elicited parents' thoughts and feelings about the NICU while their infant was acutely ill during the initial hospitalization, reducing potential recall biases influenced by the passage of time and the infant's ultimate outcome. The findings appear to confirm what many of us have noted anecdotally: parents appear to place value on having tried all available interventions to save their infant, even when the statistical likelihood of survival is low and/or the ultimate outcome is death.

S. Kukora, MD

Providing parents with individualised support in a neonatal intensive care unit reduced stress, anxiety and depression

Cano Giménez E, Sánchez-Luna M (Universidad Complutense, Madrid, Spain)

Acta Paediatr 104:e300-e305, 2015

Aim.—This study assessed the effectiveness of an individualised intervention to reduce parental stress, anxiety and depression in a neonatal intensive care unit (NICU).

Methods.—Parents of infants admitted to the NICU for a minimum of 4 weeks underwent a five-step individualised intervention programme delivered by a psychologist.

Results.—The study population comprised 40 mothers and 25 fathers in the intervention group and 40 mothers and 29 fathers in the control group who received the standard support. Similar stress levels were observed in both groups before the intervention. However, after 15 days, the group that received the individualised intervention showed a statistically significant lower level of anxiety, with none of the mothers and fathers in the intervention group reporting anxiety, compared with 2.5% of mothers and 10.3% of fathers in the control group. At discharge, 50% of mothers and 80% of fathers in the intervention group reported no level of depression, compared to all the mothers and fathers in the control group.

Conclusion.—An intervention programme individualised to the needs of mothers and fathers with infants admitted to a NICU for at least 4 weeks was effective in reducing anxiety and depression compared to the standard care.

▶ As I read this study of a randomized psychological intervention to decrease the incidence of stress among parents of neonatal intensive care unit (NICU) patients by Gimenez et al, I marveled at how far we've come in neonatology. In only a few decades, we've moved from incubated preterm infants as a side-show curiosity to fully embracing rigorous scientific investigation of neonatal disease processes and care from the petri dish to the NICU. Our colleagues, once divided into lab scientists and clinical trialists, now include health services researchers, qualitative methods experts, sociologists, and anthropologists, and our scope of interest has broadened from the systematic effects of medical interventions to include the psychologic and emotional impact of NICU hospitalization on the families of our tiny, imperiled patients. I fully admit, this study presses the boundaries of my own intellectual comfort zone—many of us don't know much about psychology, and we know even less about how to systematically study psychologic intervention, but this group, working in a NICU in Madrid, Spain, has done just that, and in so doing brings us a glimmer of hope that maybe we really can do something to lessen the blow of a prolonged and overwhelming NICU admission.

I would have liked to know a little more about the patients' medical conditions and outcomes, and I had some unanswered questions about the recruitment and study methods. Most importantly, I'd like to know more about what it takes to really do this. I'm not the first to call for more cost-effectiveness analysis in randomized control trials, but in this case, I'd really like to know whether this is a pie-in-the-sky intervention that we have no hope of implementing in a wide scale, or whether this is easy and accessible for everyone.

But that shouldn't take away from the larger message here: helping the parents of our most vulnerable patients cope with the unfathomable ordeal of a prolonged NICU admission is within reach.

N. Laventhal, MD, MA

Supporting Parental Decisions About Genomic Sequencing for Newborn Screening: The NC NEXUS Decision Aid

Lewis MA, Paquin RS, Roche MI, et al (Ctr for Communication Science, Research Triangle Park, NC; Univ of North Carolina at Chapel Hill; et al)
Pediatrics 137:e20153731E, 2016

Advances in genomic sequencing technology have raised fundamental challenges to the traditional ways genomic information is communicated. These challenges will become increasingly complex and will affect a much larger population in the future if genomics is incorporated into standard newborn screening practice. Clinicians, public health officials, and other stakeholders will need to agree on the types of information that they should seek and communicate to parents. Currently, few evidence-based and validated tools are available to support parental informed decision-making. These tools will be necessary as genomics is integrated into clinical practice and public health systems. In this article we describe how the North Carolina Newborn Exome Sequencing for Universal Screening study is addressing the need to support parents in making informed decisions about the use of genomic testing in newborn screening. We outline the context for newborn screening and justify the need for parental decision support. We also describe the process of decision aid development and the data sources, processes, and best practices being used in development. By the end of the study, we will have an evidenced-based process and validated tools to support parental informed decision-making about the use of genomic sequencing in newborn screening. Data from the study will help answer important questions about which genomic information ought to be sought and communicated when testing newborns.

▶ "Imagine that the genome is a book.
There are twenty-three chapters, called CHROMOSOMES.
Each chapter contains several thousand stories, called GENES.
Each story is made up of paragraphs, called EXTONS, which are interrupted by advertisements called INTRONS.
Each paragraph is made up of words, called CODONS.
Each word is written in letters called BASES."
—Matt Ridley, *Genome: The Autobiography of a Species in 23 Chapters*

In 1953, more than 50 years ago, James Watson and Francis Crick described the structure of DNA in a 1-page report in *Nature*. Scientific progress in the field of genetics has expanded rapidly since then, and in 2007, James Watson made history again as the first individual to have his entire 6-billion-nucleotide genome sequenced. As in many areas of scientific and technologic advancement, knowledge in this area has outpaced a thorough consideration of significant ethical and legal implications. Genomic sequencing technology, for example, has advanced to the point where it may be performed routinely as part of newborn screening. In this article, Lewis and colleagues examine how to support parental decisions about genomic sequencing for newborn screening. They describe an evidence-based process to develop validated ways to support parental decision making through the use of decision aids such as online programs that go far beyond the brochure that is often handed to parents. With the "average" American reading at a seventh-grade level,[1] it is imperative to develop methods to convey complex genetics topics in a format understandable to the average parent, and the authors are to be commended on their scientific approach to improving health literacy in this complex area of medicine.

J. M. Fanaroff, MD, JD

Reference

1. *A First Look at the Literacy of America's Adults in the 21st Century.* 2006. National Center for Educational Statistics; 2006.

Recommendations for palliative and bereavement care in the NICU: a family-centered integrative approach

Kenner C, Press J, Ryan D (The College of New Jersey, Ewing; Crouse Hosp, Syracuse, NY; Elmira College, NY)
J Perinatol 35:S19-S23, 2015

Technological advances have increased our ability to detect a life-threatening, life-limiting or lethal problem early in pregnancy, leaving parents months to anticipate a death or a prematurely born infant. Babies can also be born with unanticipated problems that could lead to death. In either scenario, perinatal palliative care should be offered as a strategy for family support. Since the preponderance of professional training focuses on saving lives, many health professionals are uncomfortable with palliative care. This article's purpose is to define best practices for the provision of family-centered perinatal and neonatal palliative care and provision of support to bereaved families experiencing anticipated and unanticipated life-limiting conditions or death of their infant. An overview of core concepts and values is presented, followed by intervention strategies to promote an integrated family-centered approach to palliative and bereavement care. The concluding section presents evidence-based recommendations.

▶ The article by Kenner and colleagues outlines and summarizes a set of core principles and recommendations to be used by professionals in obstetric practice and neonatology when faced with the challenges of fetuses and newborns who cannot, do not, or will not survive without aggressive medical and surgical care. Their summary and conclusions, aimed at best ways to help these babies and their parents, are clear and well supported. Particularly valuable is the emphasis on comprehensive prenatal conversations between parents and all involved specialists, the role of family participation in parenting, memory-making, and their very important stress on bereavement support.

An evolving area of discussion among palliative care specialists concerns the best approaches to decision making in the critical situations described in the article. This guideline appropriately emphasizes "including families as part of the decision-making process without overwhelming them" and that families "must be included in the decision-making process to the degree they deem themselves able to participate, guided by their understanding of their child's best interest." Best decisions that will minimize both suffering and decisional regret continue to be an area of both research need and professional education. An official practice guideline would be helped by adding advice about the framing of decisions based on 4 core questions at the center of all palliative care encounters: What is your understanding of what your baby is up against? What are you hoping for? If that hope does not become possible, what else is important? What are you most afraid of? The answers to these questions will frequently lead to the professional being able to present the best decision without overly burdening the parent. The decision, framed in either the passive voice (what needs to be done is ...) or the collective voice (what we should do is ...) should always be followed by silence and active listening for acceptance, clarification, or further discussion.

K. Pituch, MD

Physicians can justifiably euthanize certain severely impaired neonates
Schuklenk U (Queen's Univ, Kingston, Ontario, Canada)
J Thorac Cardiovasc Surg 149:535-537, 2015

Clinicians in a scenario involving a neonate with heterotaxy syndrome would not have included euthanasia as an option for the parents had they believed surgical procedures would likely be successful and permit the infant to live a reasonably healthy life.

Legislators in the jurisdiction where the case scenario played out concluded that there are circumstances where infanticide is morally acceptable. They legislated that physician-assisted death be made available in their jurisdiction for certain severely impaired neonates, including apparently the infant under consideration. A majority of practicing neonatologists in Europe concurs that intensive care is only acceptable if it will result not merely in the survival of an infant but also in an acceptable future quality of life. In the United States the President's Commission for the Study of Ethical Problems in Medicine and Biomedical and Behavioral Research also concluded that there can be conditions sufficiently serious "that continued existence would not be a net benefit to the infant."

There appear to be some cases, then, where continuing existence is not in a severely impaired neonate's best interest. Terminating its life, based on parent choice, seems a prima facie reasonable option.

▶ In including this article in the Year Book, the editors bring a frank, even jarring, analysis of what is likely to be one of the next big debates in neonatal ethics. Foregoing or withdrawing neonatal intensive care for infants with little or no hope for meaningful survival is commonly accepted as falling within the specter of mainstream neonatology, and providing compassionate comfort care to these infants, alone or in conjunction with palliative care specialists, is a necessary skill set for all of us. So whereas the previous question was "May we (or should we) allow this baby to die?" the question now is, "Is it permissible for us to actively and consciously hasten this baby's death?"

Dr Schuklenk says, emphatically, "Yes," and although I have no hope of resolving this debate, today or in my lifetime, what I would say is, "Not by Dr Schuklenk's arguments." This article is methodical, researched, and clearly written and takes a fearless approach to a difficult and complex issue, but it glosses over some important nuances of the Groningen protocol. The Groningen protocol, as it applies to infants with a certain prognosis (not the case here[1]), and—in my interpretation—exists as a safeguard for when compassionate care fails to achieve its objective. In this case, Dr Schuklenk suggests euthanasia as a way to bypass potential "hopeless and unbearable suffering,"[2] or worse, as a way to alleviate ourselves of anticipated emotional distress. As Dr Meilaender puts it in his opposing view commentary in the same issue, we would "try to eliminate suffering by eliminating the sufferer."[3]

In addition, the arguments ultimately rely on a seemingly outdated and, for many of us, unacceptable view of neonates: that they are not people. Although Annie Janvier and others have written about seemingly prevalent biases against the personhood of neonates, I would argue that Dr Schuklenk's arguments will lack traction with contemporary neonatologists. They harken back to the time when we thought that neonates could not feel pain or that infants with trisomy 21 were not worthy of simple surgery for duodenal atresia. I suspect that even parents who choose euthanasia in a case like this would bristle at the notion that their son was not a person.

N. Laventhal, MD, MA

References

1. Sade RM. Can a physician ever justifiably euthanize a severely disabled neonate? *J Thorac Cardiovasc Surg.* 2015;149:532.
2. Verhagen E, Sauer PJ. The Groningen protocol—euthanasia in severely ill newborns. *N Engl J Med.* 2005;10:959-962.
3. Meilaender G. No to infant euthanasia. *J Thorac Cardiovasc Surg.* 2015;149: 533-534.

Elective ventilation to facilitate organ donation in infants with anencephaly: perinatal professionals' views and an ethical analysis

Jivraj A, Scales A, Brierley J, et al (Univ of London, UK; Great Ormond Children's Hosp, London, UK)
Acta Paediatr 105:494-498, 2016

Aim.—Following the elective ventilation and referral for organ donation of an infant with anencephaly, we sought local perinatal professionals' views of this practice.

Methods.—Anonymous online survey: demographics, ethical viewpoints and potential public/maternal perceptions (standard 5-part Likert scale and free text).

Results.—Demographics: 49 replies (38 female): 4 obstetricians, 14 neonatologists, 6 foetal clinicians, 23 nurses, 1 anaesthetist and 1 reproductive specialist. Experience: 0.5—33 years (average 12). Twenty-one had experience of anencephalic delivery, and 10 reported pregnancy continued for religious reasons. Ethics: (i) 73% thought anencephalic donation acceptable, of which 64% supported elective ventilation, 20% neutral and 16% disagreed. (ii) Provision of treatments not in infant's strict best interest to facilitate donation: 22% strongly agreed, 36% agreed, 33% neutral and 9% disagreed. (iii)Accept ventilation to permit donation if societal benefit: 53% agreed, 33% neutral and 13% disagreed. (iv) Public opinion: 59% disagreed anencephalic donation would harm public opinion about donation and 19% agreed.

Conclusion.—We found a supportive local environment for donation in the setting of anencephaly, including support for elective ventilation.

Given this, and our ethical analysis, we recommend provision of organ donation information as part of palliative care counselling for women carrying a foetus with a condition likely to be fatal in infancy.

▶ "Act in such a way that you treat humanity, whether in your own person or in the person of any other, never merely as a means to an end but always at the same time as an end."—Immanuel Kant, Groundwork of Metaphysic of Morals

"Taylor was only 7 years old when she passed away, and she had brought so much happiness to our family. Our family decided to give her entire life an overall meaning by donating to others who desperately needed the gift of life."—The Family of Taylor Freeman, Organ Donor

Controversy over appropriate care for infants with anencephaly has confounded neonatologists for decades. In the 1980s, Loma Linda implemented a program to facilitate organ donation that was "short-lived" due to ethical concerns and practical difficulties meeting brain death criteria. In the 1990s, a hospital uncomfortable that a mother's demands to repeatedly intubate her infant with anencephaly was futile care went to court and was told by the Federal Fourth Circuit Court of Appeals that they were legally obligated to stabilize Baby K just like any other unstable patient.[1]

In this article, Jivraj et al reexamine elective ventilation to facilitate organ donation in infants with anencephaly. The authors use a number of methods including an anonymous online survey, literature search, and ethical analysis. The issues over the years have not fundamentally changed. To some, taking organs from an infant with anencephaly violates the Kantian imperative not to use a person as a means to an end. But from a narrative ethics perspective, organ donation often allows families to find meaning in their child's life and to allow their child to "live on" in the recipients of their precious gift. There is also valid concern about the public and media perspectives, especially in the Internet era. It is highly unlikely that there will ever be real consensus about this issue, but this well-written article provides current perspectives and may open additional professional and public discussion.

J. M. Fanaroff, MD, JD

Reference

1. In the Matter of Baby "K" (The Baby K Case), 16 F.3d F. Supp. 590 (E.D. VA 1993).

End-of-Life Care in the Neonatal Intensive Care Unit: Experiences of Staff and Parents

Cortezzo DE, Sanders MR, Brownell EA, et al (Cincinnati Children's Hosp Med Ctr, OH; Univ of Connecticut School of Medicine, Farmington)

Am J Perinatol 32:713-724, 2015

Objective.—The aim of the study is to determine the perceptions of end-of-life care practices and experience with infants who have died in the NICU among neonatologists, advanced practitioners, nurses, and parents, and also to determine perceived areas for improvement and the perceived value of a palliative care team.

Study Design.—This descriptive, exploratory cross-sectional study using surveys consisting of 7-point Likert scales and free response comments was sent to all neonatologists ($n = 14$), advanced practitioners ($n = 40$), and nurses ($n = 184$) at Connecticut Children's Medical Center's neonatal intensive care units (NICUs) in April 2013 and to all parents whose infants died in these NICUs from July 1, 2011, to December 31, 2012 ($n = 28$).

Results.—The response rates were 64.3% for physicians; 50.0% for practitioners; 40.8% for nurses; and 30.4% for parents. Most providers reported they feel comfortable delivering end-of-life care. Bereavement support, debriefing/closure conferences, and education did not occur routinely. Families stressed the importance of memory making and bereavement/follow-up. Consistent themes of free responses include modalities for improving end-of-life care, inconsistency of care delivery among providers, and the importance of memory making and follow-up.

Conclusion.—End-of-life experiences in the NICU were perceived as variable and end-of life practices were, at times, perceived as inconsistent among providers. There are areas for improvement, and participants reported that a formalized palliative care team could help. Families desire memory making, follow-up, and bereavement support.

▶ In their pilot survey study investigating end-of-life care practices in 2 affiliated neonatal intensive care unit (NICUs), Cortezzo and colleagues have tapped into some of the most pressing and salient challenges that NICU providers face in the 21st century. Gone are the days that we can be everything to everyone. Practice variation, once lauded as a way for dedicated and reflective physicians to provide individualized care based on their own personal experiences and intuition is now considered to be a marker of worse care. Handoffs—dreaded, but inevitable—necessitate consistency across care providers. Whereas individual physicians, themselves overworked and unsupported, used to expect unquestioning and subservient assistance by support staff whose own emotional needs went unacknowledged, we now know that this is not how multidisciplinary teams should work. Physicians, house officers, nurses and nurse practitioners, and families too all have their own contributions and own needs, and coordinating this delicate symphony requires us to outsource certain skills (writing total parenteral nutrition orders, monitoring drug levels) and acquire new ones—eliciting parental values, offering staff debriefing, coordinating negotiated death in the NICU after months of intensive care. This article points out an important, and perhaps irreconcilable, tension for providers of end-of-life care in the NICU: is palliative care a skill to hone or to outsource? The interesting paradox shown in the results is that even though we think we're good at this (and we probably are), we don't think we're good enough. Despite taking pride in doing the right things for our patients, we recognize that our parents' needs don't end when they leave the NICU. Bereavement is complicated and longitudinal—our families want more from us than we have to give. This article also tells about the evolving role of palliative care teams—we need them to take care of our patients, but we also need them to take care of us.

There's still work to be done—as the authors acknowledge, this survey isn't perfect, and the impact of implantation of integrated palliative care services needs to be rigorously assessed. Will our patients be better off? Will we? Will we get better at this by virtue of surrounding ourselves with experts, or will increased reliance of end-of-life specialists result in a deskilling of neonatologists that we all come to regret? I look forward to seeing what this group does next.

N. Laventhal, MD, MA

Genomic intensive care: should we perform genome testing in critically ill newborns?

Wilkinson DJC, Barnett C, Savulescu J, et al (Univ of Oxford, UK; Women's and Children's Hosp/SA Pathology, North Adelaide, Australia; et al)
Arch Dis Child Fetal Neonatal Ed 101:F94-F98, 2016

Background.—About 5% of all infants admitted to the neonatal intensive care unit (NICU) die, with most deaths preceded by decisions to withdraw or withhold life-sustaining treatments made by the family and clinical team. These decisions are based on information regarding the infant's chance of survival, the duration of survival, and the nature of survival should treatment be provided. Many clinical, biochemical, genetic, and radiological tests are used in compiling this information. As new genetic and genomic tests become available that could help in making these critical care decisions, the clinician is faced with the ethical issues associated with their use.

Genomic Testing.—Many genomic tests are already being used in newborn intensive care. These are being joined by newer methods such as multiple gene sequencing panels using next-generation sequencing (NGS) techniques, whole exome sequencing (WES), and whole genome sequencing (WGS). With the lower costs and faster speeds of NGS techniques, clinical use is now possible. Genomic tests that can diagnose multiple genetic conditions in a single exposure are especially applicable in the NICU, when congenital and genetic disorders often become apparent.

The uses of genomic testing after birth include diagnostic applications and prognostic estimates for critically ill infants. In addition, treatment modification is possible to identify specific treatments likely or unlikely to be of benefit given an infant's outcome. Anticipation or information uses provide patients with advance knowledge of potential future problems and the risk of recurrence in future offspring. Treatment limitation can also be determined. Some results may be of minimal value to decisions about treatment, whereas others may strongly indicate the need to continue or discontinue treatment.

Ethical Issues.—The benefits and risks of genomic testing of critically ill infants raise ethical considerations for clinicians. Clinicians may choose to refraining from using them until their clinical usefulness and validity are better demonstrated. In the NICU, however, the use of genomic testing is at least sometimes justified. For instance, genomic testing may lead to an avoidance of nonbeneficial treatment. Many ethical issues with the new methods are the same as with previous genomic tests.

Genomic testing used for targeted diagnostic testing involves the careful selection of patients for whom such tests are most likely to identify a pathogenic mutation. Genomic testing could and probably should also be undertaken to provide additional prognostic information that would potentially be actionable. In making these decisions, parents and clinicians must weigh the benefits against the burdens of providing treatment. Some families will choose one interpretation and provide treatment, whereas others will choose another and not continue treatment. Neither choice is wrong; it is a matter of parental discretion and consideration of what is relevant to the family.

Parents should have the opportunity to make an informed, considered decision before agreeing to genomic testing. Pre-test counseling should provide parents with the range of information that is relevant to the decision about treatment, including the possibility of identifying variants of unknown significance and incidental findings. If serious abnormalities are identified on antenatal ultrasound, it may be preferable to perform genomic tests as part of prenatal care and provide counseling before birth. This prepares the clinician to intervene.

Because of the large number of incidental and uncertain findings, results should be stratified based on the likelihood of them relating to the child's current or imminent clinical status. Information about illness or function in later life should be shared based on a discussion of what the parents consider important for their child's best interests.

Conclusions.—Determining whether, when, and how new genomic testing results should influence treatment decision-making in the NICU may be done by using existing ethical frameworks set up for clinical decisions in this setting. Clinicians should be cautious with evaluating test results. Parents will need counseling to understand the results and their implications. Further information will be needed about which tests to order and how to handle the sharing of information and its impact on neonatal care.

▶ This is an interesting and important review of genomic testing in critically ill newborns. Neonatologists currently use several modalities to help make decisions about withdrawal of support, withholding life-sustaining treatment that are not genomic tests. For example, cranial ultrasound is used extensively to determine whether a neonate has a severe intracranial hemorrhage (with likely poor neurodevelopmental outcomes). This information may be important in terms of decision making for a child who may require surgery for necrotizing enterocolitis or other life-threatening emergent condition. Similarly, results of genomic testing can offer important information about concomitant genetic conditions the child is likely to develop, such as autism or schizophrenia. This genomic information, similar to the ultrasound information, may be helpful in deciding whether to operate for the necrotizing enterocolitis. Similarly, patients who have serious congenital heart disease, such as hypoplastic left ventricle or truncus arteriosus, which may require major surgery and perhaps even cardiac transplantation, may be aided in terms of decision making depending on the results of genomic testing. This still leaves serious questions about where the lines for such decisions should be drawn. This article offers a nice summary of general ethical considerations for and against genomic testing in the neonatal intensive care unit. It may not provide the answers, but several important questions are asked that will need to be addressed as these technologies emerge.

J. Neu, MD

16 Behavior and Pain

The implementation of systematic pain and sedation management has no impact on outcome in extremely preterm infants

Deindl P, Giordano V, Fuiko R, et al (Univ Med Ctr Hamburg Eppendorf, Germany; Med Univ of Vienna, Austria; et al)

Acta Paediatr 105:798-805, 2016

Aim.—This study compared the short-term and neurodevelopmental outcomes of extremely preterm infants before and after the implementation of a protocol to manage neonatal pain and sedation.

Methods.—Our study cohort comprised 140 extremely preterm infants from two neonatal intensive care units. We retrospectively analysed opiate exposure, time on mechanical ventilation, inotropic support, nutritional aspects and growth 12 months before (controls) vs 12 months after (intervention) the implementation of the Vienna Protocol for Neonatal Pain and Sedation. Infants were evaluated at the corrected age of 12 months using the Bayley Scales of Infant Development – Second Edition.

Results.—After the protocol was implemented, the cumulative opiate dose increased from a baseline of 14 mg/kg ± 39 to 84 mg/kg ± 222 morphine equivalents. Time on mechanical ventilation, inotropic support, length of parenteral nutrition, growth, length of stay and in-hospital morbidity were similar before and after the implementation, with no differences between the groups in mental, motor and behavioural development at the one-year follow-up. However, opiate exposure was a possible risk factor for lower behaviour rating scores (estimate $= -0.39$; $p = 0.012$).

Conclusion.—Implementing a neonatal pain and sedation protocol increased opiate exposure, but had no effect on the in-hospital and neurodevelopmental outcomes of extremely preterm infants.

▶ The debate about whether opioids harm the developing brain is ongoing. Nevertheless, guidelines from several international organizations promote a systematic approach to treating and preventing pain in acutely ill and medically fragile newborn infants, using protocols based on the regular assessment of pain and sedation.[1,2] In this retrospective single-center observational study, the authors compared the short-term neurodevelopmental outcomes of very low birth weight (VLBW) infants before and after the implementation of the Vienna Protocol for Neonatal Pain and Sedation, a treatment strategy based on continuous infusions of morphine or fentanyl.[3] The control group included 75 VLBW infants admitted 12 months before the implementation of the Vienna

Protocol and the intervention group comprised 65 VLBW infants admitted after the protocol was put in place. The percentage of infants who received continuous infusions of opiate did not differ between the 2 periods (40% before the protocol introduction and 37% after protocol initiation); however, the cumulative dose of opiates was 6-fold higher after the protocol was introduced. The percentage of infants receiving midazolam or chloral hydrate remained the same (11% vs 12%; 37% vs 35%) as did the total exposure to both drugs.

At 12 months' corrected age the rate of neurodevelopmental impairment was 20% in the control cohort and 28% in the intervention group. Because of the small number of infants studied, a follow-up rate of only 62% and the early age at which the infants were evaluated, the results need to be interpreted cautiously.

L. A. Papile, MD

References

1. American Academy of Pediatrics, Committee on Fetus and Newborn, Committee on Drugs, Section on Anesthesiology, Section on Surgery, Canadian Paediatric Society, Fetus and Newborn Committee. Prevention and management of pain and stress in the neonate. *Pediatrics.* 2000;105:454-461.
2. Playfor S, Jenkins I, Boyles C, et al. Consensus guideline on sedation and analgesia in critically ill children. *Intensive Care Med.* 2006;32:1125-1136.
3. Deindl P, Unterasinger L, Kappler G, et al. Successful implementation of a neonatal pain and sedation protocol at 2 NICUs. *Pediatrics.* 2013;132:e211-e218.

Cohort Analysis of a Pharmacokinetic-Modeled Methadone Weaning Optimization for Neonatal Abstinence Syndrome

Hall ES, Meinzen-Derr J, Wexelblatt SL (Cincinnati Children's Hosp Med Ctr, OH)

J Pediatr 167:1221-1225, 2015

Objective.—To evaluate neonatal abstinence syndrome (NAS) treatment outcomes achieved using an optimized methadone weaning protocol developed using pharmacokinetic (PK) modeling compared with standard methadone weaning.

Study Design.—This pre-post cohort study evaluated 360 infants who completed pharmacologic treatment for NAS with methadone as inpatients at 1 of 6 nurseries in southwest Ohio between January 2012 and March 2015. Infants were initially treated with a standard methadone weaning protocol (n = 267). Beginning in July 2014, infants were treated with a revised methadone weaning protocol developed using PK modeling (n = 93). Linear mixed models were used to calculate adjusted mean primary outcomes, including total duration of methadone treatment, total administered methadone dosage, and length of inpatient hospital stay, which were compared between weaning protocols. The use of adjunctive therapy for NAS treatment was examined as a secondary outcome.

Results.—Infants who received NAS treatment with the revised protocol experienced a shorter duration of methadone treatment (13.1 vs 16.4 days; $P < .001$) and shorter duration of inpatient treatment (18.3 vs 21.7 days; $P < .001$) compared with infants receiving standard methadone weaning. No difference was observed in total methadone dosage administered (0.52 vs 0.52 mg/kg; $P = .97$) or in the use of adjunctive therapy (22.6% vs 25.5%; $P = .68$) between groups.

Conclusion.—Refinement of a standard methadone weaning protocol using PK modeling was associated with reduced duration of opioid weaning and shortened length of stay for pharmacologic treatment of NAS.

▶ Neonatal abstinence syndrome (NAS) continues to dramatically increase in prevalence in the United States and is associated with a high rate of intensive care unit admissions and high inpatient costs. Optimized pharmacotherapy for this condition has the potential to reduce length of stay and cost, as well as to improve the outcomes of these high-risk infants. The Ohio Perinatal Quality Collaborative is an example of the power of combining strong clinical collaboration and scientifically rigorous continuous quality improvement. Previously, this group demonstrated the ability to reduce the duration of therapy and length of stay through adherence to a stringent NAS treatment protocol. In an effort to further refine their approach, the current study examined the pharmacokinetics of methadone to develop an optimal weaning protocol. The efficacy of this protocol was evaluated in 93 infants with NAS compared with 267 historical controls. Infants treated per the revised protocol had a shorter duration of therapy (13 vs 16 days, $P < .001$) and length of stay (18 vs 22 days, $P < .001$). No difference was observed in the use of adjunctive therapy, further supporting sustained efficacy with improvements in duration of therapy. The authors estimate this reduction in treatment duration to be associated with an average of $9000 in potential cost savings.

The Ohio Collaborative represents a model for quality improvement for NAS and many other neonatal conditions. Unique strengths of this collaborative include the ability to evaluate alterations in therapy given the existence of a large historical cohort of infants for whom NAS previously was treated with a strict, consensus-based protocol. Future directions of research might include comparison to alternative pharmacologic agents or personalized treatment based on pharmacogenetics and/or individual exposure profiles. Given regional variation in demographics and common exposures, similar statewide collaboratives in Alaska, Massachusetts, Michigan, New Hampshire/Vermont, and Wisconsin provide additional systems that may prove vital to advance the care of infants with NAS.

C. McPherson, PharmD

Detection and Management of Delirium in the Neonatal Unit: A Case Series

Groves A, Traube C, Silver G, et al (Weill Cornell Med College, NY)

Pediatrics 137:e20153369, 2016

Delirium is increasingly recognized as a common syndrome in critically ill children, but in our experience, it is rarely considered in the NICU. Delirium is independently associated with prolonged length of stay and adverse long-term outcomes in children. We report the cases of 3 infants cared for in our NICU at corrected gestational ages of 4, 11, and 17 weeks who presented with classic symptoms of delirium. All 3 children had complex medical problems and were receiving multiple analgesic and sedative medications. All 3 children exhibited agitation that was unresponsive to increasing doses of medications, and they all appeared to improve after treatment with quetiapine, allowing weaning of other medications. It is possible that with increased vigilance, delirium will be increasingly recognized in newborns, thus allowing tailored intervention. Further research is needed to investigate the prevalence and associated risk factors for developing delirium in the NICU and to explore possible treatment options.

▶ This article caught my attention at a time when I was caring for a baby with advanced bronchopulmonary dysplasia (BPD) who was receiving multiple sedative and analgesic agents, including lorazepam, fentanyl, morphine, dexmedetomidine, and chronic steroid therapy. His sensorium was very much as described in these 3 patients, and he seemed to display a form of steroid psychosis as well, having almost rage-like behavior shortly after receiving boluses.

The movement disorder described in this short case series sounds reminiscent of a syndrome first described by Perlman and Volpe in 1989.[1]

Severe BPD is a frustrating disorder for both care providers and parents. There is a strong temptation to try to keep the babies comfortable, to promote sleep when they are restless, and to adequately treat pain. Unfortunately, our knowledge and understanding of the effects of pharmacologic agents—and their interactions—on the developing brain is extremely limited. Similarly, although the 3 patients presented in the article had a clinical response to quetiapine, it too is an untested agent in this population and deserves a cautionary note at the very least.

As the prevalence of severe BPD continues to increase, this is an area that is sorely in need of further investigation. In the meantime, we should all remember "primum non nocere."

S. M. Donn, MD

Reference

1. Perlman JM, Volpe JJ. Movement disorder of premature infants with severe bronchopulmonary dysplasia: a new syndrome. *Pediatrics*. 1989;84:215-218.

Children with congenital colorectal malformations often require special education or remedial teaching, despite normal intelligence

van den Hondel D, Aarsen FK, Wijnen RMH, et al (Erasmus MC – Sophia Children's Hosp, Rotterdam, the Netherlands)

Acta Paediatr 105:e77-e84, 2016

Aim.—This study prospectively evaluated neuropsychological functioning in 8-year-old patients with anorectal malformation (ARM) and Hirschsprung's disease (HD).

Methods.—School functioning and behaviour were assessed in a standardised interview. Intelligence, attention, self-esteem and quality of life were evaluated with validated tests and questionnaires. The following predictors were assessed: socio-economic status, number of episodes of general anaesthesia, laxative treatment and premature birth. Severely intellectually disabled patients were excluded.

Results.—In total, twelve of the 23 (52%) patients with ARM and 11 (55%) of the 20 patients with HD received special education or remedial teaching. The intelligence quotient was normal: mean (standard deviation or SD) was 98 (17) and 96 (17), respectively. However, sustained attention was below the norm: mean (SD) Z-score was −1.90 (1.94) and −1.43 (1.98) for ARM and HD patients; both $p < 0.01$. Self-esteem was normal: mean (SD) Z-score was 0.10 (1.29) and −0.20 (1.11) for ARM and HD patients. Quality of life was normal in ARM patients and slightly impaired in HD patients. No predictors for neuropsychological outcome were identified.

Conclusion.—Despite normal intelligence, more than half of these patients received special education or remedial teaching. In addition, problems with sustained attention were found. These findings are important for long-term care.

► This small follow-up study of children with Hirschsprung's disease or colorectal malformations who have had surgery shows interesting outcomes. Despite showing normal intelligence, half of the patients received special education or remedial teaching and had problems with sustained attention. Levels of self-esteem were normal. The reasons for these findings are unclear, but there are several shortcomings to this study that include a large number of children who were excluded and many lost to follow-up. The authors suggest that the children's problems involved visual-spatial sustained attention and perceptional organization. They speculate that this issue may be related to the extensive medical treatment most patients with these problems undergo to obtain the best possible anorectal function. The authors further speculate that this issue may be caused by attachment disorders with the parents. Although a larger study would help clarify these results, it is suggested that these children have early socio-behavioral testing included as part of their follow-up care.

J. Neu, MD

Article Index

Chapter 1: The Fetus

Chapter 2: Epidemiology and Pregnancy Complications

Chapter 3: Genetics and Teratology

Chapter 4: Labor and Delivery

Chapter 5: Infectious Disease and Immunology

Chapter 6: Cardiovascular System

Chapter 7: Respiratory Disorders

Chapter 8: Central Nervous System and Special Senses

Chapter 9: Gastrointestinal Health and Nutrition

Chapter 10: Hematology and Bilirubin

Chapter 13: Pharmacology

Chapter 14: Postnatal Growth and Development/Follow-up

Chapter 15: Ethics

Chapter 16: Behavior and Pain

Author Index

U

V

W

Y

Z

Kolibri 360 GmbH
Ferdinand-Jühlke-Straße 7
99095 Erfurt, Deutschland
produktsicherheit@kolibri360.de